P9-APG-763

AIDS

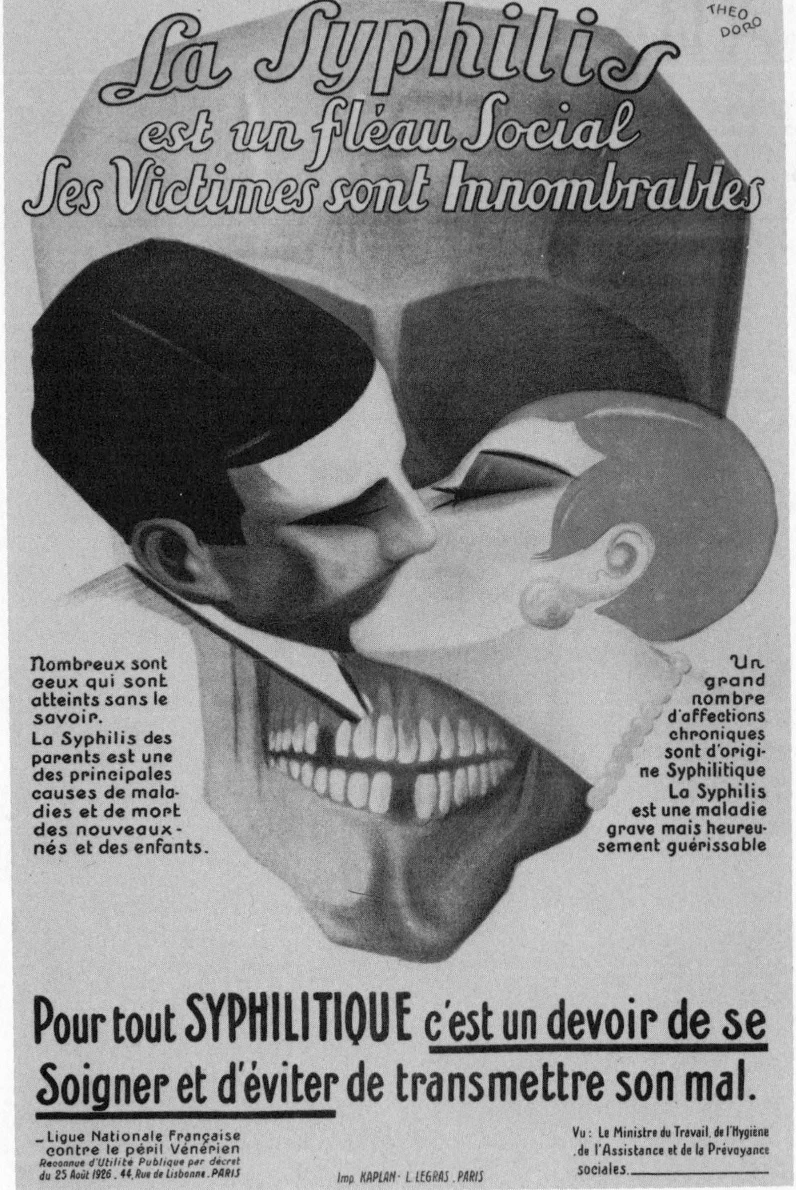

"Syphilis is a social disease. Its victims are beyond reckoning." French poster by Theodoro, c. 1930. Courtesy of the Collection of William H. Helfand, New York.

AIDS

The Burdens of History

Edited by

Elizabeth Fee and
Daniel M. Fox

UNIVERSITY OF CALIFORNIA PRESS
Berkeley · Los Angeles · London

University of California Press
Berkeley and Los Angeles, California

University of California Press, Ltd.
London, England

Printed in the United States of America

1 2 3 4 5 6 7 8 9

LIBRARY OF CONGRESS
Library of Congress Cataloging-in-Publication Data

AIDS : the burdens of history / edited by Elizabeth Fee and Daniel M. Fox.
p. cm.
Includes index.
ISBN 0-520-06395-3 (alk. paper). ISBN 0-520-06396-1 (pbk. : alk. paper)
1. AIDS (Disease)—History. 2. AIDS (Disease)—Social aspects.
3. Medicine—History—Research—Methodology. I. Fee, Elizabeth.
II. Fox, Daniel M.
RA644.A25A32 1988
362.1'9697'92009—dc19 88-040242
CIP

We have learned very little that is new about the disease, but much that is old about ourselves.

Frederick C. Tilney, M.D.,
on the polio epidemic of 1916,
New York

Contents

Acknowledgments

We would like to thank Robert Padgug and Bert Hansen, who initially helped to formulate the plan of this book, and David P. Willis and Ronald Bayer, who commissioned several of the papers. Barbara Gutman Rosenkrantz, Gerald N. Grob, and an anonymous reviewer provided useful editorial suggestions. Lynne Withey and Marilyn Schwartz of the University of California Press were generous and effective editors.

Our names are listed in alphabetical order on the title page.

E.F.
D.M.F.

Acknowledgments

[illegible]

Introduction: AIDS, Public Policy, and Historical Inquiry

Elizabeth Fee and Daniel M. Fox

Acquired Immune Deficiency Syndrome—AIDS—has stimulated more interest in history than any other disease of modern times. Since the epidemic was first identified in 1981, scientists, physicians, public officials, and journalists have frequently raised historical questions. Most often these questions have been about contemporary social and epidemiological history: Why did the disease emerge when and where it did? How has it spread among members of particular groups? Others have asked how societies have responded to epidemics in the past, and still others have questioned how the past will affect the future: What does the history of medical science and public health in this century suggest about our ability to control the epidemic and eventually to cure the disease?

These urgent historical questions are being asked at a time when the study of history often appears less relevant to public affairs than it did in the past. For more than a generation, men and women who rely primarily on historical methods have been losing influence as educators and as advisors to public officials. Practitioners of historical methods once dominated the social sciences. Historical inquiry was also essential for the study of epidemiology and public health. In recent decades, however, historical methods have become subordinate to experimentalism and model building in university curricula for the social sciences and public health and in the priorities of most of the organizations that sponsor research in the hope of ameliorating social problems. Some historians have helped create this situation by insisting on professional detachment, but, in fact, most people who use historical methods have had little choice but to do research for its own sake, whether their discipline is history itself, sociology, economics, political science, literary studies, or epidemiology. Historians, increasingly, have been writing for other historians, with little hope that they can help inform or shape the directions of public policy.

A full discussion of the complicated causes of the decline of history as a basic discipline of public policy is outside the scope of this volume. These causes include changes in priorities at all levels of education, a widely shared assumption in our culture that all problems will ultimately be solved by "hard" (quantitative, experimental) research, and, not least, a loss of interest in the relevance of their work among many scholars who use historical methods.

The diminished status of historical methods of analysis has not, of course, meant that history has disappeared from public discourse. Most people have continued to behave as if interpretations of the past are important to them. Generalizations about history abound in learned journals and in the press and public documents. This history is usually drawn from institutional memory (a euphemism for long-time employees); often it is oral tradition—particularly in the professions. Sometimes the generalizations are derived from a hurried reading of a few books or articles or from several telephone calls to historians.

Examples of this superficial use of history have been plentiful during the AIDS epidemic. Lack of serious attention to historical analysis leads to quick and crude generalizations. Here are a few problematic statements that have been made many times:

> Basic research should receive more funds because in the past this has been the path to discovering the causes and cures for diseases.
>
> There is a long historical record of public health workers protecting the confidentiality of the people they screen and test.
>
> Authority has always prevailed over liberty during periods of social terror about infectious disease.
>
> Medical progress for more than a century has made plain the fundamental biological origins of disease.

Some readers, even some historians, who read these statements quickly may wonder what is wrong with them. Each is only a partial account of evidence from the past and is therefore a dangerous basis for action in the present. Each statement, moreover, caricatures the complex ways that our descriptions of the past shape our sense of possibilities in the present. Each is a simplistic statement; people who know the pertinent historical data would respond: "not quite."

The authors in this volume offer a more thorough reading of the history of infectious diseases. The chapters exemplify some of the ways that the rigorous application of historical methods can contribute to public understanding of the AIDS epidemic.

The phrase *historical methods* requires more precise definition. It is a way of thinking and acting on information to create a nuanced description of events in the past. The information is invariably primary data: the records left by contemporaries. These records are usually words and numbers (both published and unpublished), images and objects. What other historians have written about these records—secondary sources—are hypotheses about the past grounded in primary data. These hypotheses must repeatedly be tested against the data in which they are grounded and for their power to explain newly discovered primary sources.

Historians create nuanced descriptions for several purposes. Some seek to recreate the past as contemporaries would have experienced it. Others try to discern patterns in events over time, and thus interpret primary sources in ways that would have astonished contemporaries. Many historians want both to discover historical patterns and accurately to reflect the lived experience of the past. In addition, historians are always conscious of the culturally specific, and hence are wary of positing universal principles.

Historical methods change as frequently as other areas of scientific discourse. At any time, moreover, people who use historical methods disagree about major issues of theory and practice. The contributors to this volume hold various views on controversial historiographic issues, some of which are evident in their papers. Nevertheless, the authors share a number of historiographic principles, no matter what their original discipline. They share them with most people who use historical methods to study health affairs in our time. The three most important of these principles are (1) cautious adherence to "social constructionism," (2) profound skepticism about historicism, and (3) wariness about "presentism." We will describe each of these in more detail.

Social constructionists, to oversimplify, hold that historical reality is created by people; that is, it does not exist as a truth waiting to be discovered. Some social constructionists include the data of the biological and physical sciences in their analysis, arguing that the institutions and procedures of these disciplines are the result of complex social interactions. The human body, they argue, has no historical existence except in primary sources about how it has been perceived and described by members of different societies at different times. Other historians, though sympathetic to social constructionist interpretations of the history of disease and medical practice, reject the radical relativism that denies that knowledge in the biological sciences can be independent of its social context. Still others remain uncertain about the proper scope of the theory of social construction.

The second principle, skepticism about historicism, is less controversial. Few historians now insist, as most of our predecessors did until a few decades ago, that societies or nations evolve or unfold toward goals that must be discerned by historical research: from, for example, authoritarianism toward democracy, from subordination to hegemony, from primitive ("underdeveloped") to mature ("developed"), even from capitalism to a classless society. Although most scholars argue that in some areas—medical knowledge, for instance—beneficial advance ("progress") has occurred in recent centuries, hardly anyone still insists that the human condition in general has been progressing as a result of inexorable historical change.

The third principle, wariness about presentism, is probably the most widely shared among those who use historical methods. Presentism means distorting the past by seeing it only from the point of view of our own time, rather than using primary sources to understand how other people organized and interpreted their lives. The AIDS epidemic can tempt historians to venture facile analogies with events in the past even though we know better. Many of us have had recent experience of reporters asking us to encapsulate in a sentence or two the history of social responses to epidemics or of scientific communication leading to the discovery of vaccines and cures. Each of the contributors to this book has struggled with the problems of pertinence, without succumbing to presentism, in his or her own way.

Each of the chapters addresses an aspect of the burdens of history during the AIDS epidemic. By "burdens" we simply mean the inescapable significance of events in the past for the present. Some of these events are familiar; others are almost unknown except among specialists. All of them, however, are in some way related to the collective response to the current epidemic, and they all help clarify the complex social and cultural responses to the contemporary crisis of AIDS. All the authors would agree that social, cultural, and moral values are important in determining how societies respond to disease. Many would also argue that these values are embedded in the biomedical and epidemiological theories of disease itself.

In the first essay, "Disease and Social Order in America: Perceptions and Expectations," Charles E. Rosenberg discusses the social historian's interest in the social construction of disease, in its cultural meanings, and in the power of the medical profession to name and to manage social ills. Rosenberg reflects on the history of the history of medicine and on the optimistic faith in science and medicine shared by a generation of medical historians in the 1930s and 1940s. Social reformers calling for a better distribution of the benefits of medicine did not then doubt the benevolence of medical knowledge itself. By contrast, in the 1960s and 1970s a new generation of historians expressed considerable skepticism about the claims of science and the social authority of physicians. Their critical struggles were fought around the definition of disease.

Rosenberg's essay provides a panoramic view of historical changes in the definition of disease—from sickness conceived in largely individual terms as an imbalance between an organism and its environment, to the idea of each disease as a specific entity, with a specific cause to be discovered by laboratory research. The increasing prestige of the medical profession in the early twentieth century led to the expansion of medical authority and to the redefinition of many forms of deviant or undesirable behavior in medical terms. When the specific disease concept did not lead physicians to deal well with the old and chronically ill, with mental disorders or such problems as alcoholism or obesity, medicine was subjected to an increasing volume of social criticism. In this context, AIDS arrived as a novel and frightening stranger, posing in stark form the questions about the cultural and biological meanings of disease. Rosenberg finds that the AIDS epidemic illustrates both our continuing dependence on medicine and the way in which disease reflects and lays bare every aspect of the culture in which it occurs.

In "Epidemics and History: Ecological Perspectives and Social Responses," Guenter B. Risse uses an ecological model to explore the dynamic relationship between the biosocial environment and the human experience of epidemic diseases. He examines the social context of epidemic disease and the ways in which political and health organizations have historically responded to crises. Risse selects three case studies for analysis: the bubonic plague in Rome in 1656, the cholera epidemic of 1832, and the 1916 poliomyelitis epidemic in New York City.

Risse's account shows how socially marginal groups, ethnic minorities, and the poor have often been held responsible for epidemic diseases: The Jews were blamed for the Black Death in Europe, the Irish were blamed for cholera in New York, and the Italians were accused of introducing polio into Brooklyn. He discusses the frequent infringement of civil liberties in the name of public welfare, from the hanging of violators of public health regulations in seventeenth-century Rome to the travel restrictions and quarantines of children introduced during the twentieth-century polio epidemic. Risse notes that draconian measures of isolation and quarantine generated considerable public panic and distress, while they generally failed to stem the progress of epidemic disease.

Perhaps the most common, and contested, health policy instituted during epidemics has been quarantine of the sick. In "Quarantine and the Problem of AIDS," David F. Musto examines the practice of quarantine in relation to leprosy, yellow fever, cholera, tuberculosis, and drug addiction. He shows that efforts to quarantine large numbers of people have never been successful—despite exorbitant costs and the suspension of individual liberties. Indeed, quarantines have often been both ineffective and cruel—especially in dealing with yellow fever, a viral infection conveyed by mosquitoes, and cholera, a bacterial infection transmitted by contaminated food and water. Musto concludes that quarantines have been more effective as ways of expressing public fears about outsiders or socially disapproved groups than as ways of dealing with or preventing disease. Throughout history, quarantines have thus been a response not only to the diseases themselves but also to popular demands for a boundary between the "kind of people" so diseased and the "respectable people" who hope to remain healthy.

Physicians have been called upon during epidemics to assume public functions as well as to treat particular patients. In "The Politics of Physicians' Responsibility in Epidemics: A Note on History," Daniel M. Fox argues that, although most physicians treated most of the patients who sought their care during epidemics, they frequently did so as the result of negotiations with civic leaders. These negotiations have addressed two issues: which physicians would treat patients in the lowest classes; and what incentives would be offered to physicians to take risks. From the fourteenth century to the present, despite enormous changes in the practice of medicine and the social position of physicians, there has been remarkable continuity in how the profession has responded to the threat of contagion.

An understanding of the need for public education about the prevention of the AIDS epidemic has been notably more evident in Great Britain than in the United States. In "The Enforcement of Health: The British Debate," Dorothy Porter and Roy Porter explore the historical conflicts between individual freedom and the public good in dealing with issues of public health in Britain. Under what circumstances could the state be justified in imposing compulsory measures intended to protect the public health? What restrictions could be placed on the "freedom to be sick, and to spread one's sickness, with impunity"? The authors trace the debates and struggles around these legal, philosophical, and ethical issues over a century and a half of British history, demonstrating the grounds for resistance to compulsory state measures.

In the process, they discuss the debates over public health regulation with respect to lunacy, vaccination, and venereal diseases, and show that when those whose liberties were threatened were least powerful or articulate—such as mental patients—the government was able to enact legislation with little or no opposition. In the cases of compulsory smallpox vaccination, venereal disease, and prostitution, however, proposed legislation collapsed in the face of widespread criticism. Analyzing the battle lines drawn over the compulsory examination of prostitutes, the Porters note the relative weakness of the alliance between the government and the organized medical profession, in addition to the deep division within each regarding the propriety and prudence of the enforcement measures. The authors thus provide a historical context for understanding the contemporary response to AIDS, where the British government, the Department of Health, and the medical profession have all supported mass-educational preventive programs and have generally resisted demands for compulsory screening.

Returning to social and sexual attitudes in the United States, Elizabeth Fee shows in "Sin versus Science: Venereal Disease in Twentieth-Century Baltimore" that the black community was held largely responsible for syphilis and that the recorded syphilis rates seemed to confirm white suspicions about the "unrestrained" sexual behavior of the black population. Syphilis was perceived as a disease of the "guilty," a consequence of immoral, improper, or promiscuous sexuality. Fee argues that health officials in the 1930s mounted a deliberate campaign to present syphilis as a disease of the "innocent," and she traces the historical conflict between the biomedical approach to venereal disease—which viewed it as just another infection by a microorganism—and the moral approach, which perceived disease as the consequence of sin. In Baltimore the biomedical approach was adopted by local public health officials and the U.S. Public Health Service, while the moral crusade was supported by the Social Hygiene Association, some local politicians, and the law enforcement campaign against vice and prostitution led by the Federal Bureau of Investigation (FBI) and J. Edgar Hoover. The two views of disease were never completely separate, however, and Fee's account shows that even the discovery of rapid and successful penicillin treatment failed to quiet concerns about the sexual morality and behavior of the citizenry.

In "AIDS: From Social History to Social Policy," Allan M. Brandt discusses the ways that social responses to venereal diseases have expressed cultural anxieties about contagion, contamination, and sexuality. He describes the early twentieth-century crackdown on prostitutes as "the most concerted attack on civil liberties in the name of public health in American history," observing that the policies of detention and internment actually had no impact on the rates of venereal disease. Brandt urges policymakers to pay careful attention to the history of sexually transmitted diseases before deciding on the health and social policies necessary for dealing with AIDS. He discusses the policy issues involved in voluntary screening and mandatory testing, and in funding research, health services, and sex education. He weighs the complexities involved in trying to change personal behavior patterns and discusses the balancing of individual rights with the public welfare. Brandt argues that any policy proposal must be evaluated according to two criteria: Will it work? and is it the least restrictive of all possible measures?

The cultural imagery of the ill is an important theme in historical accounts examining the social responses of health officials and the general public. The construction of AIDS through popular images and language and the creation of scientific descriptions are examined in three chapters. Daniel M. Fox and Diane Karp describe how artists have represented the impact of infectious diseases, including AIDS, using the conventions of their time and their medium. Two chapters explore the cultural imagery particular to AIDS. Paula A. Treichler applies linguistic analysis to discourse about AIDS as reflected in both popular and scientific literature. Gerald M. Oppenheimer then examines the cultural ideas embedded in epidemiological categories and biomedical research.

In "Images of Plague," Daniel M. Fox and Diane Karp present selected images from an exhibition they recently mounted in New York City. The sixteen prints and photographs they feature here are arrayed to tell two stories. One story is about changing conventions among artists for depicting the effects of physical afflictions that have invisible causes. The other is about the impact on artists of the gradual emergence of the concept of infectious disease. Despite the optimism that the germ theory generated about the control of disease by scientific measures, many artists continued to depict disease as a mysterious and intense personal experience and often as a generalized threat to society.

In "AIDS, Gender, and Biomedical Discourse: Current Contests for Meaning," Paula A. Treichler analyzes the language of AIDS from a feminist point of view. She examines the ways in which medical discourse constructs sex, sexuality, and the human body, arguing that it functions to reinforce entrenched cultural notions about gender. Tracing the early discourse on AIDS, Treichler notes that women were almost invisible, being grouped only as "Other." Women were discussed as "inefficient" or "incompetent" transmitters of an AIDS virus that was more effectively passed between men. Women entered the discussion as special, exotic categories: prostitutes, intravenous-drug-using mothers, Africans. Only with the shift in concern to heterosexual transmission, and the declared threat that the virus might pass to the majority (read white, middle class) population, did the discourse turn to women. Treichler criticizes the reassuring and self-congratulatory tone of magazine articles directed at women, and urges feminists to take a much more active role in articulating the nature and meaning of the AIDS crisis.

Where Treichler concentrates on popular media discourse about AIDS, Gerald M. Oppenheimer turns his attention to scientific studies of the disease. "In the Eye of the Storm: The Epidemiological Construction of AIDS" contrasts the roles played by epidemiologists and virologists in the scientific construction of AIDS. As Oppenheimer notes, the power of the multicausal epidemiological model is its ability to incorporate nonbiological variables. This power introduces the danger of reading social and moral judgments into our scientific models—perhaps best reflected in the frequent use of the term *promiscuity* in the scientific journals. Oppenheimer traces the early studies of homosexual men; the articulation of the "life-style" hypothesis; the discovery of cases among heterosexual Haitians, hemophiliacs, female partners of intravenous-drug-using men, and their children; and the subsequent search for a biological agent of the disease. He notes that the discovery of the human immunodeficiency virus (HIV) transformed the disease into a problem of virology, one open to chemical resolution in the form of drugs or vaccines. The biological complexities of the virus mean that such solutions will not be easy to achieve. Oppenheimer concludes that, despite the successes of virology, the multicausal epidemiological model still offers the best possibilities for primary prevention.

Despite evidence of heterosexual and nonsexual transmission, early epidemiological studies firmly linked AIDS to homosexuality. In "Legitimation through Disaster: AIDS and the Gay Movement," Dennis Altman poses the paradox of AIDS in relation to the gay movement. Although the epidemic has meant increasing stigmatization of gays, it has also brought a much greater recognition of the homosexual community and has bolstered the emergence of the gay movement as a recognized political pressure group: Gay leaders and organizations have gained prominence through their involvement with AIDS education, counseling, and policy-making. In examining the political impact of AIDS on the gay movements in Australia and the United States, Altman expresses some ambivalence about the increasing dominance of professionals in leadership roles—a marker of the new respectability of gay organizations, which may also moderate the energy of grass-roots activism.

Altman provides a useful analysis of national differences in dealing with the AIDS epidemic. He notes the tension between two kinds of approaches, one focusing on testing and screening efforts, the other on large-scale education and service programs. The emphasis in each country reflects differences in political cultures and ideologies in addition to the strength and degree of political organization of the gay community in each nation. Altman argues that in areas where gay struggles have already carved out a place for them in the political process, gay organizations have made their strongest contributions to health policy.

In the concluding essay, "AIDS and the American Health Polity: The History and Prospects of a Crisis of Authority," Daniel M. Fox uses the response to the AIDS epidemic as a lens through which to view the structure of the American health care system and the health policy process. He argues that when the AIDS epidemic was first recognized in 1981 the American health polity was undergoing a profound crisis of authority. Fox analyzes the shifting emphasis from infectious to chronic diseases, from collective to individual responsibility for health, and from access and equity to cost containment and fiscal restraint. He argues that the growing centralization of authority in the 1940s and 1950s was replaced by fragmentation and localization in the 1970s and 1980s. The decline in federal health authority was then only partially offset by an increased role for the business and private sector, encouraged by the Reagan administration. Fox argues that these events created a health polity that was both leaderless and ill-equipped to address the AIDS epidemic. The epidemic thus highlights the particular weaknesses of American health policy and poses the challenge to create a more unified, more effective collective response to disease.

This book is a beginning effort to take a more historical approach to the AIDS epidemic. While we do not claim to offer direct answers to questions of public policy, we do hope to bring new perspectives to bear on the debate. In emphasizing the contributions of historians, we hope to bring new voices into the discussion of public policy and to share some insights of historians with colleagues, students, and general readers.

The chapters in this book necessarily constitute an incomplete account of the bearing of history on the AIDS epidemic. We left out important subjects either because the scholars who write on them had commitments that prevented them from meeting our deadline, or because we could not identify appropriate contributors. These omissions include the historical context of the epidemic in Africa, Asia, the Caribbean, South America, and continental Europe; the historical epidemiology of infectious disease; and the recent history of research in virology and in the prevention and treatment of infection. We hope that the work presented in this volume will stimulate discussion and further research and that the subjects we were unable to include will soon be addressed by historians who share our interest in the application of their work to contemporary questions of public policy.

Disease and Social Order in America: Perceptions and Expectations

Charles E. Rosenberg

During the past two decades Americans have participated in a series of debates about the appropriate social response to disease. At first glance the issues seem to differ widely. What were the appropriate responses to hyperactivity in children? premenstrual syndrome in women? homosexuality? drug and alcohol addiction? Were any of these in fact diseases or simply labels for socially defined deviance? What should or could have been done about John Hinckley and other possibly insane offenders? Are diagnosis-related groups an appropriate mechanism for rationalizing the costs of inpatient health care?—does sickness come in neat and categorically distinct units? What are appropriate governmental and individual responses to AIDS? One could continue to add examples, but the point seems obvious. Despite their diversity, these controversies are bound together by several themes. One is the way that relationships between the medical profession and society are structured around interactions legitimated by the presumed existence of disease.[1] A second theme is the negotiated aspect of disease as social phenomenon. A generation of social scientists and social critics has emphasized that there is no simple and necessary relationship between disease in its biological and social dimensions. Some ills have a well-understood physical basis, others none that can be demonstrated. Meaning is not necessary, but negotiated, the argument follows; disease is constructed, not discovered.[2]

Critics have turned the delegitimating tools of cultural relativism on medicine as they have on so many other areas in which knowledge and power are closely linked. For such scholars, Michel Foucault, not Robert Merton, has become the sociologist of choice. "I assert," a recent student of cholera—and of Foucault—argues, "that 'disease' does not exist. It is therefore illusory to think that one can 'develop beliefs' about it or 'respond' to it. What does exist is not disease but practices."[3] Medical knowledge is not value-free to such skeptics, but is at least in part a socially constructed and determined belief system, a reflection of arbitrary social arrangements, social need, and the distribution of power.

The medical profession's institutional power has long been an object of reformist concern, but during the 1960s and early 1970s medicine's conceptual foundations have come under increasing attack. This relativist point of view has sought to undermine not only the apparent objectivity of particular disease entities but also, by implication, the legitimacy of the social authority wielded by the medical profession, which has traditionally articulated and administered diagnostic categories. The physician is not above social interest, but is a social actor whose mission of defining and treating disease can express and legitimate professional, class, or gender interests. This is obviously as much a political as an epistemological position. The marriage of cultural criticism and antipositivism became an influential, if never a majority, view during the past generation.

These relativist arguments are familiar and have become, in fact, a cliché among social historians and social scientists. Yet it is a point of view that seems increasingly sectarian. The weight of scholarly opinion has in the past decade shifted toward an emphasis on biological factors in the understanding of disease and human behavior. We have seen this in a growing interest in the roles of heredity and constitutional factors in disease and behavior, a growing somaticism among students of mental illness. The perceived failure of deinstitutionalization has, for example, underlined the intractability and presumed biological underpinning of the psychoses. Such views are, at least in emphasis, a rejection of once-fashionable sociological formulations that tended to dismiss the diagnosis of mental illness as an exercise in the labeling of deviance.

But no single event has had a more dramatic and illuminating impact than AIDS. It has proved an occasion for labeling, but it is not simply an exercise in labeling. Gay leaders who had for decades urged the demedicalization of homosexuality now find their community anxiously attuned to the findings of virologists and immunologists.[4] This is not to say that the social perception of AIDS and the definition of policy choices are not shaped by preexisting social attitudes; the deviant are still stigmatized, victims still blamed. But the biomedical aspects of AIDS can hardly be ignored; it is difficult to ignore a disease with a fatality rate approaching 100 percent. AIDS has, in fact, helped create a new consensus in regard to disease, one that finds a place for both biological and social factors and emphasizes their interaction. Students of the relationships between medicine and society live in a necessarily postrelativist decade.

But as we accept our dependence on the laboratory and its findings, a number of thoughtful Americans still find it difficult to remain optimistic about society's ability to harness that knowledge; increased understanding of the natural world does not bring automatic and unalloyed benefits. We have been made too conscious of the complex and problematic relationship between medical knowledge and its application. Our decade may be increasingly postrelativist, but we are still products of a generation of relativism, conscious of the costs as well as the benefits of scientific medicine, of the provisional yet indispensable quality of medical knowledge. The meaning of disease has in the recent past become more rather than less ambiguous. It is therefore hard to embrace the clarifying simplicity of either extreme: the reductionist view that concerns itself with verifiable pathological process alone, or the uncompromising relativist position that chooses to ignore that same pathological process in shaping specific social responses.

MEN OF GOODWILL

This postrelativist ambivalence about medical knowledge is an uncertain position, one that would have made little sense to men of goodwill who sought to understand the social role of medicine in the 1930s and 1940s. This generation thought very differently about disease and the doctor's role. They shared an optimistic faith in science and medicine; superstition and social injustice had, and would, impede the accumulation and distribution of knowledge—but the ultimate trend was toward a more humane, healthy, and enlightened society.

No one was more prominent in that generation than the historian Henry Sigerist, a prolific author, defender of Soviet medicine, and a self-consciously irreverent gadfly of the American medical establishment. "Disease as we conceive it today," he wrote in 1943, "is a biological process. . . . Disease is no more than the sum total of abnormal reactions of the organism or its parts to abnormal stimuli."[5] It constituted a failure of the organism to adapt to its environment; disease could, that is, be socially induced, but it was not simply a social construct. It was a real pathological phenomenon. In fact, this very lack of ambiguity underlay the role of disease as a tool of social criticism; the etiology of pellagra (a disease resulting from dietary deficiency) tells us something specific about mill villages and welfare institutions. The etiology of lice-borne typhus tells the epidemiologist something very precise about cleanliness and even the price of clothing in communities with a high incidence of the disease. The persistence of typhoid in the early twentieth century constitutes a telling critique of those communities that tolerated a contaminated water supply. Medical knowledge could serve as both tool and rationale for social intervention.

Sigerist, like almost all of his contemporaries of whatever political persuasion, always maintained an enormous faith in the ultimately positive role of science in human affairs. "The more I study history," he concluded during the darkest days of World War II, "the more faith I have in the future of mankind, and the less doubt as to ultimate result of the present conflict. The step will be taken from the competitive to the co-operative society, democratically ruled on scientific principles."[6] Science and scientific medicine were necessary aspects of the solution, not part of the problem. Such assumptions were widespread. Pioneer students of the social history of medicine, for example, tended to see as fundamental the ways in which society could stimulate, or, too frequently, impede, the autonomous and ultimately liberating development of science and medicine.[7]

Certainly scientific ideas could be misused. The Nazis' use of a racist eugenics is an obvious example; but, as Sigerist put it, eugenics was a "socio-biological experiment that deserves to be watched carefully, even if the present Nazi regime has made it subservient to a thoroughly reactionary—and unscientific—politico-racial ideology."[8] The German advocates of a racist biology were, in other words, false priests of a true religion. It seemed inconceivable to him that science would, in the long run, not stand with the forces of enlightenment and egalitarianism.

To reformers of Sigerist's generation, disease incidence was often the result of particular social arrangements, especially economic inequalities. Disease could also become part of a vicious cycle, miring families and individuals in poverty. Such ideas were widespread among advocates of what contemporaries called "social medicine,"[9] a point of view that recognized the limits of therapeutics and emphasized instead the ways in which disease reflected environmental conditions. The preservation of health therefore often required the modification of social and economic relationships. Therapeutic intervention, according to this view, was not the answer. "Medical care cannot alone eradicate pellagra and rickets," as two leading authorities explained, citing particularly telling instances: "These conditions are for the most part diseases of poverty and ignorance," they stated, "and their prevention and cure lie with the economic and social system." "Health," they continued, "can be achieved only as a part of a high standard of living, in which good medical care is only one of a number of essential elements." It must be emphasized that their study was not a call for radical social change but a plea for the more effective and equitable distribution of medical care. The point is, of course, that the authors could not envisage a conflict between these goals.[10] In the 1930s the fundamental problems in health care were not perceived as intrinsic to scientific medicine; instead they lay in maldistribution of the real benefits that medicine could provide. The establishment of hospitals and the provision of well-trained physicians for the poor and isolated were moral and practical necessities. And such convictions were shaped before the availability of antibiotics and the array of therapeutic and diagnostic tools that have transformed medical care in the past half-century.

Perceptions of medicine are rather different today. Despite two generations of enormous technical change, we have become aware that medical progress implies other than monetary costs. We have allowed an increasing number of men and women to live longer, yet often more incapacitated, lives. We have seen an expanded and generally more accessible medical system accused of insensitivity and physicians charged with greed and inhumanity. We have seen Sigerist's future, and in some ways it seems not to have worked. Few would-be reformers of medicine in the 1980s have been able to share his generation's confident belief in the ultimate and unambiguous benevolence of scientific medicine—no matter how impressive its technical achievements.

Yet as a social institution and body of ideas medicine has never been more central to American society. In the past half-century we have devoted an increasing proportion of our resources to medical care. Public expectations have increased proportionately, along with a widespread resentment at medicine's inability to comply with these imperial expectations. Malpractice suits are only one—indirect—index of the pervasiveness of such hopes.

Definitions of disease have come to play a particularly prominent role at the margins of medical competence—where the authority of medical practitioners and medical ideas is most obviously subject to negotiation. We tend not to question the appropriateness of an orthopedic surgeon's role in treating a broken kneecap, although we might his or her exclusive role (until recently) in legitimating and controlling third-party payment for that treatment. A good many more of us would question the physician's role in defining behavioral deviance. Others would question the appropriateness of contemporary medical priorities in setting health care policy in regard to the very young, the chronically ill, and the very old. We are happy to have immunologists study AIDS; we disagree about the policy implications of their findings. Americans have, in fact, asked, or have been willing to allow, physicians to play a variety of gatekeeping as well as therapeutic roles. They have been rewarded with both power and resentment. Perhaps it was inevitable that disease-definition would become a key battleground in the debate surrounding the prerogatives of physicians and the responsibilities of government.

EVOLVING CONCEPTIONS OF DISEASE

Ideas about the nature of disease have been fundamental both to the internal evolution of medicine and to the profession's complex interactions with society. But even if that centrality has remained consistent over time, the specific nature of those concepts and interactions has changed; Sigerist's confident view of disease as a discrete pathological process had already substantially evolved from traditional concepts.

Perhaps the most significant difference between his ideas and those of his late eighteenth- and early nineteenth-century predecessors lay in the areas of *boundaries* and *specificity*. In 1800 sickness was still viewed in largely individual terms; true, there were well-marked ills that experience had come to define as relatively specific—smallpox, for example. But even in such ailments, idiosyncracy and predisposition could shape an individual's response. Most sickness was not understood in specific terms, even if its ultimate manifestations fell into accustomed patterns. Even epidemic disease was understood to result from an unbalanced state in a particular individual—an imbalance resulting from the sum of interactions between an individual's constitutional endowment and the environment; thus the conventional and persistent emphases on regimen and diet in the cause and cure of sickness. It was natural for physicians to assume connections between physical and psychological environment and sickness; they imposed no rigid boundaries between body and mind or between individual and environment.[11]

It is tempting to see such systems from a functionalist point of view, to underline the ways in which this flexible explanatory system could serve both as behavioral sanction and as a basis for legitimating the physician's social role. Physicians could provide explanations for the inexplicable, reassure those still well that reason guaranteed their continued health, and at the same time reinforce society's moral assumptions. Individuals could and often did play a role in the development of their own ailments; volition and, thus, social norms explained why the drunkard, the financial speculator, and the glutton succumbed. But volition could also be used to explain the role of crowding, poor diet, and economic exploitation. The sick man was both actor and acted upon. Like an assortment of bricks, the elements of this speculative pathology could be put together in different forms according to the builder's requirements. Freethinkers could thus see enthusiastic religion as a cause of sickness, while the more evangelical could indict irreligion. The prominent role accorded to volition implied the possibility of control.

Disease ultimately expressed itself through physiological and anatomical mechanisms; but these pathological mechanisms were activated by a unique configuration of interactions between the individual and his or her environment. Significantly, however, the form of such explanations was always material and rationalistic, no matter how strained and speculative, no matter how transparently they incorporated social norms and attitudes.

Even epidemic disease could be made to fit into the same rationalistic framework, despite the obvious fact that some general factor had to be at work. The case of cholera is particularly enlightening. The most frightening and novel of nineteenth-century European and American epidemics, cholera is the closest modern analogy to AIDS.[12] Asiatic cholera was unknown in Western Europe before 1831; it killed roughly half of those it attacked, and did so, moreover, in particularly rapid and dramatic fashion. No other pandemic had so focused popular and professional fears since plague had receded from Europe in the late seventeenth and early eighteenth centuries.

Lacking an understanding of the etiological agent, contemporaries framed a picture of cholera that sought to reduce the threat of randomness while it articulated social values and status relationships. The dirty, the gluttonous, and the poorly nourished alike were predisposed to the disease. Predisposition was, in fact, a key term in attempts to explain this and other epidemic ailments, for it served to explain the selective exactions of what was at some level a general stimulus. Physicians played a necessary role, providing what reassurance they could in a rational, if, in retrospect, speculative, form. With no consensus regarding the pathology of the disease or the understanding of its etiology, social variables necessarily played a prominent role in fashioning a usable framework that enabled regularly trained physicians and their middle-class patients to cope with the disease.[13] All this was soon to change. By the end of the nineteenth century, disease had become a more specific, yet at the same time more expansive, concept.

During the first thirty or so years of the nineteenth century, elite physicians began to assimilate the idea—associated with the so-called Paris clinical school—that disease was a specific, ordinarily lesion-based entity that reenacted itself in every individual sufferer. Lesions discernible at postmortem could be correlated with symptoms exhibited during the patient's life. Disease could also be (and often was) construed as a disturbance of physiological function that induced an anatomical lesion over time. The study of physiology could—some of the discipline's nineteenth-century pioneers claimed—be a study of disease causation. But whether one emphasized anatomical change or physiological function, symptoms were the consequence of specific material mechanisms. Idiosyncracy was by no means banished; the predisposition to sickness, the clinical expression of a particular ailment, and the response to therapeutics were still seen in terms of an individual's constitution and personal habits. Physicians and laypersons alike instinctively preserved a role for choice and individual responsibility in explaining the selective exactions of disease.

The cause of these newly distinct entities remained a mystery, however. Some medical thinkers even contended that the ultimate cause of disease would always remain beyond human understanding; speculation could lead only to self-delusion. Degenerative or constitutional ailments might be assumed to be implicit in the design of the human body and the aging process. Acute infectious ailments, however, could not be so easily explained.

As we are all aware, an explanation was soon forthcoming. The germ theory, first plausibly articulated in the 1870s, promised to illuminate both the transmission of infectious ills and the particularity of pathological mechanisms. Thus, the evolving model of disease should be seen as having taken two linked steps in the nineteenth century: The first emphasized the specificity, the somatic, and mechanistic aspect of disease, the second provided a discrete cause for those changes. The legitimacy of the new style of conceptualizing disease entities was related closely to both the specificity and the tightness, or unity, of individual entities. Change was gradual, especially among laypersons. Well into the twentieth century, for example, the common cold was widely regarded—and feared—as the first stage of an illness culminating in tuberculosis.

The history of nineteenth-century pathology and clinical medicine seems only to underline the explanatory value of this new way of seeing diseases. Syphilis and tuberculosis, for example, so protean as clinical phenomena, gradually came to be seen as having fundamental unities based on cause and consequent pathology. Truth lay in discerning a more real (more universal and fundamental) causal reality beneath the elusive and ever-changing surface of their appearance in particular individuals.[14] The intellectual tools for constructing an understanding of that underlying truth came increasingly from the insights and techniques of the laboratory.[15] A minority of early twentieth-century physicians did protest the tendency toward mechanistic reductionism in diagnosis and treatment. Their successors have continued. But such warnings could not compete with the laboratory's allure; they still cannot.[16]

Even before medicine possessed resources for treating these newly elucidated clinical phenomena, the gradual acceptance of the notion of specific disease entities by laypersons and practitioners helped reshape the physician's role—underlining the importance of the technical, and increasing the gap between lay and professional medical knowledge. Early twentieth-century reforms in medical education and the standardization of hospitals were both, to an extent, responses to this emerging consensus. Sickness was now a discrete, material phenomenon, best understood by the tools of science and best treated by individuals who had mastered those tools.

But if medical knowledge was gradually becoming segregated in credentialed hands, laypersons were compensated with greater expectations and an increasing faith in medical ideas and medical experts. It was a kind of implicit contract: Society received a measure of emotional reassurance and clinical efficacy in exchange for the increased status and autonomy of medicine. Beginning in the 1880s the laboratory provided a series of dramatic insights. The discovery of the causes of cholera, tuberculosis, typhoid, and diphtheria were not esoteric events isolated in the pages of technical journals, but front-page news. And to laypersons and physicians alike, much of medicine's new explanatory power was construed in terms of specific ills and the ability to understand, diagnose, prevent, and, in a minority of cases, treat conditions previously intractable and mysterious. Even if the demographic impact of rabies immunization and diphtheria antitoxin was minor, these treatments provided striking public evidence of medicine's new powers.

The problem, of course, with this vision of disease is not that it was wrong—although in retrospect it appears incomplete and prematurely reductionist—but that it was, in fact, so powerful and seductive. No group in society was more impressed than the medical profession itself. Professional status and prestige were soon recast in these new forms. Scholarship had always been important in elite medical circles. But now that scholarship had increasingly to be expressed in the form of laboratory research or systematic clinical investigation; the library and bedside no longer defined the boundaries of professional excellence. This shift in values was also effective in helping to recast the institutional shape of the medical profession, legitimating and providing content for a proliferating specialism and an increasingly self-conscious hospital and academic elite. It is true that an appropriate role remained to be defined for the so-called basic sciences in clinic and medical school; but this is irrelevant. As we are well aware, an acute-care, specific-disease-oriented approach came to characterize both the twentieth-century hospital and the career priorities of doctors. Insofar as the laboratory and basic-science disciplines were incorporated into the hospital and academic medicine, they were most frequently bent to the purpose of elucidating and monitoring pathological mechanisms.

DISEASE AS BEHAVIORAL SANCTION

In the last third of the nineteenth century a related, yet potentially inconsistent, development was taking place in that contested cultural terrain where society's tendency to prescribe and proscribe behavior intersected with the prerogatives of medicine. Disease boundaries were expanded to include behavior patterns that might have been dismissed as perverse or criminal in earlier generations. Most conspicuous was the way in which deviance was increasingly, if by no means universally, being defined as the consequence of a disease process and, thus, appropriately the physicians' responsibility. Toward the close of the nineteenth century, for example, neurologists widened the categories of ailments they chose to treat: Phobias, anxieties, and depression could now be classed as symptoms of neurasthenia, and alcoholism, drug addiction, and homosexuality became potential diagnoses rather than culpable failures of volition.

What is particularly striking here is the way that the contemporary prestige of somatic models gradually redefined these behaviors as appropriately within the purview of medicine. The very fact that these novel but omnipresent "ills" manifested themselves exclusively in the form of behavior only emphasized the need to presume an underlying physical mechanism; without one, they could hardly be seen as acquired ailments or constitutional proclivities (the only presumed bases for genuine sickness).

The boundaries of medicine were expanding in the late nineteenth century and, to an articulate minority of self-consciously progressive physicians, that expansion constituted progress toward a more just and enlightened society. A growing secularism paralleled and lent emotional plausibility to this framing in medical terms of matters that had been previously construed as essentially moral. Science, not theology—most physicians believed—should be the arbiter of such questions.

The physician, not the priest or judge, was now viewed as the most appropriate guardian of the rights of society and the individual. The sufferer from phobias and anxieties, the victim of sexual incapacity, the man or woman consumed with desire for a socially unacceptable love object could be seen as the product of his or her material condition rather than as an outcast. By no means all contemporaries accepted such views. But to the stigmatized themselves these hypothetical diagnoses may well have been palatable; given the choice, an individual might well prefer to regard his or her deviant behavior as the product of hereditary endowment or disease process. It might well have offered more comfort than the traditional option of seeing oneself as a reprehensible and culpable actor. The secular rationalism so prevalent in the late nineteenth century freed many Americans from a measure of personal guilt at the cost of being labeled as sick. Not until the second half of the twentieth century, however, has this come to seem a problematic bargain.[17]

Late nineteenth-century medical practitioners became active in another area, apparently reflecting the laudable and inexorable expansion of medical responsibility. This new area was public health and, in particular, the shaping of an interventionist social agenda. These reformist and environmentally oriented policy guidelines seemed no more than appropriate responses to the findings of contemporary epidemiology. Sickness was repeatedly connected with poverty and deprivation. The conclusions seemed obvious to reformers. An enlightened society should purify its water, provide pure milk for its children, inspect its food, and clean its streets and tenements. The expansion of public medicine was connected in a score of ways with the style of self-consciously and self-righteously enlightened government we have come to associate with progressive reform. Moreover, there appeared to be no inherent conflicts among the expansion of medical authority, the clothing of that authority in the guise of scientific reductionism, the proliferation of disease entities—and the vision of a good society. In fact, this confluence of factors seemed necessary and necessarily benevolent. This optimistic and activist tradition still informed the assumptions and hopes of most advocates of social medicine in the 1930s and 1940s.

CONTRADICTIONS AND CRISIS

In the past two decades, however, this configuration of views has appeared to many social critics as neither necessary nor unambiguously benevolent. Medicine has been confronted with a multisided crisis in public expectation. Even those Americans least critical in their attitude toward the benefits of continued medical progress are concerned about the monetary cost. Others who are more skeptical, but still willing to concede the real equities of contemporary medical practice, deplore the ethical and human costs of bureaucratic, episodic, high-technology care. Again and again these concerns focus on the definition of disease.

The first widely expressed concern arose in regard to mental illness; it constituted what I have called elsewhere a "crisis in psychiatric legitimacy."[18] It might with equal justice have been termed a crisis in the cognitive and administrative management of deviance. Beginning in the early 1960s sociologists and social critics began to emphasize the arbitrariness of psychiatric categories and to contend that they were in essence labels, culturally appropriate ways of stigmatizing deviance. Psychiatric thought was in good measure a mechanism for framing, and thus controlling, deviant behavior. The force of this radical critique was underlined by a nagging truth.

Medicine had already come to play a prominent role in relation to just those areas—such as sexual deviance, addiction, and even criminality—where supposedly pathological behaviors fit least comfortably into the pathological model that has explained and legitimated conventional categories of somatic illness. Psychiatry still lacks a mechanism-specific understanding of the great majority of the syndromes it treats.

A dramatic tension thus remains between psychiatry's cognitive legitimacy and clinical responsibilities. Nor is it an accident that the specialty fits uneasily into medicine's status hierarchy. The recent expansion of interest in somatic approaches to psychiatric ills demonstrates these inconsistencies as much as it does the accumulation of new knowledge and new techniques.

A second area of disease-related conflict has turned around the dominance of acute, interventionist models in medical-career priorities and institutions. The prestige of medicine and the personal health expectations of Americans have increasingly come to turn on the efficacy of scientific, interventionist medicine—a system of values and expectations that has been built into the economic as well as intellectual basis of American health care in the past half century. Yet it is a system that is widely perceived as having failed to provide adequate care for the old and chronically ill, or even humane death for the moribund.

Third-party, employer-based insurance has also been structured around the hospital and explicit disease entities. So have federal health insurance schemes. Disease has served as a moral and logical rationale for these bureaucratic reimbursement systems even though payments correspond to days of hospitalization, physician visits, or particular procedures. Specific disease entities have come to mediate between the conceptual world of medicine and the expectations of laypersons. Interactions between doctor and patient ordinarily take place in units defined and bureaucratically justified by the existence of real or presumed sickness. Health insurance has provided a measure of care and emotional security for millions of Americans and a steady flow of income to hospitals and hospital suppliers. But the levers controlling that cash flow can only be pressed by physicians. The language of diagnostic categories at once helps to expedite and to legitimate this special relationship among physicians, patients, and health insurers. Physicians in the mid-1980s complain of the growing influence of cost accounting and bureaucracy and their decreasing role in making care decisions. Diagnosis-related groups seem an obvious justification for such fears. Yet these diagnostic categories are product and symbol of, and condign punishment for, the rigid and unresponsive aspects of our cost-plus, disease-legitimated system of third-party payment. It is a system, moreover, in which physicians and the values of scientific medicine have played a pivotal role.

Rising costs have helped remind us that sickness as experienced comes in units of people and families—and not of discrete, codable diagnostic entities. It is significant that socially minded physicians throughout the first half of this century repeatedly cautioned that patients had families, that managing an acute episode of sickness or trauma did not exhaust the possible universe of medical care options.[19] As early as the 1920s a minority of clinicians warned that chronic and geriatric problems would become increasingly significant as the incidence of acute infectious ills declined; they warned as well that episodic, hospital-based treatment was inadequate for the optimum care of such ailments. Few contemporaries bothered to disagree, yet such concerns became, in fact, increasingly marginal to the actual work routine of many physicians—especially the specialized and often research-oriented academic elite.

A third kind of conflict grew out of the success of medicine itself in helping banish the randomness of acute infectious illness from the perceived life chances of most Americans. The great majority of our children live to adulthood. We enjoy a greater confidence in predicting our future, but at the cost of granting enormous social power to medical practitioners and institutions. It was in some ways a mutually advantageous contract—like that between the psychiatrist and the depressed or deviant patient. But even the most dramatic and undeniable achievements of medicine have their social costs.

One such cost lies in the growing problem of chronic and degenerative ills. Another lies in our cultural habit of dealing with a diversity of elusive social problems by reducing them to technical terms—holding out the promise of neat solutions. Even the most dramatic technical achievements may simply redefine problems, not solve them; or they may create new difficulties in the process of solving old ones. The neonatal intensive care unit is a case in point; so are renal dialysis and cardiac transplants. The elusive phrase, "quality of life," has become increasingly familiar in the past decade. It is hardly an accident.

As the economic and emotional stakes increase, so does the likelihood of conflict. The social meanings of disease have become increasingly the subject of debate and negotiation. Matters of cost are in some ways simple enough. Questions of value can be even more evasive. Is the prevention of sickle-cell anemia through genetic counseling a blow for equal rights or an opportunity for masked genocide? Does a collective social interest require that individuals be forced to use seatbelts? Does calling premenstrual syndrome a disease liberate or enslave women? Does the imposition of mandatory maternity leave constitute justice or handicap women in the economic marketplace? Things were much simpler for the majority of reformers in progressive America. The control of women's hours and conditions of labor seemed to them an unambiguous social good, and woman's role seemed ultimately and unambiguously domestic.

In still another area, dominance of the disease entity has left the profession ill-prepared to address other medical problems that are not as easily construed in such terms. This is certainly one reason for the comparative lack of interest in geriatrics, chronic care, and maternal and child health. The old and chronically ill cannot—except episodically—be seen as sufferers from discrete and meliorable ills. Neither conceptually nor actuarially do they fit comfortably into contemporary practice patterns. The monitoring of particular organs, or intervention in acute episodes have already become the responsibility of one specialty or another; the patient constitutes a residual category. Similarly, victory over the most important and accessible causes of infant and early childhood mortality has left the profession little concerned with the "lingering" aspects of the problem, which are politically sensitive and not easily amenable to exclusively technical solutions. It is clear, for example, that the neonatal intensive care unit is not an all-sufficient answer to the problem of low weight and prematurity, but it is a more congenial and prestigious approach, and seemingly less elusive than the economic and political measures that are its natural counterparts. Similarly, the laboratory response to AIDS has been better funded and more focused than logically parallel efforts in the sphere of education and prevention.

The status of the medical profession, like the meaning of disease, has in the past decade become more rather than less ambiguous. As the technological capabilities of medicine become ever more dramatic, as we transplant hearts and fertilize ova in vitro, we have seen the parallel growth of skepticism and even hostility among laypersons. Such ambivalence is in fact an important component of attitudes toward medicine, technology, and the bureaucracies that embody and administer medical care. At the same time, we have by no means banished disease, even if we have altered the forms in which it is most likely to become a part of our lives. We still have to construct frameworks of understanding and reassurance within which we make sense of its inevitable exactions. Scientific medicine provides a fundamental, and to many individuals well-nigh exclusive, element in shaping that understanding—even in those ailments for which no effective treatment is available.

For many Americans, the meaning of disease is the mechanism that defines it; even in cancer the meaning is often that we do not yet know the mechanism. To some, however, the meaning of cancer may transcend the mechanism and the ultimate ability of medicine to understand it. For such individuals the meaning of cancer may lie in the evils of capitalism, of unhindered technical progress, or perhaps in failures of individual will. We live in a complex and fragmented world and create a variety of frameworks for our manifold ailments. But two elements remain fundamental: one is a faith in medicine's existing or potential insights, another is personal accountability.

The desire to explain sickness and death in terms of volition—of acts done or left undone—is ancient and powerful. The threat of disease provides a compelling occasion to find prospective reassurance in aspects of behavior subject to individual control. Mental illness was, for example, commonly explained in the past as a possible consequence of habit patterns gradually hardened into uncontrollable pathologies. Those who avoided even occasional lapses would have little to fear. In the nineteenth-century epidemics of cholera, as we have seen, there was much talk of predisposition. The victims' behavior or place of residence explained why they, in particular, succumbed to a general epidemic influence. With decreasing fear of acute infectious disease in the mid-twentieth century, Americans have turned increasingly to a positive concern with regimen—to diet and exercise—as they seek to reduce their real or sensed risk, to redefine the mortal odds that face them. The other side of the coin is a tendency to explain the vulnerability of others in terms of their acts—overeating, alcoholism, sexual promiscuity.

CONCLUSION: THE SOCIAL CONSTRUCTION OF AIDS

It is into this world that AIDS arrived—almost as novel and frightening a stranger as cholera a century and a half ago. We were not entirely prepared. Antibiotics had removed much of the fear traditionally associated with acute infectious ills. Most laypersons have come to assume that such afflictions had succumbed to the laboratory's insights. Children no longer died of diphtheria; plague and cholera no longer killed masses of men and women. Tuberculosis, too, had declined, along with typhoid and other water-borne diseases. Penicillin had robbed syphilis of much of the fear that had so long surrounded it.[20] The age of great and intractable epidemics seemed to have passed, and most laypersons assume—whether accurately or not—that medical therapeutics deserved the credit.

But AIDS is both mortal and intractable. It provokes memories of the fear that helped create cautionary and reassuring explanations for plague or cholera in earlier centuries. An ailment that combines sexual transmission with a terrifyingly high mortality, AIDS was bound to attract extraordinary social concern (in clear contrast with a more shallow and transitory social response to herpes; despite the media attention showered abruptly on herpes, it could not mobilize the same level of social concern). It reminds us of the way society has always framed illness, finding reasons to exempt and reassure in its agreed-upon etiologies. But it also reminds us that biological mechanisms define and constrain social response. Ironically, this new disease reflects both elements—the biological and cultural—in particularly stark form. Only the sophisticated tools of modern virology and immunology have allowed it to be defined as a clinical entity; yet its presumed mode of transmission and extraordinary fatality levels have mobilized deeply felt social attitudes that relate only tangentially to the virologist's understanding of the syndrome. If diseases can be seen as occupying points along a spectrum, ranging from those most firmly based in a verifiable pathological mechanism, to those, like hysteria or alcoholism, with no well-understood mechanism but with a highly charged social profile—then AIDS occupies a place at both ends of that spectrum.

The social response to AIDS also reminds us that we live in a fragmented society. To a substantial minority of Americans, the meaning of AIDS is reflected in, but transcends, its assumed mode of transmission. It was, that is, a deserved punishment for the sexual transgressor; the unchecked growth of deviance was a symptom of a more fundamental social disorder. "Where did these germs come from?" a writer to an urban newspaper asked in the fall of 1985. "After all this time, why did they show up now? . . . God is telling us to halt our promiscuity. God makes the germs, and he also makes the cures. He will let us find the cure when we straighten out." It is significant that this same correspondent felt compelled to add that he was not "a religious fanatic,"[21] for the great majority of Americans accept the authority of medicine and the reality of its agreed-upon knowledge. They look to the National Institutes of Health, not to the Bible, for ultimate deliverance from AIDS.

The meaning of scientific knowledge is determined by its consumers. When certain immunologists suggest that predisposition to AIDS may grow out of successive onslaughts on the immune system, it may or may not prove to be an accurate description of the natural world. But to many ordinary Americans (and perhaps a good many medical scientists as well) the meaning of such a hypothesis lies in another frame of reference. As was the case with cholera a century and a half before, the emphasis on repeated infections explains how a person with AIDS had "predisposed" him or herself. The meaning lies in behavior uncontrolled. When an epidemiologist notes that the incidence of AIDS correlates with numbers of sexual contacts, he may be speaking in terms of likelihoods; to many of his fellow Americans he is speaking of guilt and deserved punishment.

Of course, it was to have been expected that patients who contracted AIDS through blood transfusions or in utero are casually referred to in news reports as innocent or accidental victims of a nemesis both morally and epidemiologically appropriate to a rather different group. The very concept of infection is and always has been highly charged; enlightened physicians have always found it difficult to make laypersons accept their reassurances that particular epidemic ills might not be infectious. The fear of contamination far antedates the germ theory—which in some ways only provided a mechanism to justify these ancient fears in modern terms. It is hardly surprising that many remain unconvinced by authoritative medical assurances that AIDS is not (or is not very) contagious.[22]

Knowledge needs to be understood within highly specific contexts. And the specific content of that knowledge itself needs to be seen as a social variable. AIDS underlines the inadequacy of an approach to understanding and controlling disease that ends at the laboratory's door. But it also emphasizes the parallel inadequacy of disregarding the specific biological character of an ailment—and the status of our understanding of that character.

Our experience with AIDS emphasizes this commonsense point. As our knowledge of the syndrome changes, so do choices and perceptions. Aspects of our culture as diverse as insurance, civil rights, education, and policy toward drug addiction have all been illuminated by our increasingly circumstantial knowledge of AIDS as a biological phenomenon. Knowledge may be provisional, but its successive revisions are no less important for that. With each revision, the structure of choices for individuals and society changes. Without a serological test for exposure to AIDS, for example, there would be no debate about screening, access to insurance, and civil rights (not to mention the dilemma of millions of individuals who seek to define their own risks and predict an unpredictable future).

There are some morals here. Perhaps we cannot return to the optimistic faith so general in the 1930s and 1940s; we are too much aware of the costs. But we can share the fundamental understanding of the need to study the interactions between society and medicine if we are to bring the benefits of medicine to the greatest number. We are products of what might be termed a generational dialectic. Most students of the social aspects and applications of medicine cannot easily return to the optimistic faith of the 1940s. But our very wariness, our need to place medical knowledge in a cost-benefit as well as cultural context, underlines an important agenda for social medicine. If the recognition of disease implies both a phenomenon and its social perception, it also involves policy. And that policy inevitably reflects phenomenon and perception. If an ailment is socially defined as real, and nothing is done, then that, too, is a policy decision. This *process* of interaction between phenomenon, perception, and policy is important not only to medicine but also to social science generally. The brief history of AIDS illustrates both our continuing dependence on medicine—for better or worse—and the way that disease necessarily reflects and lays bare every aspect of the culture in which it occurs.

NOTES

An earlier version of this paper appeared in *The Milbank Quarterly* 64, suppl. 1 (1986): 34–55. I should like to thank Barbara Bates, Renee Fox, Stephen Kunitz, Dorothy Nelkin, Rosemary Stevens, and Owsei Temkin, and the editors of *The Milbank Quarterly* supplement for their helpful comments as well as audiences at Cornell, Harvard, Johns Hopkins, and Columbia universities, who tolerated and criticized earlier versions.

1. "Presumed," because disease does not exist as a social phenomenon until it is somehow perceived as existing. This perception can have any one of many relationships to a possible biological substrate.

2. For a useful—if eclectic—collection of case studies reflecting this point of view, see Peter Wright and Andrew Treacher, eds., *The Problem of Medical Knowledge: Examining the Social Construction of Medicine* (Edinburgh: University of Edinburgh Press, 1982). The sociological literature of the 1960s and 1970s on the "social construction" of mental illness was particularly influential in questioning the value-free, positivist conception of sickness categories.

3. François Delaporte, *Disease and Civilization: The Cholera in Paris, 1832,* tr. Arthur Goldhammer (Cambridge: MIT Press, 1986), 6.

4. For an analysis of the demedicalization movement, see Ronald Bayer, *Homosexuality and American Psychiatry: The Politics of Diagnosis* (New York: Basic Books, 1981).

5. Henry Sigerist, *Civilization and Disease* (Ithaca: Cornell University Press, 1943), 1.

6. Ibid., 244.

7. See, for example, the work of Bernhard Stern, *Social Factors in Medical Progress* (New York: Columbia University Press, 1927); *Society and Medical Progress* (Princeton: Princeton University Press, 1941), esp. chs. 8–10; and Richard H. Shryock, *The Development of Modern Medicine* (Philadelphia: University of Pennsylvania Press, 1936).

8. Sigerist, *Civilization and Disease,* 85.

9. See, for example, George Rosen, "What Is Social Medicine?" *Bulletin of the History of Medicine* 21 (1947): 674–733; René Sand, *Health and Human Progress: An Essay in Sociological Medicine* (New York: Macmillan, 1936) and *The Advance to Social Medicine* (London: Staples, 1952).

10. R. I. Lee and L. W. Jones, *The Fundamentals of Good Medical Care,* Publications of the Committee on the Costs of Medical Care, no. 22 (Chicago: University of Chicago Press, 1933), 15. State hospital reform in this period provides another parallel. Albert Deutsch's widely read exposés, for example, constituted a plea for the renovation and medicalization of these neglected institutions—but the therapeutic options then available inspire no great confidence today (Deutsch, *The Shame of the States* [New York: Harcourt, Brace, 1948]).

11. Charles E. Rosenberg, "The Therapeutic Revolution: Medicine, Meaning and Social Change in Nineteenth-Century America," *Perspectives in Biology and Medicine* 20 (1977): 485–506.

12. The analogy is obviously not exact. So far as we are aware, clinically identifiable cases of AIDS have a mortality rate of nearly 100 percent—but over a clinical course that is far more extended than that of cholera.

13. Etiological speculations reflected and rationalized real or potential social conflict in particular national contexts. See, for example, Charles E. Rosenberg, *The Cholera Years: The United States in 1832, 1849, and 1866* (1962; rev. ed. Chicago: University of Chicago, 1987); Roderick E. McGrew, *Russia and the Cholera, 1823–1832* (Madison: University of Wisconsin Press, 1965); R. J. Morris, *Cholera 1832: The Social Response to an Epidemic* (New York: Holmes and Meier, 1976); Michael Durey, *The Return of the Plague: British Society and the Cholera 1831–32* (Dublin: Gill and MacMillan, 1979).

14. Owsei Temkin, "The Scientific Approach to Disease: Specific Entity and Individual Sickness," in *Scientific Change: Historical Studies in the Intellectual, Social and Technical Conditions for Scientific Discovery and Technical Invention from Antiquity to the Present,* ed. A. C. Crombie (New York: Basic Books, 1963), 629–647.

15. For an influential if rather categorical statement of this point of view, see N. D. Jewson, "The Disappearance of the Sick-Man from Medical Cosmology, 1770–1870," *Sociology* 10 (1976): 224–244. See also Rosenberg, "Therapeutic Revolution."

16. A significant antireductionist tradition has always existed among clinicians. For a recent statement of this continuing tradition, see Richard J. Baron, "An Introduction to Medical Phenomenology: I Can't Hear You While I'm Listening," *Annals of Internal Medicine* 103 (1985): 606–611.

17. The psychodynamic models of behavioral disorder so influential in the first half of the twentieth century shared the determinism of their somatic forerunners, although differing in etiological emphasis. Dynamic psychiatry,

however, remained a minority and in some ways atypical aspect of American medicine—even when it loomed prominently in the world view of educated laypersons. In any case, the areas of its greatest clinical responsibilities were ones that had already been claimed for medicine before 1900.

18. Charles E. Rosenberg, "The Crisis in Psychiatric Legitimacy: Reflections on Psychiatry, Medicine, and Public Policy," in *American Psychiatry: Past, Present, and Future,* ed. G. Kriegman, R. D. Gardner, and D. W. Abse (Charlottesville: University of Virginia Press, 1975), 135–148.

19. See, for example, H. B. Richardson's pointedly titled *Patients Have Families* (New York: Commonwealth Fund, 1945).

20. The most recent history of venereal disease in twentieth-century America emphasizes a continuity in social attitudes that rendered sexually transmitted ills impervious to eradication campaigns (Allan M. Brandt, *No Magic Bullet: A Social History of Venereal Disease in the United States Since 1880,* expanded ed. (New York: Oxford University Press, 1985).

21. Charles Realdine, letter to the editor, *Philadelphia Daily News,* 31 October 1985.

22. During the first nineteenth-century cholera pandemic in the early 1830s, ironically, laypersons also tended to dismiss advanced medical opinion that reassured them the disease was not contagious.

Epidemics and History: Ecological Perspectives and Social Responses

Guenter B. Risse

Current discussions concerning the AIDS epidemic contain references about its possible African origin and hypotheses regarding the introduction and spread of the disease in the United States. It seems plausible to postulate that a set of biological factors, perhaps a viral mutation, had to find a favorable ecological niche—made possible by new attitudes toward homosexuality and widespread drug abuse—to trigger the appearance of AIDS. At the same time, our social reaction to the epidemic, presently undergoing painful reexamination, needs to be considered carefully. Why do sufferers of disease have to be stigmatized? What is all that moral judging for? Voices urge that AIDS cease to be a civil rights problem and become instead a public health issue. The implicit message to the authorities is quite simple: cease quibbling about civil liberties and start protecting public health even if it means returning to previous measures of screening, reporting, and isolation deemed successful in controlling other diseases. How can history help us understand AIDS?

To study past and present disease patterns, including AIDS, we need to employ an ecological model that allows us to discover and integrate the multiple factors involved in the arrival of epidemic disease. The dynamic relationship between the biosocial environment and humans—an "ecology" of disease—helps explain the appearance, spread, and departure of specific health problems.[1] As we establish certain webs of causality, attention inevitably focuses on the cultural environment and how human activities before and after the emergence of epidemics predispose or inhibit such dreadful events. History can furnish a valuable perspective from which to view our present predicaments.

The first task of historians is to discover reasons for the shifts that have occurred in the ecology of disease over time, allowing the emergence of successive epidemics of plague, syphilis, smallpox, yellow fever, cholera, polio, and influenza. What biological and social factors could have been responsible for such diseases? Second, we need to examine how past societies have coped with the problem of pervasive disease. What belief systems, institutions, and strategies did they develop when faced with such threats? How did such ideas and actions affect both the healthy and sick?

In order to highlight such ecological and social issues, I have eschewed the frequently employed "panoramic" view, because in my opinion each epidemic—including AIDS—presents a unique blend of ecological circumstances and social responses that develop within highly specific political, economic, and cultural contexts. Instead, I have selected three past epidemics in order to better present the relevant ecological questions and discuss in more detail human reactions to mass sickness.

PLAGUE

The first case study is the final outbreak of bubonic plague among the inhabitants of Rome, which occurred in 1656. For a variety of political reasons—not least the vanity of the reigning pope—this episode was well-documented.[2] The epidemic was fought with measures developed during the Renaissance, refined over nearly two centuries of organized responses to plague in cities of northern Italy. These measures were widely adopted elsewhere in Europe and in the ensuing centuries became the prototype for public health regulations regarding other diseases, notably yellow fever and cholera.

Although contemporary observers had detected a gradual decrease in the frequency and intensity of plague epidemics in Western Europe, authorities of the Papal States, which included Rome, were nevertheless carefully monitoring the health situation in the Mediterranean. This watch focused especially on the movement of potentially infected ships and their supposedly lethal cargoes. One may ask why the plague was retreating in the face of growing urbanization and increased commercial contacts among nations. Was public health policy on epidemics gradually bearing fruit? Probably not. The quarantine system simply stemmed the flow of goods, humans, and ships, only indirectly hampering the movement of the real culprits, namely, infected rodents and their fleas. In fact, the regular recurrence of plague epidemics after 1349 owed more to contacts between urban rodents and their increasingly plague-ridden cousins in the countryside than to the movements of ships with their contaminated cargoes. Today we know that, in spite of millions of human victims, plague remained foremost a disease of rodents.[3]

Significant environmental transformations in seventeenth-century Europe were also affecting the ecology of plague. One of the most critical changes was the gradual separation of urban centers from the surrounding reservoirs of plague-infected rural rodents. Such transformations included deforestation because of preindustrial demands for wood, draining the marshlands, and increasing the acreage under plow; all were designed to feed and shelter the population. These activities unwittingly managed to destroy wild rodent habitats, interposing agricultural cultivation between the teeming urban rat populations and their rural cousins. Even the more mobile brown Norwegian rat, capable of transcending the clearings, was unable to rekindle a decimated rodent population, which indirectly affected humans.[4]

By the mid-seventeenth century, however, bubonic plague was again spreading from North Africa to Spain and southern France. It arrived in Sardinia, then under Spanish control, in 1652. In spite of trade barriers against the island, the plague smoldered for four years, erupting in Naples in 1656, eventually killing an estimated 100,000 people in that city—about a third of the entire population.[5] Unfortunately for Rome, the Kingdom of Naples supplied grain shipments to the holy city as part of a feudal tribute. These imports were particularly welcome in view of the poor harvests that year in regions throughout Italy.

Knowing of Naples' serious epidemic, Roman officials in the spring of 1656 began to patrol the border, making careful inspections of all incoming ships, looking for sick crewmen and travelers. In spite of such precautions, however, a Neapolitan fisherman from the Roman port of Ripa—the destination port of all grain shipments—fell ill on May 10 in a rooming house in the Trastevere district of the city, a slum across the Tiber River. Although suspected of suffering from bubonic plague, the man and his landlady denied or pretended to ignore its true nature until she herself and her family came down with the disease. The fisherman was then sent to a nearby hospital, where he soon died of the plague.

His demise prompted an official report announcing the presence of the plague in Trastevere.[6] Within days, new cases appeared in the adjacent Jewish ghetto as well as in numerous other parts of the city.

According to the Easter census of 1656 Rome had a population of 120,695. In the ensuing months, the city suffered approximately ten thousand deaths directly attributable to the plague. This mortality rate reflects a lower incidence of disease than, for example, reported by the city of London nine years later, where 80,000 people perished out of a total population of 500,000. The discrepancies are difficult to explain, although it is possible that Rome's death rate was underreported because the city's 1657 census counted only 100,119 inhabitants.[7] Perhaps Rome's rat population, in frequent contact with wild rodents in the adjoining, depopulated marshes, was already partially resistant to plague.

In any event, Rome was a densely crowded city still confined within its medieval walls. Its streets were a disorderly jumble, blocked by stalls with a variety of vendors and by slow-moving carriages. Few inhabitants obeyed the municipal instructions to deposit their rubbish at the appointed heaps along the banks of the Tiber River; most garbage was simply thrown into the streets. "What's the use of living in the grandeur of Rome," wrote one critic, "if one is to walk like beasts rather than human beings. . . . Raise, Holy Father, the poor from the excrement."[8] A busy Congregazione della Strada—the department charged with the cleaning, repair, and improvement of the city's lanes—fought a losing battle, bedeviled by traffic congestion, lack of parking, and after each sweeping, the inevitable recurrence of garbage.

As in other cities, the poor bore the brunt of crowding and lack of hygiene. Their slums were located in humid, low-lying areas of the city that were periodically flooded by the Tiber, and most of their houses were in advanced stages of decrepitude, with holes in the walls and roofs and "nests of spiders, mice, scorpions and geckoes." Rents were exorbitant and people were forced to live in "cubicles, garrets and holes in the wall"; others were homeless, begging on streets, engulfed in the stench from rotting garbage and animal and human excrement. "Good Shepherd," complained the same critic, "by your leave, we no longer live in Rome but in a pigsty."[9]

The city was ruled by Fabio Chigi, or Alexander VII, a native of Siena elected pope the previous year. Alexander's passion was architecture on a grand scale. His stated goal was the restoration of Rome to its previous splendor through the completion, renovation, and construction of piazzas, palaces, and churches. With a highly developed sense of public relations, the pope tried to give the city an image of ample squares, long open streets, attractive buildings, decorative fountains, and renovated monuments. The new look was designed to bolster his personal popularity as well as to attract foreign visitors to a city that had long lost its political importance and was still feared for an insalubrious climate associated with endemic malaria in the surrounding countryside.[10]

Thus, the 1656 outbreak of plague in Rome could not have come at a less opportune time for the pope. Nevertheless, Alexander VII immediately contacted the Congregation of Health, a municipal bureaucracy created in 1630 by Pope Urban VII to monitor and fight disease. Its leader, the prefect cardinal Giulio Sacchetti, counted in turn on the assistance of another cardinal, Francesco Barbarini, who had successfully organized public health measures against the plague in Bologna twenty years earlier. For the next few months, the group met daily and implemented a traditional series of regulations.[11]

Following the fisherman's death, the health authorities ordered the immediate suspension of trade with Naples and the Campagna region surrounding Rome. Most city gates were closed, and military guards were posted at all entrances. Temporary stockades were erected in front of gates and remained only partially open to the movement of goods and people; health certificates were demanded from those trying to enter. Jews had to present a special passport. Money and mail were fumigated, and goods and animals placed in quarantine.[12] At two gates, authorized supplies of grain and wine were transferred through pipes across the fences. Large chains were placed across the Tiber to block all ship traffic to Ripa. Trastevere and the Jewish ghetto, districts where the plague found its first victims, were sealed off and patrolled by guards.[13]

Having secured Rome's borders, the authorities went on to issue a set of rules to deal with plague inside the city. Traffic was severely restricted, and the streets were cleaned of filth and garbage. Schools were closed. City functions attracting crowds such as markets, parades, and religious processions were altogether banned. Indulgences were offered for people praying at home each night while the church bells rang. Prostitution was officially quashed, and vendors, beggars, and otherwise idle folk were put to work on Alexander VII's construction projects. Many of them were marched off to pesthouses opened for people suspected of harboring the plague.

Police were also prominently involved in the handling of individual victims. Suspected cases reported by relatives or physicians were brought to a number of first-line lazzarettos (quarantine hospitals) for screening.

If clinical signs of plague appeared, the sick were quickly sent on with an escort of soldiers to the larger pesthouse on the island of St. Bartholomeo. Their homes were immediately sealed off by officials; large signs reading "SANITA" (Sanitary Service) were nailed across doors and windows. Surviving relatives could not leave the building under threat of death, remaining there quarantined for several weeks until they could prove their lack of infection.[14]

After usual periods of isolation, buildings that had housed plague victims could be "purged" of the disease through fumigation. Cleansing smoke came from burning sulfur as well as logs of pine, juniper, and laurel. Cleaners dressed in special vests, their faces covered with sponges soaked in vinegar, entered the contaminated premises and hauled out the furniture and other belongings. Some items were promptly fumigated on the spot through placement on racks while the clothing was sent to special laundries set up in nearby monasteries. Some establishments cleaned the woolens, others the linens. Before the belongings were taken away, elaborate inventories of removed household goods were taken in the presence of a notary.[15]

After recovery, survivors were placed in a convalescent category and transported to another lazzaretto for further recuperation. Following a prudent period of observation there, these asymptomatic people were conveyed to another makeshift quarantine station in a jail before their final release. In turn, the dead were promptly loaded onto wagons or boats and conveyed downriver to St. Paolo's churchyard and adjacent meadows. Here all naked corpses were buried in mass graves, their clothing burned to prevent gravediggers from recycling it and getting infected. Once in the ground, the bodies were covered with lime soaked in vinegar and fresh soil.[16]

Each ward in the city organized its own local health commission composed of two physicians and a priest. These individuals went from house to house, the doctors checking for disease while the priest held confessions and administered last rites. They were all considered tainted because of their contact with plague victims and were thus forced to live in isolation during the epidemic. On their appointed rounds, these men were forced to display wooden crosses, a sign of their contamination. Other doctors worked in the lazzarettos. In the course of these duties many of them contracted plague and died.[17]

The epidemic of 1656 unquestionably caused a great deal of fear and panic in the population. Many inhabitants, including physicians, immediately fled the city, while others simply denied the existence of the disease. After the slum of Trastevere was cordoned off by authorities, its impoverished inhabitants complained bitterly about the enforced isolation, which took away their livelihood and "freedom of action from all." Although the pope and a deputy—his brother, Mario Chigi—repeatedly crisscrossed the city handing out money to the needy and especially the shut-ins, complaints about these "guardians" (military guards) only increased, as if "the remedy was the true illness," not the plague.[18] Others were angry with physicians who took advantage of the panic to peddle profitable prescriptions.

In turn, "many sick carried illness without revealing it, hoping to cure the pestilential lungs secretly."[19] Causes given for such lack of reporting were fear of job loss, terror of being severely punished for disobeying quarantine laws, and just plain embarrassment among the well-off, who refused to confess their defilement by a disease usually associated with poverty and filth. Individuals considered tainted through contact with plague victims, and thus guilty of breaking the law, were shot.[20]

Most seventeenth-century public health measures were rooted in the widespread lay and medical belief that filth and organic decay generated poisonous vapors that contaminated the urban atmosphere. Floating in the form of invisible particles, these vapors were thought to either penetrate the skin or be inhaled; occasionally they passed from one person to another as contagion. Once in the body, such matter could disturb the victim's humoral balance, but only if his or her constitution was already compromised and thus predisposed to illness.[21]

Based on such a system of explanations, most public health measures focused on two objectives: eliminating the sources of poisoned air, or miasma, and keeping the healthy away from the sick. Environmental cleanups and quarantines, trade bans, and isolation of suspected victims were the central aims. Representing the values and concerns of a healthy elite, the public health authorities took an energetic and heavy-handed approach to protect its long-term political and commercial interests. Privacy was invaded, suspects forcibly removed from their homes, lists of victims published, houses closed, relatives shut in, beggars expelled. Violators of public health regulations were fined, summarily executed by firing squads, or hanged from gallows erected in piazzas around the city. Those committing serious crimes were actually torn apart, and their limbs publicly displayed. Informers usually received a third of the levied penalties.[22]

Scapegoats were easily found. First, of course, there were the foreigners, especially those who had arrived from plague-ridden Naples and could therefore be blamed for introducing the disease. The first victim was thought to have imported tainted "feminine ornaments—silk ribbons,"[23] thereby starting the epidemic. As always, there were the Jews, more than four thousand of them, already crowded into an unhealthy and densely populated ghetto less than a square mile in diameter near the Tiber. As a result of their strict confinement, nearly 20 percent of the ghetto inhabitants died during the epidemic.[24] The poor, who inhabited the slums like the Trastevere district, were also convenient scapegoats. Initially they suppressed information about the presence of plague in their midst out of fear of being quarantined; later they were also less than forthcoming about presenting themselves to the magistrates who were trying to screen them for disease. According to statistics, more than half of Trastevere's three thousand residents died during the epidemic.[25]

Whether the public health measures actually hampered the progress of the epidemic throughout the city remains questionable. In the Jewish ghetto and Trastevere, however, the quarantines served to facilitate human contact with plague-infected rats, thus significantly increasing morbidity and mortality in those areas. Although the papal authorities tried hard to portray their determination to care for all Romans and to mitigate individual hardships, the powerless, as usual, bore the brunt of the disease. They were the scapegoats, deprived of jobs, food, and adequate shelter, and herded into disease-infested places separated from the rest of the population. The observation of a contemporary that the "judgment of the masses was ungrateful regarding the charity of their rulers"[26] would indicate that those who suffered most during the epidemic were not very impressed with Alexander VII's public health measures. It was "as if the evil [plague] was imaginary and the cure the real evil," admitted one official.[27]

CHOLERA

Less than two hundred years later both Europe and America faced a new disease—cholera—although a number of historians argue that cholera has been around since the sixteenth century. Speculation about its origin continues. A recent hypothesis argues that a relatively harmless water-borne bacterium, easily destroyed by acid in the stomach, mutated in India early in the nineteenth century, suddenly acquiring the ability to produce a powerful toxin responsible for the severe diarrhea and vomiting, resulting in an enormous loss of fluids and high death rates.[28]

Once launched, cholera spread quickly in successive epidemics affecting virtually every country in the world. Its transmission was possible because of increased and more rapid means of transportation. Moreover, the industrial revolution promoted an accelerated and poorly planned urbanization that frequently allowed the mingling of human wastes with water supplies—ideal conditions for a disease like cholera.[29]

Reports from West Bengal suggest that the first cholera pandemic originated there in 1817, spreading throughout Asia and East Africa. A second wave began in 1829, quickly moving into Russia (1830), Germany and Britain (1831), and France (1832). Having effortlessly crossed the seas and three continental landmasses, there was a justified fear that cholera would also travel to the New World, given the high volume of transatlantic traffic. Although the demographic effect of cholera's deaths was relatively small compared with the great killers of the past—nevertheless, in Britain alone about thirty thousand people died of the disease in 1831–1832—its sudden evolution and spectacular symptoms caused considerable horror and panic.[30]

In the spring of 1832, therefore, Americans warily awaited cholera's leap across the Atlantic. Even before cholera broke out in Quebec and Montreal on June 15, New Yorkers had braced themselves for the onslaught by reorganizing the city's sanitation system. Money was made available to erect hospitals should cholera strike.

Although holding infrequent meetings, the city's permanent Board of Health had been in operation since the yellow fever epidemic of 1822.[31] When cholera erupted in Europe, board members—including New York Mayor Walter Bowne and city aldermen—gathered information about the disease. By the fall of 1831 quarantine regulations went into effect for the screening of all incoming passengers and goods first from Asia and Africa, and then from southern Europe as cholera spread to that continent. By June 1832 a blanket quarantine against all European and Asian travelers went into effect. No vessel could approach within three hundred yards of the docks if suspected of carrying cholera victims. American physicians, in turn, went to Canada to observe the newly arrived disease and returned to issue recommendations for preventing the scourge. Cleanliness and temperance were considered critical.[32]

New York had a population of about 250,000 at this time. With the greatest port on the continent, the city was a thriving but densely populated commercial center. Thousands of European immigrants—especially the Irish—crowded into the humid, marshy areas of Lower Manhattan, occupying unfinished cellars and back rooms. Located near the docks and common sewers, these slums furnished a highly favorable ecology for cholera. Horse stables as well as pens for cows and swine dotted the alleys; more than a thousand pigs roamed through the streets. Following the news from Canada about the arrival of cholera, perhaps as many as a hundred thousand inhabitants left the city. Driven by fear, people fled in stagecoaches, steamboats, carts, and even wheelbarrows.[33]

In spite of all precautions, an Irish immigrant named Fitzgerald became ill on June 26, 1832, complaining of stomach pains. His wife and two children were similarly affected, and although he recovered, they died a few days later. Perhaps there had been previous victims of cholera, hidden from authorities or deliberately unreported by officials to avoid panic. In any event, within days the news circulated that the disease had appeared in various areas of the Lower East Side, and in the notorious "Five Points" area in the Sixth Ward, Greenwich Village, and the Bellevue almshouse. Before it was over in September the epidemic killed nearly 3,500 inhabitants, claiming most of its victims—perhaps 2,000—among the poor.[34]

On July 2 the Medical Society of New York announced that nine cases of cholera had already occurred, expecting to prod the municipal authorities into greater action.[35] Although the Board of Health considered the medical declaration an "impertinent interference" in its affairs, members agreed to appoint a special medical council, composed of seven prominent physicians, to look into the matter. Like the Roman Health Congregation, this group promised to meet daily and, if necessary, to issue public health regulations. Predictably, the medical confirmation of cholera in New York merely exacerbated the exodus already in progress. "Oceans of pedestrians" were reported on roads leading out of the city. Farm and countryhouses within a thirty-mile radius quickly filled up with panic-stricken refugees.[36]

Despite professional opinion that cholera had indeed reached the city, the Board of Health and especially the newspapers continued to question the assertion. Fearful passengers on steamboats landing in New York resented the medical announcement as "injudicious and premature" by "unauthorized and meddling doctors which have filled the nation with such groundless apprehensions."[37] No matter—the alarm had been sounded. In the eyes of one observer, the Fourth of July holiday lacked the "usual jollification." Stores were closed and the official parade was canceled, although some troops marched on their own and "the places of public amusement were filled in the evening."[38] Although the Board of Health was forced to report twenty new cases and eleven deaths for that day, all presumed to be cholera victims, one newspaper tried to soften the impact of such tidings by explaining that festivities associated with national holidays caused fatigue and notoriously encouraged intemperance in eating and drinking. Only such preconditions, it suggested, would allow the appearance of the disease if combined with environmental pollution.[39]

Over the next few weeks the press tried to minimize the importance of the epidemic. The Board of Health required that practitioners who were reporting cases also disclose the sex, age, occupation, and former health of their patients. It not only published daily the names and addresses of new cholera victims but also the number of individuals brought to the various city hospitals suspected of having the disease. In addition, the board now included on its lists the names of the doctors reporting the cases. Reporters quickly realized that most attending physicians reporting cholera cases were not among the professional elite then practicing in the city, many of whom had obviously left with their rich clients; this created further skepticism about the seriousness of the cholera epidemic. "The alleged visitation of the Asiatic cholera seems to have brought an entirely new fry of doctors into existence as a shower of summer rains brings out a new race of frogs and toads," mused one paper.[40] The unknown doctors could not be entirely trusted, the paper suggested, to provide an accurate picture of morbidity. "We have some cholera in the city," concluded the article, "and a great deal of humbug."[41]

Although not among the elite, the physicians who cared for cholera patients took considerable risks. Theirs may not have been household names gracing the social pages, but these practitioners "who pass[ed] swiftly up and down the streets in their gigs" tried to find early cases of the disease when in their eyes treatment still had a chance to succeed. By contrast, prominent members of the medical profession who were advising the Board of Health expressed "fear of contagion," and in fact dared "not to enter the room in which a patient lies suffering from that affection which these very medical advisors deny to exist."[42]

Errors in reporting by the Board of Health continued to generate skepticism about the true impact of cholera. Alarmed neighbors found one presumed victim busily engaged over her washtub; a barber in the Bowery was quietly shaving customers when the newspaper announcing his illness was thrown through his doorway.[43] In any event, the lists chiefly disclosed "the intemperate, the dissolute, and the poor creatures who are too ignorant to know what to do, or too destitute to procure needful attention."[44] Because most casualties indeed occurred among marginal members of society, the "causes of apprehension" concerning cholera were, according to press reports, "greatly diminished." Perhaps because of this, the authorities were slow to promote the usual public health measures. "What in the name of common sense is the reason the Corporation will not do their duty?" someone wrote in the physicians' *Cholera Bulletin* of July 13.[45] Indifference to the citizens' welfare was the charge; the officials were told to resign. In an utterance reminiscent of contemporary statements on AIDS, the same author wrote: "Public health is now at stake, and if prompt and efficient measures be not immediately adopted to secure it, in a short time it will be too late, for thousands of our citizens will have been consigned to the tomb."[46]

Finally, time-honored public health measures were indeed implemented, including a vigorous campaign of street cleaning. Instead of merely dampening the refuse with water, workers actually deprived many streets of knee-high manure, garbage, and dead animals—only to dump it, however, on other city roads. Cesspools were covered with quicklime, and "nuisances" around slaughterhouses were discarded. Houses that had harbored the sick were fumigated and purified using chloride of lime and sulphuric acid. Walls were whitewashed. Fire destroyed clothing and bedding belonging to cholera victims. Tar and pitch were burned to purify the atmosphere. "Let us learn from the past," stated the *Cholera Bulletin,* "and by improving the present, diminish the danger to the future."[47]

As one resident of Five Points—that "hotbed of contagion"—complained, such public health measures were not equally enforced in all areas of the city. In that neighborhood, rubbish continued to be thrown into the streets with impunity. At night, beds and bedding belonging to cholera victims were also burned outside. Hemmed into a crowded ward that now reported thirty to forty cases of the disease daily, residents produced enough refuse at Five Points "to feed the cholera for the next forty years." Not even the Fire Department dared send their trucks there. Referring to the slumdwellers at Five Points, one critic felt that unless some action by the authorities was forthcoming, "at the end of that time (forty years) there will be no occasion for their interference."[48] In a word, it was hoped that, if left sufficiently alone, the susceptibles would all die and the disease would burn itself out.

Instead of neglect, others advocated harsh measures. "The Five Points and their vicinity are inhabited by a race of beings of all colors, ages, sexes and nations, though generally of but one condition, and that beneath the nature almost of the vilest brute," wrote one reader.[49] The cure was easy: "Turn out the inmates of the place, ventilate and purify the beastly hovels, guard effectively against their return, fence up the streets."[50] In certain instances compulsory evacuation of the poor to makeshift shanties was actually carried out.

In the meantime, New Yorkers witnessed a rampage of vandalism in dwellings belonging to those who had left the city. Carpets were cut to pieces and furniture broken; some homes were completely ransacked from top to bottom. Lacking a sufficient security force, the authorities seemed unable to control the crime wave. In response, many homeowners quickly procured insurance against theft. "At the present crisis, those who are leaving town would find it a measure of prudence to effect an insurance," advised the New York Equitable Insurance Company.[51]

Those suspected of harboring cholera were quickly taken to makeshift hospitals for observation and treatment. Because the Medical Council had concluded that "the disease in the city is confined to the imprudent, the intemperate, and to those who injure themselves by taking improper medicines,"[52] hospitals classified their admissions "according to habit" into "temperate" and "intemperate," with an intermediate category of "irregular"; unconscious or dying patients were termed "uncertain."[53] Drunks were often reported as cholera patients. The dead were buried with indecent haste in mass graves dug at Potter's Field, robbing families of traditional wake practices. Instances of resistance to such public health measures were reported, with angry mobs attacking and beating up city officials and even some physicians.

The practices described above reflected the widely held belief in the atmospheric origin of the disease.[54] Because of cholera's erratic epidemiological patterns, the issue of direct contagion was frequently debated but generally deemphasized. In spite of repeated pronouncements that they were useless and bad for business, traditional quarantines continued to be imposed by apprehensive officials. Poisonous particles from urban decay were thought to rise from streets, cellars, and tenement houses. Such vapors were presumed to irritate both stomach and bowels but led to cholera only if the individual's constitution was already weak because of dietary deficiencies and excessive consumption of alcohol. Cholera and rum traveled together: "Short is the transition from the grog-shop to the hospital, to the grave, and to perdition."[55] Critics questioned such medical assumptions, pointing out that cholera cases frequently appeared in almshouses and jails where no liquor was available.

Indeed, the association of cholera and intemperance filled the pages of medical books, pamphlets, handbills, and newspapers. "It is now universally known that cholera has a most peculiar affinity for the system of a drunkard, so much so that it is a very rare thing for the intemperate to escape," wrote one physician.[56] "Well-appointed nurses" at hospitals were instructed to obtain a "correct" history from newcomers regarding their drinking habits. Even small amounts of port, brandy and water, or wine taken as cholera preventives were considered harmful.[57] Taverns ("abominable styes of pollution") and liquor stores ("visible nuclei around which the epidemic raged with unwonted fury") were especially singled out as sources for a habit that now could lead to the dread infection. Cholera victims were perceived to include "the poorest class of Irish, many of them have for years (as they themselves confessed) been almost daily intoxicated."[58]

Not coincidentally, cholera claimed most of its victims among New York's poor, those who received the lowest wages but were forced to pay high rents for the humid and filthy cellars they called home. Among the women, there were poor seamstresses driven into prostitution, their susceptibility to the disease explained by the combination of "filth, crowded rooms, irregular diet, intemperance, and the debasing vice to which they are addicted."[59] Others were "hard-working women whose constitutions had been broken by years of incessant toil."[60] When cholera broke out among "carefully conducted" middle-class people, however, physicians were perplexed. In one boardinghouse on Broad Street, stumped public health inspectors pondered the death of the respectable owner and her daughter. Finally, a "local mischief" was found: a large quantity of cattlehides and bones rotting in the cellar of an adjacent warehouse.[61]

In the eyes of most contemporaries these were "innocent" victims of cholera. Most were thought to have willfully weakened their bodies through unwholesome ways of life and were now being punished for their sins. According to religious leaders, the three prominent abominations of the time were sabbath-breaking, intemperance, and debauchery, and cholera was viewed as a disease of "mental and corporeal debility."[62] The best preventive measure was a prudent life emphasizing temperance in eating and drinking, avoidance of garden vegetables and fruits, abstention from ardent spirits, and sexual moderation.

Among practitioners there was pessimism regarding compliance among the poor. "The mass of mankind are, and there is reason to fear, ever will be insensible to the operation of great moral principles," wrote one physician.[63] Cholera was therefore viewed as a just punishment for people who were unwilling to change their lives. For many contemporary observers cholera was a godsend: It gave the temperance movement a formidable impulse by exposing the danger of ardent spirits. Providence had brought "good out of evil" and taught a valuable lesson to civil and municipal authorities. The sacrifice of cholera victims had not been in vain!

By the end of July the worst seemed over. The number of reported cholera cases was down, ostensibly unrelated to public health measures.[64] With all the accusations of intemperance and vice in relation to cholera, criticisms were voiced about the role of "newsmongers," writers, and even newspaper readers who were accused of prolonging the terror. The press was blamed for displaying an "unruly passion for publishing this heaping of trifling matters" in response to demands by eager consumers of print, who became confused "from such a heterogenous assemblage" in blanket size, as they "devoured [it] in a constant panic."[65]

Medical professionals raised another issue: the official reporting of cases by the Board of Health. Indisposed patients reported by their attending physician could be listed twice if any of them got admitted to a hospital and appeared the next day among hospital cases. If the victim died, there was the possibility of being listed a third time. "Is this not humbugging the public and most unjustifiably magnifying our distresses?" asked one practitioner.[66] To make matters worse, the Health Board apparently never checked the truth of such reports, although physicians providing incorrect information could be fined. Because of the suspected and proved inaccuracies in reporting the epidemic, the public at large remained ambivalent about the seriousness of the epidemic, an uncertainty not conducive to allaying their fears.

By August 27 thousands of refugees returned to New York City in spite of warnings by the Special Medical Council that the streets and city air were still polluted. Those coming back were invited to "contribute in preserving the commercial and trading interests from destruction."[67] Among them were physicians "who, impelled by the desire of avoiding the unprofitable labours which such calamities impose on our profession, deserted their posts in time of danger or sought refuge from their personal fears by inglorious flight."[68] Devoid of patients, some of the cholera hospitals closed their doors. As one contemporary observed, "business has revived, the streets are lively and animated, and everything seems to be resuming its wonted appearance."[69] The sky, clear because of idle factories and unused domestic fireplaces, gave way again to "the dense cloud of smoke which always lays over the city."[70]

As in the previous case of plague, the cholera epidemic of 1832 constitutes another paradigm for social responses to disease. Here again, the poor—often immigrants—were the primary victims both of the disease and of the blame. In this view, moral failings thought to be responsible for poverty and dissipation provided a fertile substratum for cholera to break out among those marginal sectors of society "different" from the hard-working, God-fearing majority. Public health measures sought to clean up the environment, thus reassuring the anxious public, but the activities were selective: Slums such as the Five Points area continued to wallow in garbage and to be without fire protection. Epidemic disease served once more as a focus for the expression of religious, political, and cultural biases within society.

POLIO

The third and final case study presented in this chapter deals with the serious epidemic of poliomyelitis, or infantile paralysis, which erupted among inhabitants of New York City in the year 1916. The disease had been rare before 1907, although minor episodes occurred in Austria (1898) and Scandinavia (Norway and Sweden, 1904). In Rutland, Vermont, an outbreak of polio was reported in 1894 which took the lives of 132 people before striking New York in 1907 and killing an estimated 2,500 persons. After 1907 polio epidemics became increasingly more frequent. Between 1910 and 1914 alone about five thousand deaths and thirty thousand cases were reported in the United States.[71]

As in previous instances, human actions contributed decisively to the creation of a favorable ecological setting for poliomyelitis. Ironically, the culprits were improved public sanitation and personal hygiene, slowly achieved after decades of cholera and typhoid fever. Such relative cleanliness presumably reduced the transmission of wild and ubiquitous polioviruses that had hitherto routinely infected most infants and young children without producing paralytic complications. As a consequence, these groups became increasingly unprotected and susceptible to the crippling form of disease. In fact, many children became polio victims soon after being weaned and thus deprived of maternal immunity.[72]

Ever since poliomyelitis had become a reportable disease in 1910, public health authorities everywhere carefully monitored its appearance. This was especially true during the summer months, when polio was known to strike. Authorities in New York were especially on alert because the city had already suffered two serious epidemics of the disease in 1907 and 1910. The new administration of Mayor John P. Mitchell was proud of its Health Department. This unit was composed of competent professionals and led by Haven Emerson, a former medical practitioner who had treated the last cases of cholera. Successful campaigns against unsanitary boarding rooms, subway and streetcar crowding, as well as trade in patent medicines had bolstered the department's morale. In the eyes of its officials, a declining infant mortality rate testified to the city's sanitary standing. Its combined population from all five boroughs was estimated at 5,570,000.[73]

All but forgotten in the midst of an election year, the war in Europe, and a Mexican-American crisis prompted by Pancho Villa's raid, the first cases of polio in New York were reported on June 6. All of the sick children came from a densely populated section of Brooklyn near the waterfront, primarily populated by Italians. Visiting nurses making a house-to-house search soon discovered another twenty-two victims of the disease, some ill for several weeks but not severely enough to demand medical attention.[74]

There was no denying it. Polio had returned to New York. In the following days 327 new cases were disclosed in Brooklyn alone, with a mortality rate of about 20 percent. Before it was all over in November, New York City reported a total of 8,927 true cases of polio and 2,343 deaths, with the two less-populous boroughs, Richmond and Queens, actually showing the highest case rates. Nearly half of the victims—4,500, were seen in or admitted to the city's hospitals. Nationwide, the poliomyelitis epidemic of 1916 affected 27,000 people in 26 states and caused about 6,000 deaths.[75]

One of the first tasks of the New York Health Department was to ascertain the dimensions and geographic contours of the new epidemic, a coordinated process based on numerous field reports provided by an army of inspectors and nurses. As one publication stated: "It is the health officer's task in an epidemic to know where all cases are in his bailiwick."[76] Detection and disclosure of new cases was paramount to achieving control of the epidemic, and it could only be carried out with the help of the medical profession and the public. Neighborhood health stations were at the forefront of these search-and-report missions. Some infants brought in for regular visits could not hold on to their bottles.

Mothers were advised to bring all febrile children, especially those with "weak legs" or to send for a doctor.[77] All physicians in affected areas were urged to cooperate. Moreover, the authorities offered diagnostic lumbar punctures and spinal fluid examinations free of charge.

As the house-to-house searches were stepped up with the help of additional inspectors and nurses, quarantine procedures went into effect to isolate the suspected victims of polio.[78] Many children were promptly and forcibly separated from their parents and removed to specially outfitted pavilions at nearby hospitals for proper diagnosis and treatment. Initially, most patients arrived at Kingston Avenue and Queensboro hospitals.[79] Only two visits to the sick by members of the family were allowed over the next eight weeks. Confirmed cases of the disease were made public, and their names as well as addresses were published daily in the newspapers. Parents were urged to read the lists and keep their children far away from the infected places. Houses yielding victims of the disease were immediately placarded. Like a scarlet letter, the clearly visible sign was placed outside on the street front and in tenement buildings on the street door, entrance hall, and apartment door. Inspectors checked on the yellow signs daily, trying to discourage their removal, which was subject to a heavy fine.[80]

Well-off parents, of course, could keep their sick children if they could provide them with a separate room and adequate nursing as well as medical care. Such isolation lasted eight weeks and required comprehensive cleaning of the premises, provision of separate bedding and utensils, and careful disposal of bodily discharges. If a child died at home, coffins were immediately sealed and burial occurred without a church ceremony. Houses were thoroughly fumigated and new wallpaper installed. All surviving siblings under the age of sixteen were quarantined in the house for the next two weeks.[81]

To ensure public support for such draconian isolation measures, Haven Emerson and his Health Department prepared half a million yellow leaflets for distribution. New Yorkers were told that polio was "a catching disease," its method of spread "not yet definitely known." Its germ was present in discharges from the nose, throat, and bowels of ill and even healthy persons, and therefore it was essential for children to stay away from crowds in parks, swimming pools, movie houses, and stores. Fresh air, wholesome food, shower baths, and general cleanliness were recommended as the best prophylaxis.[82]

The role of filth in poliomyelitis and its implications for public and personal hygiene was ambiguous but attractive to public health officials.

Because the spread of the disease was unpredictable—ignoring class distinctions and geographical boundaries—the idea of an environmental factor responsible for transmission of the disease was quite appealing. Moreover, experiments carried out in 1912 by Milton Rosenau, a professor of preventive medicine at Harvard, suggested that flies, especially the biting stable fly, could transmit polio. Although the importance of this possible vector was still under investigation, the Health Department could not ignore it.[83] All scientific studies concerning infantile paralysis were problematic at this time. Although a virus believed responsible for the disease had already been isolated in 1909, virology was still in its infancy; given the contemporary climate of fear, no one could take any chances.[84]

The New York Health Department therefore embarked on a vigorous cleaning campaign. Four million gallons of water were dumped daily on the city's streets, paradoxically *before* the garbage was hauled away. Refuse and ash piles accumulating in halls of tenement houses and on sidewalks had to be removed. All stray cats and dogs were collected; according to the Society for the Prevention of Cruelty to Animals, three hundred to four hundred fifty cats and dogs were put to death daily in early July. Flyswatters and screens to fend off the gregarious stable fly and its less aggressive domestic cousin were widely dispensed. Parents were urged to keep their homes spotless, and to go over all woodwork daily with a damp cloth, sprinkling floors with damp tea leaves or shredded newspaper before sweeping; to take daily baths; and of course, to keep covers over each garbage pail.[85]

Homeowners caught depositing refuse on the streets were fined. Brooklyn, an early locus of the epidemic, became the black sheep in the eyes of Commissioner Emerson. He accused its citizens of lacking enough civil pride to keep their streets clean, suggesting that perhaps they were responsible for the abundance of cases there.[86] An army of thousands of volunteers began patrolling the neighborhoods on foot and on motorcycles, checking for violations of the Sanitary Code. By July 11 the authorities had already charged 148 individuals with violations; eventually 2,266 such summonses were listed.[87]

As most public health measures increasingly focused on environmental filth and garbage, polio began to be viewed as another plague of poverty primarily affecting the same marginal slumdwellers who had been blamed for previous epidemics. "If we could get rid of ignorance and the filth and superstition that go with it, there would be little need to hunt down the mysterious germs that no filter can stop and no microscope disclose," wrote one editorialist.[88] Indeed, the poor lacked the airy, clean, and cheerful rooms which Emerson recommended for the domestic treatment of polio cases. They seemed unable or even resistant to following the rules of hygiene which presumably contributed to a disease-free environment. "Defilers of the streets are to blame," commented one writer.[89] Even New York's mayor stressed cleanliness. "There is no occasion for alarm or panic," read Mitchell's statement published July 9 "Careful observance of the simple directions given by the Health Department as to personal and household cleanliness will go far to prevent further spread of or exposure to infection."[90]

Not surprisingly, poor Italian families bearing the early brunt of the epidemic were suspected of having introduced polio from their homeland, although inquiries by Emerson to the quarantine station at Ellis Island failed to confirm such an impression. Both the immigration authorities and American consular staff in Italy declared that no polio cases had been reported in that country. In spite of such reassurances, suspicion lingered and quickly included Lower East Side Jews and Poles, who also furnished a disproportionate number of polio cases. Certain neighborhoods appeared to be especially dangerous. One of them was "Pigtown," an Italian section of Brooklyn around Albany Avenue and Maple Street.[91]

As the toll from the epidemic mounted in July, the New York Health Department increased its "war" against the crippling scourge. Among the newly recruited "forces" were 21,000 citizens organized by the city's police commissioner under the banner of "Home Defense League." Its members spread out to every precinct, where they worked thirteen-hour shifts accompanying policemen on patrol and searching for violations of the sanitary code. Grocery stores, fruit markets, and street vendors came under strict surveillance. One hundred and fifty gangs with water trucks were placed into service. All theaters and movie houses were closed to children under the age of sixteen.[92]

Public acceptance of and cooperation with such a health campaign were critical, and Emerson was quite aware of the difficulties awaiting him if he failed to persuade the community through educational means about the importance of sanitary and quarantine measures. "Anything which causes antagonism of the public to the policy of reporting and removal to isolation hospitals, develops deception, hiding of cases, and such methods of obstruction as to frustrate to a great degree any approach to successful separation of the sick from the well."[93] But how could the public be convinced? Repeated visits by public health nurses trying to educate families at risk proved only partially successful. The pitch was directed to the children of immigrants themselves, who apparently grasped the importance of the measures before their parents; because of cultural and language barriers, these parents were less amenable to the sanitary gospel. "Results obtained among adults were largely due to fear of authority and the force of the department and not to voluntary action on their part," commented one newspaper editorial.[94]

There was, of course, resistance to the actions of the Health Department. As the seemingly conflicting messages of environmental hygiene and personal contagion took hold, fear began to grip the wary. "Many a family of children was housed for weeks, often in tight-shut rooms, the children's pale faces pressed against the window panes, mute evidence of their unreasonable imprisonment," recalled Emerson.[95] Others slammed the door in the faces of visiting nurses, who were suspected of carrying polio from one family to another. One nurse stationed at a pediatric clinic in Brooklyn, who had repeatedly reported cases of the disease as well as violations of the sanitary code in "Pigtown," received a life-threatening "black hand" letter and from then on had to be escorted by a policeman between her home and place of work.[96]

The Red Cross, in turn, provided its nurses for home visits because they apparently generated less fear among mothers who worried that their children would be summarily confiscated and removed to hospitals. The latter were rumored to be hotbeds of polio infection easily transmitted to arriving children and health personnel. Even many private schools and colleges refused to admit students on trivial grounds.[97]

By mid-July publicity surrounding the polio epidemic in New York City prompted a major effort by neighboring communities and indeed the rest of the nation to confine the city's children within the metropolitan area, thus avoiding a possible spread of the disease to other cities and villages. Towns on Long Island, a favorite summer destination for countless New York families, placed billboards at their city limits urging city dwellers with children to return home. Hotel-owners admitting them overnight were heavily fined. At numerous railroad stations families traveling with children were turned back or placed under observation.[98]

With assistance from the U.S. Public Health Service, the New York Health Department agreed to issue one-day health certificates or traveler's identification cards, certifying that the child was free of symptoms and did not come from an infected household. The same document could also be obtained from a private physician after an examination.

The certificate was routinely requested from all children under the age of sixteen before embarkation for travel at all ferry and rail terminals as well as steamboat piers. Those who managed to leave without such cards were not allowed to disembark at their destination.[99]

Although thousands of certificates were issued in the following weeks, many communities around New York City refused to accept them. Some demanded similar documents from the accompanying adults, and other communities, such as those in Connecticut, quickly escorted arriving families out of town and abandoned them in open fields. One child from Brooklyn, who possessed a health certificate, came down with polio in Rochester, forcing Emerson to reiterate that the examination given prior to issuance of a permit card could not detect disease during the early stages of incubation.[100]

Given the presence of large numbers of healthy carriers, Emerson actually questioned the ban on travel out of New York City. In his view, such quarantine measures were futile and had no effect on the spread of the epidemic. "I know that nothing has developed so many automobile detours, such ingenuity in the violation of the laws, and such wholehearted disrespect for reasonable sanitary law and its enforcement."[101] Strangely enough, Emerson's opinion about quarantines outside New York was totally at odds with his strong belief in their utility within the city.

Emerson's reference to travel detours was pertinent. Anxious parents planning summer outings or more extended vacations flooded the Automobile Club of America with requests for routing around the more than five hundred quarantines imposed by towns and villages bordering New York City. In many instances guards with red flags were posted at the entrance of such towns, stopping every automobile and carefully searching for concealed children. Those carrying anybody under the age of sixteen had to report to police stations or health offices.[102] "I hardly need to recall the countless instances of inconvenience, hardship, yes, real brutal inhumanity which resulted from the application of the general quarantine," admitted Emerson.[103] No wonder so many people "developed a most perverse ingenuity in discovering automobile detours."[104]

During the month of August, reported cases of polio began to ebb, and doubts were increasingly voiced concerning the success of Emerson's quarantine measures. The vector theory of the stable fly was discredited;[105] dissemination of polio was now thought to occur mostly via unrecognized carriers through person-to-person contacts. It was also thought that the decline in polio cases resulted from the depletion of susceptible children who lacked natural immunity.[106] "Perhaps twenty-five years from now our present prophylactic efforts may appear to have been too troublesome, over strenuous, or even ill advised," conceded one editorial in a medical journal.[107] With the epidemic now abating, it was safe to criticize such measures. In nearby Oyster Bay irate fathers interrupted a town council meeting on August 28 demanding the return of their children who had been removed to isolation hospitals. The local quarantine was branded as another instance of "propaganda to terrify the people."[108]

One cannot avoid noticing a sobering skepticism which overtook public health officers, medical practitioners, and scientists as the polio epidemic of 1916 came to an end. The New York City Health Department had tried in part to control the outbreak by teaching the public everything known about the disease with the help of professional groups, volunteer organizations, the press, and leaflets. After all, responsibility for infectious diseases had significantly shifted in the twentieth century from the environment to individuals, their way of life, and behavior. But public education alone was certainly not enough; it only heightened the fears of many, failed to reach others because of ethnic and social barriers, and, moreover, failed to stem the epidemic.

Emerson was persuaded to adhere to sanitary principles and isolation methods employed since the Renaissance. As he wrote: "Health of the individual is a public asset in which the civil government has an interest and for the protection of which broad police powers may be exercised."[109] Such functions were specifically authorized by law, then executed and enforced for the public good at the expense of individual rights. Environmental sanitation, quarantines, and isolation of the sick were among the key objectives of such a campaign.

None of the approaches was entirely successful. "As to the lessons we have learned during the epidemic," declared one physician, "we have learned very little that is new about the disease, but much that is old about ourselves."[110] Scientists were still debating the nature of the agent causing polio and its method of transmission. Physicians, while expressing appreciation for the great clinical opportunities furnished by the epidemic, argued about the usefulness of spinal fluid examinations and convalescents' serum treatments.[111] Five hundred children with varying forms of paralysis presented formidable challenges to those entrusted with their rehabilitation.

And then there was public health. Isolation and quarantine had appeared to help stem the onslaught of polio. But, did they really, or was the waning of the epidemic during autumn just part of a natural cycle? No matter. Again ethnic minorities and the powerless poor had been stigmatized in the name of established public health dogma.[112] "The sanitary code is a body of sanitary law passed by the Board of Health in the last fifty years," asserted Haven Emerson, "it is the substance of the best that the medical profession has been able to produce for the community control of disease."[113] Residents of Oyster Bay saw it differently. Their resolutions lifting the local quarantine concluded with the statement that "both profane and modern history are replete with the medico-politico barbarism of which we are now receiving a sample as anyone who knows the history of quarantine must understand and acknowledge."[114]

CONCLUSION

What are some of the implications of each case study presented in this chapter? Is there anything about these epidemics that could inform our approach to AIDS? Are there "lessons" here we cannot ignore? In the first place, we need to be aware that epidemics are the result of a complex interplay of biological and social factors which at certain points in our history create favorable ecological niches for given diseases to thrive and therefore decimate humankind. As we observed with epidemics of plague, cholera, and polio, the appearance of such illnesses was facilitated by bacterial and viral mutations, voyages and migrations, wars and trade, as well as the development of cities and social classes.

Most of these events were components of an intricate web of causality imperfectly understood even today. As epidemics erupted in history, the contours of such relationships were not only dimly perceived but also frequently completely misunderstood, particularly when the etiological agent remained unknown. Yet it is important for us to review the ecology of past infectious diseases and to reconstruct it as well as possible. Although often speculative, these studies allow us to see the ebb and flow of disease as inevitably complex and even erratic events. Such a perspective may provide encouragement to those who are constructing an epidemiological model for AIDS—an essential step if we are to control the disease.

Perhaps just as important for our understanding of the social dimensions of AIDS are the reviews of previous responses to mass disease. Our public memory has grown dim and we need to remember the social reactions to other epidemics, particularly because, with AIDS, we are already repeating them, despite all of our perceived sophistication. Although each disease has its own clinical characteristics, it often targets social groups which are more vulnerable to it because of genetic, cultural, and political factors.

In the face of epidemic disease, mankind has never reacted kindly. Collective fears, anxiety, and panic prompted a number of measures designed to protect the still healthy by cleaning up an environment deemed to be harmful, and by identifying, removing, and isolating those already found to be sick. As we saw in the epidemics discussed above, these rational self-protection measures formed the core of a sanitary code that has been legislated, executed, and enforced for centuries in different societies around the world.

That these sometimes drastic measures emerged at the same time that city states consolidated their political power and established complex bureaucracies to control the economic resources of their respective states is by no means coincidental. Healthy citizens were needed to achieve the goals of state sovereignty and commercial success. Epidemics created emergency conditions in which civil rights were suspended in the name of public survival. As all three case studies demonstrate, freedom of movement, privacy, and confidentiality were rescinded by authorities struggling to control the effects of disease.

Organized responses to epidemics were obviously not totally heartless exercises in power politics or economic self-interest. Health officials often risked their own lives in the implementation of sanitary laws and at times sought to ameliorate the economic impact of quarantines. Given the lack of knowledge about the causes and mechanisms of disease, these measures may have been reassuring to a majority of the population in a climate of panic and fear. As visible testimonies of society's obligations to protect the public health, these rules received broad approval and support.

Finally, we should also remember that the response to disease is a powerful tool to buttress social divisions and prejudices. All three examples demonstrate some of the stereotypical responses of anxious and frightened individuals and groups confronted by the ravages of disease. Flight and denial come first, followed by the scapegoating of those who are judged to be different by virtue of religious beliefs, cultural practices, or economic status. These social reactions reveal our ambiguities about the meaning of such diseases while furnishing convenient targets for projecting responsibilities and blame. The stranger, the Jew, the poor, the immigrant—all were victims of discrimination in the cases presented in this chapter, their deviance vindicated by the fact that the epidemics claimed a disproportionate number of casualties among them. Here the parallels to AIDS are not difficult to see. If history has a role to play in the present AIDS crisis, it is to restore public memory about our behavior during past epidemics and to continue to raise questions about the meaning and consequences of disease.

NOTES

1. The literature on disease ecology is extensive. For some basic views consult L. L. Klepinger, "The Evolution of Human Disease: New Findings and Problems," *Journal of Biosocial Science* 12 (1980): 481–486; Macfarlane Burnet and David O. White, "The Ecological Point of View," in *Natural History of Infectious Disease,* 4th ed. (Cambridge: Cambridge University Press, 1974), 1–21; and Frank Fenner, "The Effects of Changing Social Organizations on the Infectious Diseases of Man," in *The Impact of Civilization on the Biology of Man,* ed. S. V. Boyden (Toronto: University of Toronto Press, 1970), 48–76.

2. Among the works describing this epidemic are the following: Paolo S. Pallavicino, *Descrizione del contagio che da Napoli si comunico a Roma nell'anno 1656* (Rome: Collegio Urbano, 1837) and two manuscripts: "Memorie diverse appartenenti alle cose di Roma in tempo del male contagioso 1656" (MSS Corsiniano 171, the library of the Accademia dei Lincei, Rome) and "A di 5 maggio 1656. Principio il contagio nella citta di Roma" (MSS Chigiano Codex E III, 62, the Vatican Library, Rome). Pallavicino's account has been translated into English by Ellen B. Wells, but remains unpublished. I am indebted to her for allowing me to study it. Wells has described the epidemic in considerable detail: see "The Plague of Rome of 1656," M.A. thesis, Cornell University, 1973.

3. This point has not been emphasized enough in most accounts of the Black Death which focus almost exclusively on the human disease. In fact, one hypothesis tries to bolster the interhuman transfer of the disease: S. R. Ell, "Some Evidence for Interhuman Transmission of Plague," *Reviews of Infectious Diseases* 1 (1979): 563–566.

4. This explanation has been proposed by John Norris, a long-time student of plague epidemiology. His paper "Final Deliverance: The Disappearance of Plague from Western Europe" (The 1986 Benjamin Lieberman Memorial Lecture, University of California, San Francisco) still awaits publication. However, he has given us a valuable insight into the origins of the disease: "East or West? The Geographic Origin of the Black Death," *Bulletin of the History of Medicine* 51 (1977): 1–24.

5. A primary source about this disastrous event is Girolamo Gatta, *Di una gravissima peste. . . . dell'anno 1656 depopulo la citta di Napoli* (Naples: Fusco, 1659). Useful mortality statistics for both Naples and Rome can be found in L. del Panta and M. Livi Bacci, "Chronologie, intensité et diffusion des crises de mortalité en Itali: 1600–1850," in *Population,* numéro spécial (1977): 401–444, reprinted in *The Great Mortalities: Methodological Studies of De-*

mographic Crises in the Past, ed. Hubert Charbonneau and André Larose (Liège: Ordina, 1980).

6. Pallavicino, *Descrizione,* 10. The most comprehensive history of Italian epidemics is Alfonso Corradi, *Annali delle epidemie occorse in Italia dalle prime memorie fino al 1850,* 8 vols. (Bologna: Gamberini e Permeggiani, 1865–1894). A new five-volume edition was reprinted in 1972–1973.

7. See Francesco Corridore, *La Popolazione dello Stato Romano, 1656–1901* (Rome: Loescher, 1906), and Roger Mols, *Introduction a la démographie historique des villes d'Europe du XIVe au XVIIIe siècles,* 3 vols. (Gembloux: J. Duculot 1954–1956). These statistics are also quoted in Richard Krautheimer, *The Rome of Alexander VII, 1655–1667* (Princeton: Princeton University Press, 1985), 159, based on another study by F. Cerasoli, "Censimento della popolazione di Roma dall'anno 1600 al 1739," *Studi e documenti di Storia e Diritto* 12 (1981).

8. The remark was made by a critic, Lorenzo Pizzati from Pontremoli, a former official at the papal court, in a memorandum to Alexander VII. Quoted in Krautheimer, *Rome,* 127, and also Chigi, C III, 71 (Vatican Library, Bibliotheca Apostolica), and other sources.

9. Krautheimer, *Rome,* 127–130.

10. For further detail consult early chapters of Krautheimer, *Rome,* esp. chap. 1, 8–14. An extensive biography by Paolo S. Pallavicino is *Della vita di Alessandro VII,* 2 vols. (Prato, 1839–1840). A brief notice can be found in the *Dizionario biografico degli Italiani* (Rome: Instituto della Enciclopedia Italiana, 1960) 2:205.

11. Not much has been written about early public health measures. The most informative account is by Carlo M. Cipolla, "The Origin and Development of the Health Boards," in his *Public Health and the Medical Profession in the Renaissance* (Cambridge: Cambridge University Press, 1976), 11–66. Also useful, by the same author, is *Cristofano and the Plague; A Study in the History of Public Health in the Age of Galileo* (Berkeley and Los Angeles: University of California Press, 1973).

12. See Saul Jarcho, *Italian Broadsides Concerning Public Health* (Mount Kisco, N.Y.: Futura, 1986), 123–125. The documents reproduced in this work applied to both Rome and Bologna.

13. Pallavicino, *Descrizione,* 15–16. A contemporary Jewish physician, Jacob Zahalon, described the events in his work, *The Treasure of Life,* published in Venice in 1683: "The Jews were forbidden to leave the ghetto and enter the city as was their custom. . . . They appointed an officer, Monsignor Negroni, who came twice a day to look after the needs of the community and to enforce rigid isolation at a great penalty; they set up gallows near the gate to hang anyone transgressing these orders." See H. A. Savitz, "Jacob Zahalon and His Book, *The Treasure of Life,*" *New England Journal of Medicine* 213 (1935): 167–176. More information about plague in the Jewish ghetto can be obtained from J. O. Leibowitz, "Bubonic Plague in the Ghetto of Rome (1656); Descriptions by Zahalon and Gastaldi," *Koroth* 4 (1967): 25–28.

14. These actions were all depicted in a series of contemporary drawings designed and produced by Giovanni G. Rossi in Rome as a tribute to Alexander

VII's efforts against the epidemic. One set of illustrations is available at the National Library of Medicine, Historical Division, Prints and Photographs, negatives 68–221, 68–222, 68–223, and 67–536. Similar scenes drawn by another artist and published by Giacomo Molinari are available at the Philadelphia Museum of Art, Ars Medica Collection. A third set is in the British Museum, London.

15. Ibid. Most of this information can be obtained from the captions accompanying the scenes. The artists even used numbers to properly identify all buildings and actions. For a summary see Ellen B. Wells, "Prints Commemorating the Rome 1656 Plague Epidemic," *Annali dell' Instituto e Museo di Storia della Scienza di Firenze* X (1985): 15–21.

16. Pallavicino, *Descrizione,* 20. See also the various pertinent drawings previously cited.

17. Zahalon recalls that "when the physician visited the sick it was customary that he take in his hand a large torch of tar, burning it night and day to purify the air for his protection." Savitz, *Zahalon,* 175. For an assessment of the perils awaiting healers who remained to attend plague victims and the rewards offered by cities for their courageous duty, see C. M. Cipolla, "A Plague Doctor," in *The Medieval City,* ed. H. A. Miskimin, D. Herlihy, and A. L. Udovitch (New Haven: Yale University Press, 1977), 65–72.

18. Pallavicino, *Descrizione,* 14.

19. Ibid., 35.

20. One of the drawings previously described contains such an execution scene. Other persons were hanged in public places on specially erected platforms. In extreme cases violators were torn apart and their limbs displayed separately suspended from scaffolds.

21. These notions were aptly summarized by a contemporary physician, Girolamo Fracastoro (1484–1553), of Verona. See his *Contagion, Contagious Diseases, and Their Treatment,* trans. W. C. Wright (New York: Putnam, 1930). For a good review of these concepts see V. Nutton, "The Seeds of Disease: An Explanation of Contagion and Infection from the Greeks to the Renaissance," *Medical History* 27 (1983): 1–34.

22. Krautheimer cites a number of decrees issued by the Health Board and Street Department regarding refuse and circulation of animals through the streets; following the epidemic there were bans against the open slaughter or display of meat, frying pasta or fish in the squares, "for the hygiene of the city," *Rome,* 190–191.

23. Pallavicino, *Descrizione,* 10.

24. Savitz, *Zahalon,* 175–176. More statistical information is available in a very detailed work by Pietro Savio, "Richerche sulla peste di Roma degli anni 1656–1657," *Archivio della Societa Romana di Storia Patria* 95 (1972): 138.

25. See Savio, "Richerche," 119. For an overview, also consult D. F. Zanetti, "Peste et mortalité differentielle," *Annales de Demographie Historique* (1972): 197–202.

26. Pallavicino, *Descrizione,* 31.

27. Ibid., 4.

28. This idea is advanced by L. A. McNicol and R. N. Doetsch in "A Hypothesis Accounting for the Origin of Pandemic Cholera: A Retrograde Analysis," *Perspectives in Biology and Medicine* 26 (1983): 547–552. The traditional view represented by R. Pollitzer and J. Chambers is that the disease has been present since antiquity. See R. Pollitzer, *Cholera* (Geneva, World Health Organization, 1959), esp. chap. 1, pp. 11–16.

29. There is no comprehensive work on the history of cholera from a global perspective. A useful sketch of the various pandemics can be found in Erwin H. Ackerknecht, *History and Geography of the Most Important Diseases* (New York: Hafner, 1965), 25–32.

30. For a chronology of cholera in Britain, see Norman Longmate, *King Cholera. The Biography of a Disease* (London: Hamilton, 1966). The impact of the disease on epidemiology and sanitation in that country is contained in Margaret Pelling's *Cholera, Fever and English Medicine, 1825–1865* (Oxford: Oxford University Press, 1978). For a review of the social reaction to cholera see A. Briggs, "Cholera and Society in the Nineteenth Century," *Past and Present* 19 (1961): 76–96. More recently, Robert J. Morris wrote *Cholera 1832. The Social Response to an Epidemic* (London: Croom Helm, 1976).

31. This epidemic has been described in great detail by Charles E. Rosenberg. See his article, "The Cholera Epidemic of 1832 in New York City," *Bulletin of the History of Medicine* 33 (1959): 37–49, and *The Cholera Years: The United States in 1832, 1849, and 1866* (Chicago: University of Chicago Press, 1962), esp. chaps. 1–4. A brief overview of the epidemic in the United States is provided by John Duffy, "The History of Asiatic Cholera in the U.S.," *Bulletin of the New York Academy of Medicine* 47 (1971): 1152–1168.

32. Dudley Atkins, "A sketch of the history of the epidemic cholera which prevailed in the city of New York and throughout the United States, in the summer of 1832," in *Reports of Hospital Physicians and Other Documents in Relation to the Epidemic Cholera of 1832,* ed. Dudley Atkins (New York: Carvill, 1832), 5–8.

33. Rosenberg, *Cholera Years,* 17–20. See also Thomas Ford, *Slums and Housing* (Cambridge: Harvard University Press, 1936), 92–93.

34. Atkins, *Reports,* 9–13; see also Philip Hone, *The Diary of Philip Hone, 1828–1851,* ed. and introd. Alan Nevins, 2 vols. (New York: Dodd, Mead & Co., 1927) 1:68–69.

35. "We do not wish to excite unnecessary alarm in the public mind—but we do believe that the only way to obviate panic and meet danger when it threatens—is to be made fully aware of its existence and extent. We deem it, therefore, our duty to announce . . . that a malignant disease resembling in every respect the Asiatic or Canadian cholera, has made its appearance in our city," as quoted in *Daily Albany Argus,* 3 July 1832.

36. Atkins, *Reports,* 10–11; see also map in David M. Reese, *A Plain and Practical Treatise on the Epidemic Cholera* (New York: Conner & Cooke, 1833), pointing out the initial cholera outbreaks. "Nearly all farmhouses and private boarding houses in this vicinity have already been monopolized by fugitives from the cholera," *New York Evening Post,* 12 July 1832.

37. Letter from a passenger on the steamboat *Boston,* writing from Providence, Rhode Island, where the ship had been diverted to, *New York Evening Post,* 6 July 1832.

38. Hone, *Diary* 1:69; see also comments in *New York Evening Post,* 5 July 1832.

39. "The day in which this mortality occurred was a national holiday—a day on which many instances of excess always occur, and that very probably a considerable portion of those who died of cholera induced that disease by a degree of intemperance in eating and drinking," *New York Evening Post,* 6 July 1832.

40. *New York Evening Post,* 11 July 1832.

41. "None of these instances of spasmodic cholera come within the range of practice of these physicians whose very names would go far to convince credulity itself," ibid.

42. *Cholera Bulletin* conducted by an Association of Physicians, vol. 1, nos. 1–24, 1832, reprinted with an introduction by Charles E. Rosenberg (New York: Arno Press, 1972). This note is printed in vol. 1, no. 2 (9 July 1832), 6.

43. *New York Evening Post,* 13 July 1832.

44. Reese, *Epidemic Cholera,* map, and 55–60. See also Atkins, *Reports,* 14.

45. *Cholera Bulletin* 1 (13 July 1832): 26.

46. Ibid., 26.

47. *Cholera Bulletin* 1 (4 August 1832): 98.

48. *New York Evening Post,* 20 July 1832.

49. *New York Evening Post,* 23 July 1832.

50. Ibid.

51. *New York Evening Post,* 21 July 1832.

52. *Cholera Bulletin* 1 (11 July 1832): 17.

53. Atkins, *Reports,* 116.

54. Charles E. Rosenberg, "The Cause of Cholera: Aspects of Etiological Thought in Nineteenth-Century America," *Bulletin of the History of Medicine* 34 (1960): 331–354. See also Atkins, *Reports,* 14–25, and Reese, *Epidemic Cholera,* 24–25.

55. Reese, *Epidemic Cholera,* 59.

56. Atkins, *Reports,* 66.

57. Reese, *Epidemic Cholera,* 62.

58. Atkins, *Reports,* 15, 93.

59. Ibid., 94; see also Reese, *Epidemic Cholera,* 59.

60. Atkins, *Reports,* 94.

61. Martyn Paine, *Letters on the cholera asphyxia as it has appeared in the City of New York* (New York: Collins and Hannay, 1832), 45.

62. Gardiner Spring, *A Sermon Preached August 3, 1832* (New York: Leavitt, 1832).

63. Atkins, *Reports,* 68.

64. From the various comments in newspapers, by health officials and individual physicians, the conditions originally blamed for causing cholera remained virtually unchanged.

65. *New York Evening Post,* 26 July 1832.

66. *New York Evening Post,* 28 July 1832.

67. *Cholera Bulletin* 1 (15 August 1832): 138. A note in the *New York Evening Post,* 4 August 1832, read: "It is proper to state for the information of those physicians who so precipitously left town in consequence of the cholera, that those resident of the west side of the city may now return as the disease is evidently on the decline."

68. Reese, *Epidemic Cholera,* pref., 4.

69. Hone, *Diary* 1:73.

70. *New York Evening Post,* 6 August 1832.

71. For a general history of the disease, see John R. Paul, *A History of Poliomyelitis* (New Haven: Yale University Press, 1971). Also see S. Benison, "The Enigma of Poliomyelitis: 1910," in *Freedom and Reform: Essays in Honor of Henry Steele Commager,* ed. H. M. Hyman and L. W. Levy (New York: Harper & Row, 1967), 228–254.

72. See N. Nathanson and J. R. Martin, "The Epidemiology of Poliomyelitis: Enigmas Surrounding Its Appearance, Epidemicity, and Disappearance," *American Journal of Epidemiology* 110 (1979): 672–892; and John R. Paul, *Epidemiology of Poliomyelitis* (Geneva: WHO, 1955), 9–30.

73. For an overview see Arthur Bushel, *Chronology of New York City Department of Health (and Its Predecessor Agencies), 1655–1966* (New York: New York City Department of Health, 1966). Also available is John Duffy, *A History of Public Health in New York City,* 2 vols. (New York: Russell Sage Foundation, 1968–1974). A brief contemporary summary can be found in the *American Review of Reviews* 53 (January–June 1916): 495–496, under the title "Mayor Mitchell's administration of New York City."

74. Paul, "The Epidemic of 1916," *History,* chap. 15, 148–160.

75. *Journal of the American Medical Association* (hereafter *JAMA*) 67 (4 November 1916): 1379, summarizing the statistics provided by the New York City Health Department in its *Bulletin* no. 43. Further additions and new totals were published in *JAMA* 67 (25 November 1916): 1609. See also Haven Emerson, "The recent epidemic of infantile paralysis," *Bulletin of the Johns Hopkins Hospital* 28 (1917): 132.

76. *Survey,* 2 June 1917.

77. *World,* 25 June 1916.

78. "Our method of fighting the disease is this: whenever a case is reported in a block not previously affected, a house to house canvas of that block is made. In this way many unreported cases have been found." *New York Times,* 1 July 1916.

79. *New York Times,* 28 June 1916; *JAMA* 67 (7 July 1916): 129–130.

80. "Dr. Emerson yesterday issued a warning to all landlords with tenants as well as owners of the tenement houses that Health Department placards on the front of the houses would stay there until the patient's room had been entirely renovated." *New York Times,* 5 July 1916.

81. *JAMA* 67 (29 July 1916): 366.

82. An extract from the leaflet distributed by the Health Department is available in Haven Emerson, "Some practical considerations in the adminis-

trative control of epidemic poliomyelitis," *American Journal of Medical Sciences* 153 (1917): 161–162. The leaflets were printed in English, Italian, and Hebrew.

83. For popular writings on the subject, see for example, "Infantile paralysis from fly-bites," *Literary Digest,* 28 December 1912, 1220–1221. Even *Good Housekeeping* warned: "The fly is literally not only as dangerous as a rattlesnake but as disgraceful as a bed-bug. He is born of filth, is attracted by filth, and breeds in filth." See W. W. Hutchinson, "An ancient enemy under a new name," *Good Housekeeping,* January–June 1916, 509. The *Good Housekeeping* pattern department even issued patterns for special clothes, "designed to protect the little lads and lassies from the sting of the deadly stable-fly."

84. For a view of contemporary scientific research on viruses, see S. Benison, "Poliomyelitis and the Rockefeller Institute: Social Effects and Institutional Response," *Journal of the History of Medicine and Allied Sciences* 29 (1974): 74–93. A brief account of work at that institution was written by H. T. Wade, "The Rockefeller Institute for Medical Research," *American Review of Reviews* 39 (1909): 183–191.

85. Some of the instructions were printed on the previously cited leaflets. One physician blamed the polio epidemic on New York City's seemingly faulty scavenger system. He felt that the garbage should be hauled away *before* street cleaning began instead of the usual practice of watering and sweeping before such removal. *New York Times,* 10 July 1916.

86. Ibid.

87. *New York Times,* 11 July 1916.

88. *New York Times,* 10 July 1916.

89. *New York Times,* 13 July 1916. The relationship between polio and dirt was not believed to be causal, although lack of cleanliness was thought to help spread the disease. "If all children who live on dirty streets and alleys or in dirty homes should have infantile paralysis, the Brooklyn sky which is now overcast with gloom would become as black as a storm sky at midnight," wrote Thomas J. Riley in an article entitled "Poverty and poliomyelitis," in *Survey,* 29 July 1916, 447. The best summary is available from the New York City Health Department: *A Monograph on the Epidemic of Poliomyelitis in New York City in 1916* (New York: M. B. Brown, 1917).

90. *New York Times,* 9 July 1916.

91. *New York Times,* 1 July 1916. See also article by T. J. Riley: "Another *first impression* was that the disease was found mostly among Italians. . . . I concluded that infantile paralysis is no respecter of nationalities," in *Survey,* 447, emphasis in original. For details on Jews see D. Dwork, "Health Conditions of Immigrant Jews on the East Side of New York, 1880–1914," *Medical History* 25 (1981): 1–40.

92. *New York Times,* 9 July 1916.

93. Emerson, "Some practical considerations," *American Journal of Medical Sciences* 153 (1917): 168.

94. New York City Department of Health, *A Monograph on the Epidemic of Poliomyelitis in New York City in 1916* (New York: Brown, 1917), 40.

95. Emerson, "Some practical considerations," *American Journal of Medical Sciences* 153 (1917): 162.

96. *New York Times,* 23 July 1916.

97. The Health Department usually employed nurses for the removal of children suspected of suffering from polio, "as it has been found that mothers would surrender their infants to other women, when they would not let men take them away," *New York Times,* 10 July 1916.

98. One such poster from Setauket, Long Island, was reprinted in the *New York Times:* "Warning—we are informed that families from the infected part of New York City and Brooklyn are offering high prices for rooms and houses here. While we sympathize fully with all who are suffering from this dread disease, infantile paralysis, we certainly should be very careful to whom we extend the hospitality of our village," *New York Times,* 8 July 1916.

99. For further details about the epidemic outside New York City, see Naomi Rogers, "Screen the Baby, Swat the Fly: Polio in the Northeastern United States, 1916" (Ph.D. diss., University of Pennsylvania, 1986). For an interesting case study of nearby New Jersey, see Stuart Galishoff, "Newark and the Great Polio Epidemic of 1916," *New Jersey History* 94 (Summer–Autumn 1976): 101–111.

100. Several stories about the quarantine around New York City can be read in *Survey,* 29 July 1916, and 5 August 1916. For an overview see Hugh S. Cumming, "The U.S. Quarantine System during the Past Fifty Years," in *A Half Century of Public Health,* ed. M. P. Ravenel (New York: APHA, 1921), 118–132.

101. Emerson, "Some practical considerations," *American Journal of Medical Sciences* 153 (1917): 170.

102. *New York Times,* 23 August 1916.

103. Emerson, "Some practical considerations," *American Journal of Medical Sciences* 153 (1917): 170.

104. *Survey,* 2 June 1917.

105. Before that time, giant flytraps had been put up at the Jefferson Market, *New York Times,* 25 July 1916. There were also suggestions for the installations of electric fans to deal with the fly problem at Washington Market, *New York Times,* 23 July 1916.

106. A pamphlet on polio prepared by Dr. Wade H. Frost and issued by the U.S. Public Health Service in late July 1916 listed unrecognized healthy carriers as the chief source of infection, *Public Health Reports* 31 (14 July 1916): 1817–1833. See also S. Flexner, "The nature, manner of conveyance and means of prevention of infantile paralysis," *JAMA* 67 (22 July 1916): 279–283. This paper was first presented at a symposium sponsored by the New York Academy of Medicine on 13 July 1916. During the discussion Dr. William H. Park remarked that "the sick person and the carrier are the chief sources of infection. There is no evidence that a fly or insect transmits the disease," 313.

107. *JAMA* 67 (26 August 1916): 687.

108. *New York Times,* 29 August 1916. In one incident, removal to the hospital of an individual suspected of having polio required four deputy sheriffs to

wrest the child from its father. The episode was viewed as an "especially flagrant offense against the freedom of the community."

109. Haven Emerson, "Relative Functions of Health Agencies: Viewpoint of the Official Agency," *Selected Papers* (Battle Creek, Mich.: Kellogg, 1949), 60. This paper was presented in San Francisco in 1920.

110. Commentary by Dr. Frederick C. Tilney during a symposium on poliomyelitis, *Long Island Medical Journal* 10 (November 1916): 469.

111. Much of the scientific research is summarized by S. Benison in "Speculation and Experimentation in Early Poliomyelitis Research," *Clio Medica* 10 (1975): 1–22, and "The History of Polio Research in the U.S.: Appraisal and Lessons," in *The Twentieth-Century Sciences: Studies in the Biography of Ideas,* ed. G. Holton (New York: W. W. Norton, 1972), 308–343.

112. The article by Thomas J. Riley in *Survey,* 29 July 1916, 448, asked: "Is not infantile paralysis one of the health problems arising among the same people and in the same conditions as give us our problems of tuberculosis and other contagious or infectious diseases, of poverty, ignorance, deformities, and defects? Perhaps one could include also delinquency and drunkenness. . . . Must we forever have these plague spots and these ill-favored folks?"

113. Haven Emerson, "The Responsibilities of the Department of Health of the City of New York," *Long Island Medical Journal* 10 (July 1916): 261.

114. As quoted in the *New York Times,* 29 August 1916.

Quarantine and the Problem of AIDS

David F. Musto

Men take diseases, one of another.
Therefore let men take heed of their company.
Henry IV, Part 2

In ancient times citizens noted that, occasionally, a disease from a distant locale was sweeping toward them from neighboring villages, or that after a ship from a foreign land reached shore with ill persons aboard, residents in the port city would take ill. Such temporal sequences could not be ignored and, if the illness were a serious one, fears escalated as the illness came closer. Knowing the cause of an illness or its mode of transmission provides the basis for some rational approach to containing the spread of the disease. Prior to the nineteenth century, however, these agents were unknown, and civil authorities were thus left with whatever means seemed reasonable in the wisdom of the time to fight the spread of diseases. Protective measures were based on what we would now consider erroneous explanations for contagion. From this era of scant knowledge comes the origin of the familiar word we use to describe the isolation of the sick or contagious from the healthy. "Quarantine" comes from the Italian word for "forty days," and refers to the period during which ships capable of carrying contagious disease, such as plague, were kept isolated on their arrival at a seaport.[1]

Today, quarantine has come to mean a marking off, the creation of a boundary to ward off a feared biological contaminant lest it penetrate a healthy population. The essential characteristic of quarantine is the establishing of a boundary to separate the contaminated from the uncontaminated. But to consider only those quarantines of diseases that are infectious or that have short periods of illness, characterized by, say, fever, would be to overlook the deeper emotional and broader aggressive character of this measure. Evidence of this elemental fear of contagion includes such instances as measures taken against yellow fever in the eighteenth century and the growing fear of the AIDS epidemic in the late twentieth century. The assumptions and psychology of quarantine are evident in restrictions against groups thought liable to degrade "racial purity" if allowed to immigrate into a "racially healthy" country. The multiple determinants of quarantine can be seen in a much earlier age also. The social history of leprosy is an enduring and dramatic example of boundaries being drawn around those with a lengthy illness that was highly feared and believed to be highly contagious.

LEPROSY

The bacillus responsible for leprosy was not discovered until 1874, one of the first bacterial pathogens to be described. In preceding centuries the early stages of leprosy had often been confused with other skin diseases, but the advanced stages of leprosy—characterized by loss of nerve conduction and bodily disfigurement—occurred frequently enough to ensure continuous alarm about physical signs that might foretell the gradual and, for all practical purposes, irreversible wasting of the body by leprous infection. Leprosy was dreaded first of all because it was frequently assumed to be incurable and eventually fatal. Second, it was thought to be contagious—somehow. The strict rules established over the millennia to quarantine lepers reveals that people commonly believed they could be infected by touching a leper or coming into contact with his or her breath.

Medical care often falls into the simple sequence of diagnosis, then treatment. For leprosy the sequence was diagnosis, then separation. Leviticus, the third book of Moses, contains detailed rules for the diagnosis of leprosy. Once the diagnosis is made, the following is commanded by the Lord:

> The leper who has the disease shall wear torn clothes and let the hair of his head hang loose, and he shall cover his upper lip and cry, "Unclean, unclean." He shall remain unclean as long as he has the disease; he is unclean; he shall dwell alone in a habitation outside the camp.
>
> (Lev. 13:45–46, RSV)

We often associate leprosy with Europe's Middle Ages, and indeed leprosy was a widespread problem then. It is estimated that thousands of individual or group asylums called *leprosaria* existed in the thirteenth century.[2] The Christian church had reaffirmed the Mosaic concern with diagnosis and separation. The Third Lateran Council (1179) mandated living provisions for lepers, and elaborate rituals were decreed for the ceremony of separation. The common image of the medieval leper is of a forlorn individual coldly isolated and seeking sustenance through begging. It was not uncommon to believe that the loathsome disease was God's punishment for sin, particularly venereal transgressions. This linkage of leprosy with sexual promiscuity, with promiscuity seen either as a cause or a consequence of the disease, is interesting in light of our present attitudes toward AIDS.

But medieval society also took a larger and more humane view of leprosy. The church, the chief instrument for dealing with disease and sin during this era, devised religious ceremonies that enlisted the leper's cooperation in his or her isolation. The ritual centered on the leper and presented separation from society as a mutually wise decision. Sometimes the leper was encouraged to regard the disease as the sufferings of purgatory here on earth; leprosy was a sign that the leper would pass directly into heaven without the intervening punishment other mortals must endure in order to attain a purified form. Buttressing this concept were the Crusaders returning to Europe with leprosy apparently acquired in the Holy Land. A link between sin and the disease in these cases was unthinkable.

The ritual varied from one diocese to another and over time—for leprosy was a problem that, unlike its victims, would not go away. Fundamentally, the ritual was a service for the dead, because lepers, in effect, were declared dead to their society and the communion of the healthy. A priest would conduct the leper to church where the leper would hear mass kneeling under a black cloth suspended over his head. After mass he would be led again by the priest preceded by a crossbearer to another site in the church where comforting passages from the Bible would be read. As the leper left the church, he was sprinkled by the priest with holy water. The whole procedure was similar to that of conducting a dead body to the church, the saying of a requiem mass, and the passage from the church to the cemetery. Indeed, some rituals specified that dirt be scattered over the head of the leper or onto his feet; in some dioceses, the leper would stand in a freshly dug grave. When at last the leper had concluded his role in these elaborate ceremonies, he separated himself from society, while the priest admonished him:

> I forbid you ever to enter the church or monastery, fair, mill, marketplace, or company of persons. I forbid you ever to leave your house without your

leper's costume, in order that one may recognize you and that you never go barefoot. I forbid you to wash your hands or anything about you in the stream or in the fountain and to ever drink; and if you wish water to drink, fetch it in your cask or porringer. I forbid you to touch anything you bargain for or buy, until it is yours. I forbid you to enter a tavern. If you want wine, whether you buy it or someone gives it to you, have it put in your cask. I forbid you to live with any woman other than your own. I forbid you, if you go on the road and you meet some person who speaks to you, to fail to put yourself downwind before you answer. I forbid you to go in a narrow lane, so that should you meet any person, he should not be able to catch the affliction from you. I forbid you, if you go along any thoroughfare, to ever touch a well or the cord unless you have put on your gloves. I forbid you ever to touch children or to give them anything. I forbid you to eat or drink from any dishes other than your own. I forbid you drinking or eating in company, unless with lepers.[3]

The priest might follow these uncompromising orders with a comforting message. At Reims the ritual included this expression:

> This separation is only corporeal; as for the spirit, which is uppermost, you will always be as much as you ever were and will have part and portion of all the prayers of our mother Holy Church, as if every day you were a spectator at the divine service with others. And concerning your small necessities, people of means will provide them, and God will never forsake you. Only take care and have patience. God be with you.[4]

Lepers took a prominent role in the diagnosis of leprosy. One or more lepers might be on the committee responsible for these fateful examinations. Within the asylums lepers took care of one another. Religious orders sometimes cared for the sick and for the farm sometimes associated with the lepers' enclosure, but such a formal mixture of lepers with the healthy was limited.

In the course of the long period during which lepers were feared and segregated, it became apparent that not only was it difficult to control lepers who remained unpersuaded that they should be isolated but also that the placement of large numbers of lepers in quarantined farms required a degree of social organization and resources lacking in many parts of Europe. Prodded by the widespread fear of leprosy, however, church and state institutions perpetuated the practice of quarantine. Although the quarantine ideally was softened by religious rituals as described above, such benign practices were balanced by other instances of brutality in some places and by extermination programs carried out by Henry II of England and Philip V of France. Eventually, leprosy became a metaphor for heresy, moral turpitude, and unnatural and excessive lust. Leprosy resisted one wave of attempted cure after another—alchemy, miracle, penance, whatever stirred hope—while disfigured people suffering its late stages continued to evoke dread, thereby promoting quarantine.

Leprosy can be contrasted with diseases whose courses are dangerous but brief, such as plague, yellow fever, and cholera. The isolation of ships coming from lands where plague was present was the classic example of quarantine. During the Black Death of the fourteenth century, when a sizable fraction of Europe's population perished through a rapidly spreading, quickly fatal infection, attempts were made both to establish quarantine, on the one hand, for habitations still spared or, on the other, to isolate the sick. Physicians and others with a need to visit the diseased wore apparel that entirely enclosed the body: gloves, shoes, headgear, and a gown with a cache under the nose for holding strong-smelling herbs to purify the air breathed in. Clearly, quarantine and such elaborate apparel carry an assumption that diseases are contagious; the means of contagion, however, remained unclear. The breath, putrefying organic matter, even the patient's gaze was suspected. With no certainty about what was the target of control, the citizenry's anxiety could quickly shift from one possibility to another, even to groups of people, as when Jews were suspected of poisoning wells and deliberately spreading plague. Frustration over their society's failure to halt a terrifying contagion led to destructive, irrational outbursts.

YELLOW FEVER

The New World was not immune to epidemics. North American port cities were subject to occasional but nevertheless disastrous onslaughts of yellow fever, a viral infection now known to be transmitted by mosquitoes. Cholera spread fear and death through several waves of infection, particularly during the nineteenth century. Cholera was later discovered to be caused by a bacterium and spread through food and water contaminated by human waste. For many years, though, both diseases confounded physicians and citizens alike. Observers divided roughly into two camps, contagionists and anticontagionists, which had considerable bearing on the issue of quarantine. Although writers on epidemic disease during the eighteenth and nineteenth centuries did not always maintain a pure belief in one or the other alternative, the differences can be simply stated. Contagionists took what appears to have been the commonsense position of most people through the ages, that a disease was transmitted from one person to another. Anticontagionists, on the other hand, believed that both yellow fever and cholera were caused by many individuals coming into contact with the products of putrefaction as a result of hot weather or the inadequate cleansing of streets, homes, and businesses.[5]

These two views postulated strikingly dissimilar conclusions not only for the origin of epidemic diseases but also for their control. When yellow fever struck Philadelphia—then capital of the United States—in 1793, government officials fled, many people died, and an acrimonious controversy ensued over the origin of the ailment. Contagionists, who were in the majority at the College of Physicians, argued that the disease had been brought into the city by a ship from the West Indies. Under this line of reasoning, quarantine of suspect ships was a wise precaution. Dr. Benjamin Rush professed the opposing view. He argued that the epidemic was caused by summer weather and the spoilage of a shipment of coffee near the wharf. He went on to assert that yellow fever was only the intensification of fever which normally "prevails every year in our city, from vegetable putrefaction."[6] This latter view was quite in keeping with Rush's assertion that all diseases were essentially the same disruption of the body's function. From the point of view of Philadelphians, however, Rush's position was a condemnation of the city itself, while the contagionists' explanation merely called for greater vigilance, with the help of quarantine, against danger from the outside such as ships from the West Indies and visitors to the city of Philadelphia.

From the perspective of the twentieth century, the contagionist-anticontagionist controversy seems paradoxical. The contagionists correctly assumed that a specific infectious agent had to be transmitted to a person in order to elicit a specific disease. But it was the anticontagionists who, although etiologically incorrect, championed sanitary measures such as clean streets and efficient elimination of human waste which we now consider essential to a healthy community. Only later in the nineteenth century would the roles of inadequate waste disposal and mosquitoes breeding in stagnant pools be seen to be links in the epidemic chain. Rush denounced the contagionists for advocating quarantines, whose "faith in their efficacy . . . has led to the neglect of domestic cleanliness." Further, he claimed, "From this influence, the commerce, agriculture, and manufacturing of our country have suffered for many years."[7]

The social effects of quarantine were equally deplorable:

> A belief in the contagious nature of yellow fever, which is so solemnly enforced by the execution of quarantine laws, has demoralized our citizens. It has, in many instances, extinguished friendship, annihilated religion, and violated the sacraments of nature, by resisting even the loud and vehement cries of filial and parental blood.

Rush maintained that yellow fever "is propagated by means of an impure atmosphere, at all times, and in all places." Do not quarantine, he admonished, but drain the marshes and clean the streets instead. His plea to reject the contagionists' solution might have been written today about conditions found with AIDS patients: "A red or a yellow eye shall no longer be the signal to desert a friend or a brother to perish alone in a garret or a barn, nor to expel the stranger from our houses, to seek asylum in a public hospital, to avoid dying in the street."[8] Benjamin Rush responded to the fear that created the imposition of quarantine, as well as to the cruelty that sometimes accompanied it. Such consequences are all the more regrettable now that we know that isolating yellow fever patients has no public health value whatsoever. The history of medicine, however, is filled with useless and even harmful remedies confidently applied to the trusting patient. Rush was one of many anticontagionists who not only believed that quarantines were useless, but also that those who advocated them were themselves obstacles to clean, airy, and sanitary cities.

CHOLERA

By 1832, when the first cholera epidemic struck the United States, enlightened physicians were much more in Rush's camp than in that of the contagionists. In fact, anticontagionism had become a mark of the educated physician, although the populace continued to hold the unsophisticated view that diseases such as cholera were transmittable from one person to another. Indeed, cities did declare quarantines, over the objections of physicians. The president of New York City's Special Medical Council, Dr. Alexander H. Stephens, privately characterized the quarantine he was supposed to help enforce as a "useless embarrassment to commerce." Politically, however, not to have enforced quarantines would have been "suicidal," according to Charles E. Rosenberg, author of the chapter on disease and social order in this book. Still, cities that did not impose a quarantine had a commercial advantage over those that turned away or detained ships seeking to enter their ports. Agitation within a city would increase if potential victims could not flee to a countryside believed to be more safe.

The first cases appeared in New York City in late June, and the epidemic was upon the city for the remainder of the summer. The Board of Health was greatly criticized for its efforts: The job of cleaning the city was too big to accomplish in such short order, the cholera hospitals were overcrowded, and it was not easy to find caretakers for the sick and dying. The public had demanded protection, and the response of government at the state and local level was quick and authoritarian. The natural response of the populace was to cordon off the healthy or to confine the sick; a show of support for the creation of boundaries overwhelmed the medical experts' assurances that the disease was not contagious and that quarantine was an expensive and useless weapon.

Cholera, as we saw in the chapter by Guenter B. Risse, was associated with the poor and the immoral. About two weeks into the epidemic the Special Medical Council stated that the disease was "confined to the imprudent, the intemperate and to those who injure themselves by taking improper medicines."[9] The highest incidence of cholera occurred in the red-light district, which the *New York Evening Post* reported to be populated by the vilest brutes whose breath would contaminate and infect the atmosphere with disease, even "be the air pure from Heaven."[10] Cholera arrived in the 1830s, and the social reaction to the ensuing epidemic was greatly complicated by the emotionally charged atmosphere of an active temperance movement in which moralizing was common. Advice for resisting the disease frequently included warnings against ardent spirits. One of the first and most prominent of American psychiatrists, Dr. Amariah Brigham, advocated in 1832 that boards of health be given "the power to *change the habits of the sensual, the vicious, the intemperate*."[11] The link between illness and morality has maintained a long and strong tradition. When an epidemic illness hits hardest at the lowest social classes or other fringe groups, it provides that grain of sand on which the pearl of moralism can form. Such was the case with a disease that has elicited alarmed calls more recently for isolation: tuberculosis.

TUBERCULOSIS

Tuberculosis resembles leprosy in that it often is a long-term illness that permits the sufferer to remain ambulatory, perhaps for years, while potentially infectious. The victim might recover, but the high mortality rate for the illness makes the diagnosis a very serious matter. By the nineteenth century tuberculosis became one of the most frequent causes of death in the Western world. If the cause and contagiousness of cholera were disputed until a bacterium was proved responsible in 1883, it is not surprising that tuberculosis, a more obscure and chronic infection, also sparked debate. The general opinion during the last century was that some people harbored a hereditary tendency toward tuberculosis that was exacerbated by poor sanitation and living conditions. The value of quarantine under these circumstances therefore seemed doubtful. But tuberculosis evoked quarantine responses once the cause was established to be a bacterium by Robert Koch in 1882.

Ten years after Koch's astounding announcement that the cause of tuberculosis had been found, the first tuberculosis association in the United States was formed in Pennsylvania. From this early effort to combine lay and professional support to battle one disease grew many other associations; eventually the National Tuberculosis Association (now the American Lung Association) emerged. The goal of the society was the prevention of tuberculosis by, first of all, "promulgating the doctrine of the contagiousness of the disease."[12] At about the same time, the New York City Health Department initiated steps toward mandatory reporting of tuberculosis cases. Beginning in 1894 institutions were required to submit such reports and three years later physicians were similarly obligated. Opposition among physicians to this requirement was substantial. Some argued that the mandatory reporting of cases of tuberculosis implied a lack of faith in the practitioners' abilities to take care of their patients. Others resented what they considered to be state interference in the patient–physician relationship, while still others believed the disease was hereditary regardless of what might be seen under a microscope.[13] Eventually, however, reporting of tuberculosis cases became compulsory throughout the nation.

Identification of tubercular patients led to requirements that the disease be properly treated. An effective antibiotic against the tubercle bacillus was not found until the 1940s, so treatment for the illness shifted from a relatively benign open-air regimen in cold climates, such as at Saranac Lake under the direction of Dr. Edward Trudeau, to a later, more drastic vogue for the collapsing of one lung and resectioning part of the rib cage. A general consensus that patients needed extended periods of bed rest and that everyone else needed to be isolated from the healthy led to the construction of tuberculosis sanatariums by state and local governments. The federal government built hospitals for native

Americans, who gave evidence of being particularly susceptible to the disease.

We have all but forgotten the terror tuberculosis aroused earlier in this century. The death rate from tuberculosis in 1900 exceeded today's death rate from cancer and accidents combined. As its contagiousness became more widely acknowledged, medical experts increasingly advocated early detection and treatment. Some potential patients, however, tried to evade diagnosis not only to avoid the bad news but also because being reported as a tubercular would make it difficult or even impossible to obtain insurance or to keep a job. Public health officials seeking authority to bring into treatment anyone who in their view was irresponsible, supported state laws to permit enforced treatment of the "careless consumptive" and to prohibit the discharge of a patient without approval of the medical staff.

Reports of involuntary-treatment laws in Connecticut suggest they were used infrequently and may have served more as a threat to obtain the cooperation of a patient. One reason appears to have been simply the expense of caring for a patient against his or her will, but it is unclear how many patients or potential patients were affected by the threat to invoke this stringent public health law. The health officer of New Britain, Connecticut, estimated he had invoked it "ten to fifteen times" in the period from 1920 to 1945.[14]

Gradually, the prevalence of tuberculosis, along with the fear it inspired, have declined until both are not even memories for many Americans today. The disgrace of having a disease often associated with unhealthy habits, not to mention the isolation from family and neighbors, has faded along with the many hospitals that were once strung across the nation for the care of the tubercular. It is clear, though, that by the time the disease reached its height, public-health-control measures had overcome many obstacles: The chest X-ray and the tuberculin skin test became so routine as to evoke hardly a comment from the patient.

Quarantine measures were also applied to other communicable diseases as their pathogens became identified. Efforts to quarantine sick persons and their households were dropped, however, when, in the light of new knowledge, it became apparent that such measures were ineffective. The infectious period of an illness, it was discovered, may occur prior to the onset of obvious symptoms; and the problem of enforcing quarantine, in any event, had always proved extremely difficult. Just as quarantine appeared to have no remarkable effect on the control of cholera in nineteenth-century America, so did the closing of schools in response to infectious diseases such as scarlet fever and diphtheria, which broke out in the twentieth century.[15] Similarly, during World War I, an equally ineffective response to disease was to hold soldiers with venereal diseases in special enclosures.[16] Still, it should be borne in mind that quarantine has been most popular when the fear or prevalence of a serious disease has been highest. The fear of a disease, as the history of quarantine indicates, is not aroused by the simple knowledge of physiological effects of a pathogen, but from an ill-informed consideration of the "kind of person" liable to become ill, and the habits thought to cause or predispose people to the disease. Likewise, quarantine is a response not only to the actual mode of transmission, but also to a popular demand to establish a boundary between the "kind of person" so diseased and the "respectable people" who hope to remain healthy.

QUARANTINE AND THE "DISEASE" OF IMMIGRATION

Creating boundaries between groups to prevent entry of undesirable agents of disease (an essential element in the concept of quarantine) can be seen in the tacit philosophy of some of the United States' immigration laws. Immigration laws have traditionally sought to prevent entry of anyone who would create a public burden. The philosophy of immigration laws early in this century, however, carried the notion of quarantine much further than the restricted entry of the diseased or disabled. Hereditarian theories of race and racial superiority were buttressed by the discoveries of Mendelian genetics and reports of animal-breeding experiments, all of which combined to create the eugenics movement. Those Americans alarmed by the influx of immigration from southern and eastern Europe late in the nineteenth century found, in what was then modern genetics, "scientific" support for their long-standing fear: Undesirable races would pollute the Anglo-Saxon germ plasm if allowed to enter the United States and to intermarry with the extant population. There were many exponents of this theory, which so closely resembled a simple view of the germ causation of disease: If a germ entered the body, a specific disease would be caused—neither the environment, nor educational efforts, nor biological variability of the individual infected by the germ were important. This racial theory surely demanded a line of defense around the racially pure, just as any quarantine drew the line against the biological contaminant, the cholera germ.

The ideas calling for a racial quarantine are summed up in Madison

Grant's *The Passing of the Great Race,* a pessimistic account, published in 1916, of undesirable immigration run amok, and of the glory of the Nordic race gradually fading into oblivion. Using eugenics theory to impart a "scientific" justification for his fears, Grant warned that such intermarriage "gives us a race reverting to the more ancient, generalized and lower type." Accordingly, racial disease could be prevented only by excluding carriers of biological contamination—the central concept of quarantine. This outlook triumphed in the Immigration Act of 1924, which drastically limited the influx of Europeans whom a person like Madison Grant would have found undesirable. The act was so effective that a year after its enactment the commissioner of immigration at Ellis Island reported that now almost all immigrants looked exactly like Americans.[17]

DRUGS AND FEARED MINORITIES

The quarantine model can also be found in American reaction to the use of drugs by feared minority groups. The United States had an almost unrestricted market in morphine, opium, cocaine, and heroin during the nineteenth century and the first decade of this century. The use of these drugs became widespread, and in the years around World War I opposition to their nonmedicinal use reached a peak. Stringent federal laws assisted a variety of partial and conflicting state statutes attempting to control the use of narcotics. Interestingly, the campaigns that led to these laws ascribed the use of certain drugs to specific feared groups. Opium was linked to Chinese immigrants; cocaine to southern blacks; and heroin to an urban, violent, and criminal underclass. In the 1930s a similar, specific assignment was made of marijuana to Mexican immigrants who had come to the agricultural regions of the nation during the booming 1920s. In the crusade to control dangerous drugs, the emotional energy released by associating drugs with feared minority groups helped pass legislation prescribing severe penalties. The contrast with drugs that might be addicting and dangerous but are commonly used by the middle class, such as barbiturates, illustrates the intense emotions that can be evoked by appealing to the kind of fears that gave rise to the immigration laws of the 1920s.[18]

By the 1960s, a time of renewed addiction problems in the United States, simply being an addict rendered a person subject to involuntary confinement for therapeutic purposes. The Supreme Court declared that "in the interest of the general health or welfare of its inhabitants," a state "might establish a program of compulsory treatment for those addicted to narcotics. Such a program of treatment might require periods of involuntary confinement."[19] Justice William O. Douglas in his concurring opinion went so far as to add that confinement might be justified "for the protection of society" and not just for the treatment of the addict. California and New York both established sites where addicts could be committed for treatment. In 1966 the federal government made provision for civil commitment through the Narcotic Addict Rehabilitation Act. All of these programs for massive detention of addicts failed legislators' expectations: Detention proved expensive and the rehabilitation rate was quite low. For our purposes—that is, to compare these latter measures with the possibility of quarantine in response to the AIDS epidemic—it is worth emphasizing that a group without an explicit ethnic affiliation but marked by a primary, and much feared, trait—addiction—was seen to deserve confinement "for the protection of society" by no less a champion of personal liberties than Justice Douglas. We have the advantage of knowing that the programs supported by such juridical sentiment proved impracticable.

The perceived role of drugs among feared minority groups was thought to be similar to that of a virus in an otherwise fairly healthy group. Eliminate the virus and the group would not only function much more efficiently but would also cease being a source of infection to the remainder of society. In a way, however, the fear of drug contagion was a little more optimistic than the eugenicists' pessimism that ascribed an unalterable inferiority to some ethnic groups. Remove the drug, or discourage its use by punishment, and the person and the group would be more easily assimilable and certainly less dangerous. Even so, some said the Chinese, for example, had a racial weakness for opiates. Broadly speaking, however, the tangible reality of the drug encouraged the hope that its removal would make a threatening group more tractable.

Early in this century, cocaine was said to cause southern blacks' hostile attacks on whites. Fear of cocaine fed the mounting racial tensions in the southern states. Cocaine was thought to improve marksmanship, while alcohol made it worse. Believing that blacks might be high on cocaine, officers in one police department traded their guns for larger calibers because they thought a mere .32 caliber revolver could not stop a "cocaine-crazed" black.

The smoking of opium by Chinese was used as an argument against Chinese immigration. Opium was said to be the means Chinese men used to seduce white women. Heroin, on the other hand, supposedly bolstered the courage of underworld figures before a robbery. Champions of the strictest and most punitive antinarcotics laws, such as Capt. Richmond Pearson Hobson, considered narcotics a "racial poison." Hobson warned that the United States was under bombardment by the rest of the world, which sought to undermine American values and government through addicting narcotics. Each continent sent its wicked poison: Africa, hashish; Asia, opium; South America, cocaine; Europe, heroin. Captain Hobson was a keen student of the notion of racial degeneration, and the parallel he drew with undesirable races who wished to "invade" the United States is clear. The solution was to establish a boundary no foreign contaminant could pass.[20]

Some drug experts consider quarantine a remedy because they believe the isolation of drug-users is a protection against contagion. The idea that drug abuse is contagious is not new. In 1915 a Tennessee state official responsible for control of narcotic use, Lucius P. Brown, wrote in the *American Journal of Public Health* that

> contagion is undoubtedly a very frequent method of spread. I have met many instances in which more than one member of a family was infected, the first case acquired accidentally or through a physician, infecting the other members of the family largely through a certain tendency on the part of the addict, particularly in the early stages, to introduce others to the delights of addiction.[21]

Addiction spread through contagion, or, as it is more commonly described now, "peer pressure," has led to some forms of isolation in the United States. During the years just after World War I, for example, addicts in New York City were brought to North Brother Island in the East River. In the 1930s a federal narcotics hospital was built in the form of a prison in Lexington, Kentucky. The major reason for these isolated locations was to ensure that the patient would have no access to drugs, although treatment and imprisonment also removed "pushers" from communities.

With the second major onslaught of drug use in the United States and other nations in the 1960s, the contagion model again proved popular, both to explain the growing use of dangerous drugs and to suggest a means of control. Dr. Henry Brill, later a member of the National Commission on Marihuana and Drug Abuse (1970–1973), described in 1968 two kinds of addicts: the medical, caused by treatment for a painful disease; and the nonmedical, or "street," addicts. The former he found to be solitary users, but the latter frequently used drugs in groups, and their primary mode of spreading addiction was through "psychic contagion," as Brill labeled it, which may assume "epidemic proportions."[22]

A prominent Swedish drug expert, Dr. Nils Bejerot, agreed that interfering with this form of spread was a key to stopping epidemics of drug abuse. In Sweden the problem in the 1960s was stimulant abuse, such as amphetamines and other "diet pills," but the principle still held, he believed, for other forms of drugs. He called this situation an "epidemic toxicomania" and recommended establishment of "treatment villages" in open locations "without the patients being able to escape at the first impulse." He favored islands or depopulated areas for the construction of treatment villages. Dr. Bejerot thought a year in a village would be the minimum required. Women would have intrauterine devices inserted to prevent pregnancies.[23] Although these villages have not been adopted in Sweden or the United States, the proposal is an interesting look at the wish to apply quarantine to a feared and massive social problem.

Quarantine boundaries are best defended if there is a clear distinction between the feared aggressors and those requiring protection. The leper had a prescribed costume and warning cry. Immigrants often looked different from settled citizenry; in the cities, the poor could be distinguished from the middle and upper classes. In the case of narcotics, Chinese, blacks, and Mexicans stood out from mainstream society; and society, threatened by their discontent and hostility, hoped to stop their use of dangerous drugs, if not to expel them and "their" drug from the nation altogether. How convenient it was to discover a contaminant among a group already held in low esteem and easily distinguishable from the majority of the population; the role that this view of addiction played in race discrimination should not be underestimated.

When such groups are quarantined, lasting psychological damage may follow. Insights into the emotional sequelae (aftereffects of disease) that would be involved in quarantining those who test positive for human immunodeficiency virus (HIV), but are otherwise unaffected by the illness may be gathered from studies of Americans of Japanese ancestry who were interned in concentration camps during World War II simply because of their lineage. About 120,000 persons—men, women, and children living in western states—were abruptly taken from their homes and settled in government camps for several years on the grounds that they presented a security risk to the United States. In recent years deep regret for this action has been expressed in Congress and by many citizens aware of what happened under the stress of war. Studies conducted on the former detainees reveal a number of reactions including denial; loss of faith in legal protections; aggression turned inward, with consequent feelings of guilt, shame, and inferiority—and identification with the aggressor.[24] We should try to learn from that era of fear and to consider the effects of quarantine on the targets of that fear. The efficacy of the quarantine procedure itself must also be questioned.

ACQUIRED IMMUNE DEFICIENCY SYNDROME

In light of the history of quarantine and its various ramifications, the position of the AIDS victim and society's response to the disease can be better appreciated. The large majority of AIDS patients in the United States are found in two groups, male homosexuals and intravenous drug users. The disease itself is caused by a virus that is transmitted by means of an infected needle or during sexual activity, especially anal-receptive sex. The disease itself occurs in an uncertain fraction of those who have been exposed to the virus. So far, the mortality rate for AIDS has been nearly 100 percent, although the patient may live a year or two after the diagnosis has been made and then mostly in the community and not in a hospital.

The question is whether AIDS possesses those characteristics that have aroused healthy citizens to call for a quarantine. It is indeed a serious disease with, so far, no cure. In this regard, AIDS patients face an irrevocable death sentence, much like the lepers of the Middle Ages. Furthermore, the groups with which AIDS is most closely associated in this country have typically been held in low esteem by the general population, the objects of discrimination in jobs, housing, and everyday social contact. Also, the disease is generally transmitted among drug addicts and homosexuals by means that have been or are still illegal in the United States. In this regard, AIDS, like other contagious diseases of the past, is associated with minorities who are considered sexually deviant and promiscuous. Like tuberculars and lepers, AIDS patients may have relapses between which life might continue outside the hospital, at home, or, at the least, in the community. During this time, however, the patient remains infectious and is therefore a source of apprehension. Recalcitrant patients who do not follow recommendations for "safe sex" evoke memories of "careless consumptives" whose presence motivated the passage of special laws permitting their involuntary isolation. Like tuberculous patients, AIDS patients have difficulty obtaining insurance and, like members of any rejected minority linked to a serious communicable illness, the group as a whole may be treated as if all its members have the most dangerous form of the disease when any one of them applies for employment or housing, an ascription similar to the widespread association of specific drugs with feared minorities. In sum, AIDS patients have reason to be concerned over the possibility of quarantine or isolation. Are there any countervailing arguments?

The first restraint against a rush to institute quarantine measures against AIDS victims is the extensive experience showing that sustained quarantine for large numbers of people has not been successful. The great efforts to control the individual behavior of drug addicts have obviously been thwarted, or drug users would not now be spreading AIDS by injecting substances into their veins. Further, the spread of AIDS has not been found to be through casual contact, and there is reason to believe that not all of those with AIDS antibodies will develop a serious illness. If, however, longer experience with patients tested positive for AIDS antibodies reveals a very high incidence of illness in later years, or that AIDS is rapidly spreading from groups now chiefly associated with it—i.e., intravenous drug users, male homosexuals, and recipients of blood infected with the AIDS virus—the general population will in all likelihood become highly anxious.

The United States has a long history of mistrust of physicians and the medical establishment. The government also has had difficulty regaining its credibility about dangerous drugs after so many excessive warnings, particularly about marijuana, in the 1960s. When authorities make pronouncements about AIDS, their comments meet with considerable public skepticism. This skepticism must be borne in mind by those trying to provide reassurance, for if their reassurance is later found to have been overstated, the public confidence, which is needed to contain destructive emotions, will be compromised.

Strong reactions to the threat of AIDS will more likely result in restrictions on individuals if the disease continues to spread and to affect many more unsuspecting citizens. Passions could be mobilized politically and could result in a program to mark or isolate persons testing positive for AIDS antibodies. Just because quarantines are not effective does not mean they will not be attempted. The 1832 cholera epidemic in New York City led to politically mandated quarantine in spite of the almost unanimous opinion of leading physicians that it was a useless expenditure of time and funds. Perhaps the most helpful counter to unenlightened outrage is public awareness of the enormous effort under way to understand and treat AIDS. This effort includes evidence of the growing success of educational programs among the groups most affected by AIDS.

If the AIDS crisis persists for some years, one can speculate that society or the groups most involved may develop ritual forms to recognize the mutual responsibilities between the healthy and the diseased. It would appear that such ceremonies for leprous persons helped both the healthy but vulnerable and the afflicted to accept their condition. Of course, with the absence of a single religious authority today, whatever ritual is developed may take on a more civic character.

If other diseases, say, multiple sclerosis and some cancers, are found to be preceded by a lengthy, asymptomatic viral infection, we may see the establishment of a new class of patients in circumstances common to AIDS victims now: A test may reveal the likelihood of death years in the future. What are these people to do in the meantime? How will they deal with the inevitable shock and grief that follow such a diagnosis? Our society may become motivated to create a sympathetic ritual not only to sustain but also to acknowledge these citizens. AIDS may be the model for ways to help both the well and the sick deal with such conditions produced by medical advances in etiology and diagnosis, but not in curative therapy.

In conclusion, the quarantine of AIDS patients remains a possibility, and depends on such factors as time until an effective vaccine or treatment is available, secondary and tertiary spread of the virus, and the faith of the public in official pronouncements regarding the illness. AIDS possesses many of the characteristics that have motivated past quarantine efforts—association with feared social subgroups, transmission through means the public has deemed unlawful or distasteful, the potential for spread outside these rejected groups to the public at large, and a lengthy infectious period outside hospital confinement. There is no assurance that quarantine will not be attempted, but awareness of its past ineffectiveness, accurate information, and understanding the irrational fears that wrongly prompt quarantine are good defenses against it.

NOTES

An earlier version of this paper appeared in the *Milbank Quarterly* 64, suppl. 1 (1986): 97–117.

1. J. Gerlitt, "The Development of Quarantine," *Ciba Symposia* 2 (1940): 566–580.

2. George Rosen, "Forerunners of Quarantine," *Ciba Symposia* 2 (1940): 563–565.

3. Saul N. Brody, *The Disease of the Soul: Leprosy in Medieval Literature* (Ithaca: Cornell University Press, 1974), 66–67.

4. Ibid., 68.

5. Erwin H. Ackerknecht, "Anticontagionism between 1821 and 1867," *Bulletin of the History of Medicine* 22 (1948): 562–593.

6. Benjamin Rush, "An Account of the Bilious Yellow Fever, as it Appeared in Philadelphia in 1793," in *Medical Inquiries and Observations,* ed. Benjamin Rush, 4th ed., 4 vols. (Philadelphia: M. Carey, 1815), 3:111.

7. Benjamin Rush, "An Inquiry into the Various Sources of the Usual Forms of Summer and Autumnal Disease, in the United States and the Means of Preventing Them," in *Medical Inquiries,* 4:138.

8. Benjamin Rush, "Facts, Intended to Prove that Yellow Fever not to be Contagious," in *Medical Inquiries,* 4:170.

9. Charles E. Rosenberg, *The Cholera Years: The United States in 1832, 1849, and 1866* (Chicago: University of Chicago Press, 1962), 30.

10. Ibid., 34.

11. Amariah Brigham, *A Treatise on Epidemic Cholera* (Hartford, Conn.: H. and F. J. Huntington, 1832), 338, emphasis in original.

12. George Rosen, *A History of Public Health* (New York: M.D. Publications, 1958), 388.

13. Daniel M. Fox, "Social Policy and City Politics: Tuberculosis Reporting in New York, 1889–1900," *Bulletin of the History of Medicine* 49 (1975): 169–195.

14. Connecticut Public Health and Safety Committee, "An Act Concerning Prevention of the Spread of TB," *Hearings,* stenographic transcript, State of Connecticut Legislative Archives, 17 April 1945, p. 178.

15. A. L. Hoyne, "Are Present-Day Quarantine Methods Archaic?", *Illinois Medical Journal* 80 (1941): 205–208.

16. Allan M. Brandt, *No Magic Bullet: A Social History of Venereal Disease in the United States Since 1880* (New York: Oxford University Press, 1985), 116.

17. John Higham, *Strangers in the Land: Patterns of American Nativism, 1860–1925* (New York: Athenaeum, 1963), 156, 325.

18. David F. Musto, *The American Disease: Origins of Narcotic Control,* exp. ed. (New York: Oxford University Press, 1987), 3–8, 219.

19. *Robinson v. California,* 370 U.S. 660 (1962).

20. Musto, *The American Disease,* 190–197.

21. Lucius P. Brown, "Enforcement of the Tennessee Anti-Narcotics Law," *American Journal of Public Health* 5 (1915): 323–333.

22. Henry Brill, "Medical and Delinquent Addicts or Drug Abusers: A Medical Distinction of Legal Significance," *Hastings Law Journal* 19 (1968): 783–801.

23. Nils Bejerot, *Addiction and Society* (Springfield, Ill.: Charles C. Thomas, 1970), 271–275.

24. U.S. Commission on Wartime Relocation and Internment of Civilians, *Personal Justice Denied* (Washington, D.C.: Government Printing Office, 1982), 295–301.

The Politics of Physicians' Responsibility in Epidemics: A Note on History

Daniel M. Fox

Current disputes about physicians' ethical responsibility to treat persons with AIDS or HIV infection have stimulated interest in how they behaved during previous epidemics. Most historical accounts have emphasized what individual physicians did or neglected to do. I ask a related, but different, set of questions about the past: How did the medical profession, collectively, behave toward patients with contagious diseases and how did public policy affect that behavior? Despite enormous changes in the practice of medicine and the social position of doctors over the past five hundred years, there has been remarkable continuity in how the profession has responded to the threat of contagion.

Recent papers by physicians ably summarize the literature about how members of the medical profession behaved in past epidemics.[1] According to this literature, during most epidemics for which records survive, most physicians seem to have treated most of the patients who sought their help, though they frequently charged higher fees. Nevertheless, many physicians fled from cities in time of plague, including Galen from Rome in the second century A.D., Sydenham from London in the seventeenth, and some leaders of the profession in Philadelphia and New York during outbreaks of yellow fever in the eighteenth and cholera in the nineteenth centuries. In addition, many physicians who did not flee reportedly refused to visit patients who were acutely ill. On balance, however, most accounts describe members of the medical profession as dutiful despite personal risk. One historian assigned physicians in late medieval Europe a "high degree of ethical and professional responsibility."[2] Another concluded that, after discounting exaggeration, American general practitioners in the nineteenth century responded to epidemics with hard work and at "great risk and sacrifice."[3] Others have concluded that patients were at more risk of overtreatment than of abandonment.[4]

The historical record is not, however, a straightforward source of ethical guidance for the present. Much of the evidence about physicians abandoning patients during epidemics, when read in context, furnishes no proof that such conduct violated prevailing ethical norms. During some epidemics, for instance, physicians followed their patients into temporary exile. Moreover, physicians have often justified abandoning individual patients. Their justifications have included powerlessness to help, threats of physical violence by distraught family members and neighbors, or, more recently, the scarcity of such resources as their time and hospital beds. Physicians have also justified not treating particular patients in order not to transmit disease themselves.[5]

NEGOTIATION AND OPPORTUNITY

Similarly, physicians who treated patients during epidemics were not necessarily acting solely or even primarily on the basis of ethical principles, secular or religious, written or implicit. Two themes stand out in accounts of the mobilization of the medical profession during epidemics between the fourteenth and the nineteenth centuries. First, civic leaders and physicians negotiated about who would treat those who were stricken, especially patients in the lowest classes. Second, these epidemics offered physicians opportunities as well as risks.

These themes are closely linked. In instance upon instance the lay and medical leadership of a city jointly chose particular physicians to carry out the most onerous duties during an epidemic. The physicians who were chosen for these duties invariably knew from the beginning of their service that they were balancing personal risks against potential benefits in status and income.

The modern history of health policy begins with the response of the leaders of Italian city-states to the epidemics of Black Death that occurred periodically for three centuries after 1348. Policies devised in Italian cities became the model for the rest of Europe and, later, the Western Hemisphere. The merchants who dominated these cities during most of this period had prospered through international trade and had devised effective mechanisms to govern large populations. These mechanisms included what one historian calls a "large and complex set of institutions which cooperated in looking after the health of [the cities'] inhabitants."[6] With each outbreak of plague, the major issue of public policy for civic leaders was how to contain its spread. Because the prevailing etiological theory connected the spread of the plague to the movement of people and goods—the basis of the cities' economies—civic leaders quickly adapted existing public policy mechanisms. In most cities, health boards, composed mainly of merchants but often including physicians as members or consultants, organized quarantines, isolated victims in homes and plague hospitals, and disposed of the dead.

Medical treatment was an important but subordinate issue for organizers of the cities' responses to plague. They used a variety of policies, often in concert or in sequence, to ensure minimum levels of palliative treatment. Physicians were forbidden to leave some cities and their hinterlands. They were offered high fees and prizes to visit patients in the lazzarettos, or, as I will call them, plague hospitals. In many cities civic officials offered contracts to physicians to care for patients with plague. Most often, civic leaders tactfully delegated to local colleges of physicians the task of selecting members to serve in the hospitals.

Sometimes local physicians as a group declined to serve, in one case suggesting that treating patients meant "certain death." These doctors then suggested that the local surgeons should care for plague patients. (Surgeons were accorded lower status than physicians everywhere in Europe until the nineteenth century.) The physicians recommended that the surgeons shout the "quality, sex, and condition of the patient and stage of illness" from an open window to a physician at a safe distance, who would then shout back a course of treatment.[7]

City officials could also coerce reluctant physicians. In 1656, for example, the cardinal who headed the health board in Rome ordered the arrest of a doctor who had denied that the outbreak was plague, and assigned him to serve in the hospital.[8]

The civic leaders and physicians who offered these combinations of incentives and disincentives to treat patients with plague regarded them as business propositions. As such, they were regulated by contracts that differed in substance but not in form from the commercial instruments that merchants in Italian cities used to regulate what had become the most affluent economies since the end of the Roman Empire. Moreover, physicians routinely contracted to provide services during normal times to guilds, religious orders, hospitals, and the state.

Here is an example of how a contract expressed the mutual self-interest of a physician and a city. In 1479 the city of Pavia contracted with a young physician, probably from the countryside, to treat plague patients at a monthly salary that was considerably more than that of a skilled laborer or university lecturer but less than the mayor or famous university professors. The doctor was also granted a salary advance, reimbursement for living expenses, and the promise of citizenship—that is, the right to practice permanently in Pavia—if he behaved acceptably. In return, he agreed to visit plague patients as frequently as necessary in the company of a man designated by the community who would make certain that the physician would not mingle with other people. As the historian who published the contract noted, "A plague doctor was regarded as a contact and all contacts had to live in isolation."[9]

In sum, a plague doctor's obligation to treat patients was the result of a contract for personal services executed in response to public policy. The plague outbreaks between the fifteenth and seventeenth centuries seem to have raised the level of professional consciousness about ethics; treatises and codes proliferated. Still, ethical consciousness was less effective a motive for action than economic interest or, more broadly, fear of loss of status. Thus the author of a sixteenth-century treatise on professional ethics said that "to avoid infamy [I] dared not absent myself but with continual fear preserved myself as best I could."[10]

By the seventeenth century, moreover, both civic and medical leaders in Italian cities could claim that by applying the best science of the time physicians could avoid getting or transmitting the plague and thus had less reason to avoid responsibility for treating patients. Physicians in France had invented a robe of fine linen coated with an aromatic paste that prevented the venomous atoms in the poisonous air—called miasmas—that allegedly caused plague from adhering to the doctor and his clothing.[11] This robe, which was widely used in Italy, apparently worked—we would probably say because it repelled fleas—and helped confirm the theory that contagion was carried by miasmas. Science now reinforced civic authority, economic interest, and moral obligation as reasons for physicians to agree to treat patients during epidemics.

EPIDEMICS IN THE UNITED STATES

The history of physician conduct in epidemics in the United States from the 1790s to the 1850s illustrates the same themes that characterize the examples from Italian cities. Physicians' behavior in epidemics has been a result of their negotiations with civic authority, and as a result of such negotiations, plague doctors—temporary specialists—often balanced their opportunities against their risks. These themes transcend enormous changes in medicine and society.

Americans may not have known the details of how physicians behaved during epidemics in Italian cities, but they reacted similarly in similar situations. Some may have drawn analogies to events in London during the outbreaks of plague in the seventeenth century.[12] More important, however, were the similarities in the conditions confronting medical and civic leaders in early modern Italy and the United States in the late eighteenth and early nineteenth centuries. In both situations, doctors were uncertain about the etiology and treatment of infectious disease. In both, city governments dominated by merchants developed policy to contain epidemics.

The most frequently described epidemic in American history before the twentieth century may be the outbreak of yellow fever in Philadelphia in 1793. Its fame derives partly from its severity but also from its occurrence in what was then the national capital, where it sharply curtailed the affairs of government, and mainly from the heroic—if in retrospect dogmatically wrongheaded—behavior of Dr. Benjamin Rush. The slightest exposure to medical history is likely to include the story of Rush racing about Philadelphia trying to bleed patients back to health while many of his colleagues in the distinguished College of Physicians fled the city.

This is caricature, of course, but it links events in the young American republic with those in the Italian city-states. The conventional American accounts of epidemics, like those generated in late medieval and early modern Europe, portray both brave and cowardly doctors against a background of descriptions of contagion, suffering, and death. The American accounts, like the earlier European ones, are misleading in their emphases, not necessarily wrong in detail.

In Philadelphia in 1793 Rush's heroics were less significant than the decisiveness of the merchants who exerted civic authority. These highly political merchants "viewed the plague with a larger perspective" than did Dr. Rush.[13] Indeed, the important medical story concerns the hospital created by these merchants during the height of the plague. The hospital, which was two miles outside the city, was initially staffed by four young physicians, who had found time to make only twelve visits, collectively, in two weeks to visit the sixty to two hundred patients in each day's census. The civic leaders, led by Steven Girard, then decided to employ a full-time physician. They found a recent refugee from Santo

Domingo, a French physician who preferred to treat yellow fever with stimulants and quinine rather than by venesection. After six days of conflict between some leading Philadelphia physicians and the merchants, the French physician's appointment was confirmed. He was soon joined by a full-time volunteer from the Philadelphia medical elite who, for whatever mixture of motives, was delighted to have allies in a dispute with his colleagues about medical policy. Again, civic authority and a negotiated contract with a physician who saw a personal opportunity in the epidemic determined the organization of medical care.

This pattern also appears in an anonymous contemporary account of a yellow fever outbreak in Natchez, Mississippi, in the summer of 1823. As usual, many affluent citizens and their physicians left the city. The author, using conventions for describing plagues that had become part of the Western literary heritage in the works of Boccaccio and Defoe, reported that the "practicing physicians of the city (one excepted) had prudently withdrawn themselves to the country with the citizens of better circumstances . . . leaving the dead to bury their dead." In contrast, civic leaders, the trustees of the Natchez hospital, "invited the sick poor to resort thither." The superintending trustee then "solicited an intelligent and well read physician to abide with the trustee's family and attend the hospital and sick poor . . . without fee or reward."[14] More than likely, internal evidence suggests, the anonymous author was himself the plague physician and took his reward in local esteem.

Eyewitness accounts of cholera epidemics in New York City in 1832 and 1849 exemplify the linkage of civic and medical authority in somewhat different ways. In 1832, the resident physician of the port—the highest-ranking public physician—denied that an epidemic of Asiatic cholera had begun. He angered the leadership of the New York Medical Society by refusing to make a night call to a patient who later died of the disease. In this instance, medical leaders, claiming that they were not "restrained" by "fear," successfully pressed the civic authorities to take action against the epidemic.[15]

In the epidemic of 1849, much of the burden of communicating with the public in New York City was carried by three physicians serving as "medical counsel" to the Board of Health. In a public notice early in the epidemic, these physicians insisted that "in this city no difficulty in obtaining the speedy assistance of a physician can exist." Nevertheless, in a report three months later, the city Sanitary Committee regretted the death, as a "result of exhaustion in attendance on cholera cases of a physician who had been appointed to the Third Ward [Police] Station

House." Despite the claim of medical counsel about the availability of speedy assistance, New York was employing plague doctors.[16]

The final example from the nineteenth century is the yellow fever epidemic in New Orleans in 1853, in which 10 percent of the population died. As in Philadelphia in 1793, overtreatment was more of a risk than abandonment for more affluent patients. Once again, the interests of the civic authorities and of individual physicians seeking opportunity converged. A group of young businessmen, calling themselves the Howard Association, raised funds and advised the city government on public health policy. According to a recent historian of the epidemic, "As the cases mounted with increasing rapidity the Howard Association eagerly hired all available medical men." He estimated that "dozens of young doctors seeking fame and fortune entered New Orleans."[17]

INSTITUTIONALIZING PLAGUE DOCTORS

The patterns of civic and medical response to epidemics established between the fourteenth and nineteenth centuries persisted, though in modified form, into the twentieth. These patterns were institutionalized as the nature of the threat changed. Civic authority was vested in permanent agencies of government rather than in temporary committees of influential businessmen and physicians. Since the late nineteenth century, state, county, and city public health departments have had responsibility for disease surveillance and prevention and, very often, for hiring physicians to work in public hospitals and clinics. During the twentieth century, the diseases of the sick poor became first a responsibility of graduate medical education and then an important source of income for medical faculty themselves. Foreign medical graduates remained the most conspicuous group explicitly seeking opportunities by caring for diseases among the poor.

Moreover, as a result of medical advances, general economic conditions, and changes in the natural history of infectious disease, devastating epidemics seemed to many people to be a matter only of historical interest, except in non-Western countries. In the twentieth century, epidemics in the United States have generally been perceived as manageable and likely to be resolved in short course by the application of modern scientific methods. I have seen no evidence that access to physicians was considered a problem during the influenza and polio epidemics earlier in the century.[18] Most physicians seem to have regarded risks to themselves from treating patients with communicable diseases as manageable, often as negligible, if proper procedures were used. An exception to this generalization, until the late 1940s, was the risk to every medical student and house officer of contracting tuberculosis.

The common law, medical practice acts, and codes of ethics seemed adequate to regulate physicians' behavior in choosing patients. This body of precedent and exhortation permitted physicians to select their patients, except in emergencies. Once having chosen a patient, in the AMA's formulation earlier in this decade, "a physician has a duty to do all he can for the benefit of his individual patient" without concern for the "allocation of scarce resources."[19]

PHYSICIANS' CONTEMPORARY OBLIGATIONS

AIDS does not raise new issues about physicians' responsibility to treat patients. Even before the AIDS epidemic caused some physicians to reexamine their obligations, a few critics were uneasy about the subtle and less than subtle ways in which physicians sometimes denied their services to patients. Such issues have a long history that is perceived more clearly against the background of previous centuries than in the context of twentieth-century optimism about the progress of medicine. It is a history of professional accommodation to civic obligation rather than simply of adherence to ethical precepts. Accommodation has been based on a sense of collective professional responsibility: Most medical communities have been intolerant of assertions that each physician could make his or her own decision about how to behave in an epidemic. Instead, civic and professional leaders have jointly chosen or recruited plague doctors. Moreover, a similar pattern has been followed for identifying physicians to treat such endemic infectious diseases as leprosy, syphilis, and tuberculosis.

The question of what should be done when contemporary physicians hesitate or refuse to treat patients whose conditions may harm them may not be resolved much differently than in the past. If the resolution is similar, however, it will result from political circumstances, not historical inevitability. A considerable number of physicians are refusing to treat persons with AIDS or HIV infection, or threatening to refuse. Leaders of the medical profession have recently joined with civic authority, both formally and informally, in setting policy. In New York, for example, where medical school faculty members treat most persons with AIDS in public and voluntary hospitals, the members of the Associated Medical Schools threatened to censure faculty members who withhold treatment. However, the civic and medical authorities who negotiate with physicians to treat persons with AIDS are more likely to offer them incentives than disincentives. In the past, many physicians' incomes improved during epidemics. Plague doctors performed the most dangerous tasks, but they were amply rewarded in cash and, if they survived, in the more important coin of social and professional status. A new cadre of plague doctors now serve in dedicated AIDS units or treat most of the persons with AIDS in particular hospitals. Their rewards are often access to research funds or academic status rather than income alone.

The new problem of our time is the potential risk to physicians who perform invasive procedures on patients potentially infected with HIV. In the past, most physicians who were uneasy about treating patients with infectious diseases did not run the risk of working inside their bodies. Moreover, physicians cannot identify HIV infections in asymptomatic patients and therefore cannot refuse to treat them without first testing. A negotiated solution to these problems may involve more widespread testing of patients upon admission to hospitals or more rigorous adherence of physicians to universal infection-control procedures.

There is—and no professional historian would say this judgmentally—continuity between the physician in Chaucer's *Canterbury Tales* who delighted in the "gold he kept from pestilence"[20] and the well-known academic physician who said in my presence two years ago that "AIDS has been good to me."[21] This continuity may be the result of a broader truth about civic behavior in Western society, at least since the late Middle Ages: It is not that every person has a price, but that, within any group, enough people's prices can be paid to achieve most goals of policy.

NOTES

Reprinted with permission, *Hastings Center Report* 18 (1988): 5–10.

1. Erich H. Loewy, "Duties, Fears and Physicians," *Social Science and Medicine* 12 (1986): 1363–1366; Abigail Zuger and Steven H. Miles, "Physicians, AIDS and Occupational Risk: Historic Traditions and Ethical Obligations," *Journal of the American Medical Association* 258 (1987): 1924–1928.

2. Darrel W. Amundsen, "Medical Deontology and Pestilential Disease in the Late Middle Ages," *Journal of the History of Medicine and Allied Sciences* 32 (1977): 403–421.

3. Donald E. Konold, *A History of American Medical Ethics, 1847–1912* (Madison: Madison State Historical Society of Wisconsin, 1962). Unfortunately, how people perceived risks in different historical periods cannot be compared, except in dangerous speculation. The reasons for this difficulty are beyond the scope of this paper. In simplest terms, we do not know much about the history of terror and anger—or even pleasure.

4. For example, John Duffy, *Sword of Pestilence: The New Orleans Yellow Fever Epidemic of 1853* (Baton Rouge: Louisiana State University Press, 1966).

5. Mary Catherine Welborn, "The Long Tradition: A Study in Fourteenth-Century Medical Deontology," in *Legacies in Ethics and Medicine,* ed. C. R. Burns (New York: Science History Publications, 1977), 204–217. Carlo M. Cipolla, *Faith, Reason and the Plague in Seventeenth-Century Tuscany* (Ithaca, N.Y.: Cornell University Press, 1979), 13. Carlo M. Cipolla, "A Plague Doctor," in *The Medieval City,* ed. H. Miskimin, D. Herlihy, and A. L. Udovitch (New Haven: Yale University Press, 1977), 65–72.

6. Katherine Park, *Doctors and Medicine in Early Renaissance Florence* (Princeton: Princeton University Press, 1985). Cf. Richard Palmer, "Physicians and the State in Post-Medieval Italy," in *The Town and State Physician in Europe from the Middle Ages to the Enlightenment,* ed. A. W. Russell (Wolfenbüttel: Herzog August Bibliothek, 1981).

7. Carlo M. Cipolla, *Cristoforo and the Plague: A Study of Galileo* (Berkeley and Los Angeles: University of California Press, 1973), 25–26.

8. Carlo M. Cipolla, *Public Health and the Medical Profession in the Renaissance* (Cambridge: Cambridge University Press, 1976), 9.

9. Cipolla, "A Plague Doctor"; cf. Robert S. Gottfried, *The Black Death: Natural and Human Disaster in Medieval Europe* (New York: Free Press, 1983), 125–126; cf. Walter George Bell, *The Great Plague in London in 1665* (1924; London: Bodley Head, 1951), 85–86, 162, 286. Dr. Benjamin Freedman called to my attention an account of plague doctors in the seventeenth-century records of the Portuguese Congregation in Hamburg in I. Jakobovits, *Jewish Medical Ethics* (New York: Bloch, 1967), 108–109.

10. Amundsen, "Medical Deontology," 411.

11. Carlo M. Cipolla, *Fighting the Plague in Seventeenth-Century Italy* (Madison: University of Wisconsin Press, 1981), 9–12.

12. Walter George Bell, *The Great Plague in London in 1665;* for references to plague doctors see pp. 86, 162, 286.

13. John Harvey Powell, *Bring Out Your Dead: The Great Plague of Yellow Fever in Philadelphia in 1793,* 2d ed. (New York: Arno Press, 1970), 148.

14. Henry Tooley, *History of the Yellow Fever as it Appeared in the City of Natchez in the Months of August, September and October, 1823* (Washington, Miss.: Andrew Marchall, 1823).

15. John Stearns, "Concerning the Cholera Epidemic, 1832." New York Academy of Medicine, MS 169–171. For a full account of the epidemic, see Charles E. Rosenberg, *The Cholera Years: The United States in 1832, 1849, and 1866* (Chicago: University of Chicago Press, 1962).

16. Samuel Smith Purple, "Manuscript Notes on Cholera in the United

States, 1849." New York Academy of Medicine. Dr. Purple saw no reason to note that the American Medical Association had recently adopted a code of ethics that obligated physicians to treat in time of pestilence.

17. Duffy, *Sword,* 164–166.

18. During the influenza epidemic of 1918–1919, most countries already had a cadre of plague doctors in military service; see Alfred W. Crosby, *Epidemic and Peace, 1918* (Westport, Conn.: Greenwood Press, 1976).

19. *Current Opinions of the Judicial Council of the American Medical Association* (Chicago: AMA, 1981), IX.

20. Geoffrey Chaucer, *The Canterbury Tales* (London: Penguin Books, 1972), 31.

21. Privileged communication with the author.

The Enforcement of Health: The British Debate

Dorothy Porter and Roy Porter

Not least among the issues raised by the AIDS epidemic is the problem of how to square individual freedom with the public good.[1] Under what circumstances, if any, would a state be justified in taking compulsory powers (screening, hospitalization, isolation, enforced treatment, etc.) to prevent the spread of a lethal disease, a disease that constitutes a threat to other people's right to health and to liberty in general? Present discussions of this dilemma in Great Britain have all too often been emotional, even hysterical, and have lacked philosophical rigor, a sense of historical context, and social realism. On the one side, certain well-meaning members of the medical profession have too readily presumed that any action is better than none, that necessity knows no law, and that medico-scientific knowledge confers a right to power.[2] On this model, "doctor's orders" should be applied on a national scale and the medical imperative should be sovereign. On the other side, radical libertarians of all political hues have equally fiercely contended that the state's assumption of any compulsory powers believed to counter AIDS would form part of a conspiratorial agenda for the creation of a police state, leading to the criminalization of illness together with all other forms of deviance, as in Samuel Butler's teasing dystopia *Erewhon*.[3]

In the heat of debate, it is easy to treat these dilemmas raised by AIDS as if they were something new, as if governments had never before been faced with agonizing problems of having to regulate lethal diseases, or (looking at it from another angle, from "below") as if individuals had never before proffered rational arguments against the unwise enforcement of health regulations. Nothing could be further from the truth. Throughout the nineteenth century the spread of what was variously called sanitary science, public hygiene, preventive medicine, and state medicine necessarily tilted the balance between public power and private liberty.

But the crises of health in that newly industrialized and urbanized society, and the availability of new medical and sanitary practices by no means led straightforwardly and inevitably toward the medicalization of life and the therapeutic (welfare) state. Dissent, pressure groups, controversy, policy reversals, and compromise formed the order of the day in Victorian England. Medical, metaphysical, legal, moral, and religious arguments all fought for mastery, and the outcome—one that endowed the administrative state with considerable powers while falling well short of the general policing, let alone the criminalization, of disease—smacked more of pragmatism than of philosophy. Amid all the noise of competing ideologies, the subtle art of the administratively possible was central to the politics of health.[4]

This chapter will survey a number of major initiatives chiefly in the fields of socially and sexually transmitted diseases in England over the last century and a half. Its aim is to focus attention on what has been a long-running debate on the relations between state powers and individual liberties, the public health and individual medical care (as classically inscribed in the one-to-one confidential contract between patient and doctor). These legal, philosophical, and ethical issues have been largely neglected by historians surveying the rise of the welfare state from Edwin Chadwick to William Beveridge and Aneurin Bevan. That history has traditionally been written either as a celebration of the march of the public health movement as progress, leading up to the National Health Service,[5] or (in more recent, "alternative" accounts) as the marginalization and expropriation of medical sects (e.g., homeopaths) by the juggernaut of state-medical imperialism.[6]

Contemporaries, however, were not deaf to such concerns, debating the connections between physic, philosophy, and politics with a clarity and a passion uncommon today. Our approach here is first to survey the Victorian ideological battleground, and then to explore the complicated relationship between what battling ideologues proclaimed, what found its way onto the statute book, and (not least) what was finally put into practice by medical officers of health, magistrates, and police. This background should afford a better understanding of what is truly at stake today in the contending ideas and policies over AIDS.

THE INDIVIDUAL AND THE STATE

One of the earliest comprehensive and systematic philosophical vindications of the fundamental rights of the individual against the state is set out in William Godwin's extremely influential *Political Justice,* published in 1793.[7] Godwin believed that existing governments improperly invaded the rightful liberty of the individual in many departments of life; the fundamental freedoms of speech, of publication, of assembly, of conscience, of moral belief and action were all unjustly impeded. Yet there is one conspicuous absence in Godwin's indictment of the state. He makes no complaint about the state's interference with the health or the medical choices of the individual. The silence is not an omission, but merely reflects the realities of England at the close of the eighteenth century. Though there was a state religion, there was no state medicine, unlike in many parts of the Continent. Indeed, the very phrase "medical police"—so common in the parlance of enlightened absolutism on the Continent as a part of *Kameralwissenschaft* (the science of bureaucracy), and known even in Scotland—was hardly even an Anglicized expression.[8]

Some two-thirds of a century later, in 1859, John Stuart Mill published *On Liberty,*[9] the classic mid-Victorian philosophical defense of the freedom of the individual.[10] Fighting what he saw as the tyranny of mass opinion, which he believed was fast being consolidated into a new legislative tyranny, Mill argued for the priority of the individual over the claims of state and society. The fundamental purpose of the state was to protect natural personal liberties, rather than (as in Edmund Burke's political philosophy) to enforce political, religious, and moral allegiance and orthodoxy within a superorganic whole. Mill brought to bear arguments partly metaphysical (individuals had the fundamental right to dispose of their lives as they pleased), and partly utilitarian (self-reliance built character, intellectual dissent stimulated the march of mind, and in the long run these benefited both individual and society). The only ground for curbing one person's liberty, he argued, was when its exercise materially interfered with the free exercise of another's.

Mill clinched his case for liberty through pious appeals to the martyrs of history—Socrates, Galileo, and so forth—and presented telling illustrations from everyday life. Suicide should be decriminalized, because in the last resort it was for the individual, not for society, to decide what to do with his or her life. Similarly, poisons should be sold freely, as should narcotics and alcohol. Society had the right to educate and caution against, but not to prohibit indulgence in, such vices. The danger of their abuse was less than the stifling evils of what then was called paternalism.

Mill is strangely and revealingly silent, however, on matters of public health. He believed that bad morals and bad practices should be permitted, because they would be destroyed by free and fair competition, and that truth would prevail. But did the same apply to bad air, bad drinking water, and contagious diseases? To what extent and under what circumstances was the enforcement of public health proper? Mill does not say.

It is hardly anachronistic of us to put this question to him, especially given that the powers of the state to enforce the public health were controversially transformed beyond recognition during his own lifetime. The General Board of Health, set up by the Public Health Act of 1848, had been granted unprecedented powers to regulate such matters as dangerous sewers and contaminated water supplies—powers that Edwin Chadwick, its only paid and chief commissioner, exploited to the hilt.[11] This board proved unpopular and short-lived, but it was succeeded by a new medical department established at the Privy Council, with additional powers of inspection and supervision of public health services, under the expert judgment of Sir John Simon.[12] The Medical Act of 1848 also empowered local authorities to establish medical officers of health, who were mandated to monitor morbidity and coordinate the provision of statutory services in local sanitary districts, and granted a broad range of legal powers under a series of Nuisance Removal acts passed in the 1850s.[13] Most radically of all, legislation of 1853 made universal childhood smallpox vaccination compulsory, carrying fines and even imprisonment for defaulters.[14]

Faced with this tide of administrative centralization, the Tory press expressed its horror at the rising tide of Whig paternalism and its interference into private property and local government. The *Herald* claimed that "a little dirt and freedom, may after all be more desirable than no dirt at all and slavery."[15] But this Canute-like gesture proved in vain. The current of compulsory public health, backed with state sanctions, was flowing powerfully. In the 1860s the Contagious Diseases acts (1864, 1866, 1869) empowered the medical inspection (under specific circumstances) of women believed to be common prostitutes. If found diseased, they could be compulsorily detained and treated.[16] Somewhat later, the whole domain of infectious diseases came under surveillance and administrative regulation. Notification of Diseases acts in 1889 and

1899 required any incidence of a listed infectious disease (smallpox, diphtheria, scarlet fever, croup, typhus, etc.) to be compulsorily reported to the medical officer of health, who then had it in his powers to remove and isolate sufferers and their families and to compel medical treatment.[17]

Looking back as early as 1868, less than a decade after Mill's *On Liberty,* Sir John Simon was loquacious about the dramatic benefits of this enlargement of the domain of public health regulation:

> It has interfered between parent and child, not only in imposing limitation on industrial uses of children, but also to the extent of requiring that children should not be left unvaccinated. It has interfered between employer and employed, to the extent of insisting, in the interests of the latter, that certain sanitary claims shall be fulfilled in all places of industrial occupation. It has interfered between vendor and purchaser, has put restrictions on the sale and purchase of poisons, has prohibited in certain cases certain commercial supplies of water, and has made it a public offence to sell adulterated food or drink of medicine, or to offer for sale any meat unfit for human food. Its care for the treatment of disease has not been unconditionally limited to treating at the public expense such sickness as may accompany destitution: it has provided that in any sort of epidemic emergency organized medical assistance, not peculiarly for paupers, may be required of local authorities; and in the same spirit it requires that vaccination at the public cost shall be given gratuitously to every claimant.[18]

Thus the high noon of free trade and individualism in the manner of Samuel Smiles's *Self Help* (1859), was also, paradoxically, a time when the state made staggering inroads on the freedom of the individual in the name of the national health. A battery of different ideologies contributed to breach the citadel of laissez-faire. Through trusty disciples such as Edwin Chadwick, Jeremy Bentham's doctrine—that it was the duty of the legislator to secure the greatest happiness of the greatest number through the deployment of science, expertise, and legal sanctions—had its impact, especially in the public health domain.[19] In other fields of abuses, particularly those concerning children and lunatics, Evangelicalism's moral paternalism overcame the dogmatic defense of hallowed individual rights. And, as recent historians have been concerned to stress, pragmatic pleas of necessity in the teeth of "intolerable" evils such as cholera disarmed opposition.[20]

Regarding particular abuses, it is important to stress the presence of a variety of distinct ideologies—in some ways complementary and in others competing—that could be used to argue for limited state action to safeguard the public health. The debates over legislation for sanitation, smallpox, or venereal disease never resulted in simple gross polarizations of opinion—Whigs versus Conservatives, religious versus secular enthusiasts, the medical establishment versus the people at large. Rather, we see internal fractionalization within each of the powerful parties, professions, and estates of the realm. Each instance—water supply, burial grounds, vaccination—brought about new alliances and allegiances, leading to a jerky, uneven development of powers that often reflected the preoccupations of a particular influential reformer (such as Lord Shaftesbury with lunacy law reform) or a pressure group of zealots.

It is in this context that we should interpret Mill's peculiar silence. Issues such as religious bigotry and humbug over private morality concentrated and united all his principles and prejudices. By contrast, the questions raised by the possibility of enforcing public health cut confusingly clean across his beliefs, as they did for many other Victorian intellectuals, physician and civil servant alike. Mill was deeply wedded both to utilitarianism and to libertarianism, and he believed that in the long run they were totally compatible. In the medium term the causes of happiness, progress, and utility, Mill contended, would best be served by maximizing liberty. Yet (in a way that might seem casuistic) he was also willing to countenance state intervention, or the infraction of liberties, in certain cases to ensure the effective operation of freedom, as he saw it. Thus, no man should be allowed to exercise the "freedom" of selling himself into slavery, because servitude itself denied human liberty. Similarly, Mill believed, the state was duty bound to compel parents to educate their children (despite the interference with the normally sovereign rights of parents), because without education no young person would be in a position to exercise freedom properly. This approach, which T. H. Green was soon to call "hindering hindrances," incorporated a certain paternalism within the philosophy of liberalism. The state could act to protect the liberty of those who could not protect themselves, or it could interfere in the lives of those who had abused their liberty. In its various ideological garbs, such a doctrine provided a key legitimation of selective state action (in allegedly exceptional or anomalous cases) for those eminent Victorians who deplored Prussian or French bureaucracy and primarily saw themselves as crusaders for liberal freedom.

STATE INTERVENTION, PATERNALISM, AND RESISTANCE

Given the strength of this prevailing liberalism, it should not be surprising that the most dramatic initial inroads on the individual right and duty to monitor one's own health came with a group particularly unable to protect themselves—the insane. The prereform-era English state had permitted the unchecked growth of a uniquely laissez-faire method of managing madness. In most of continental Europe from the seventeenth century onward, some form of state authorization was required for the legal confinement of a mad person by his or her relatives or friends (in France, for example, it was by royal *lettre de cachet,* in the United Provinces, by order of town councils).[21]

In England, by contrast, the state had kept completely clear of the trade in lunacy. Through most of the eighteenth century anyone could be indefinitely confined in a privately owned madhouse by the agency of friends or family willing to pay the fee; the transaction was purely private. In 1774 medical certification of the insane and licensing of private madhouses were introduced for the first time.[22] Inspection, however, remained rudimentary until the establishment of the Lunacy Commission, set up for the metropolitan area in 1828 and extended to the whole country in 1845.[23] Thereafter, a state-appointed board, chaired for fifty-three years by the indefatigable Evangelical, Lord Shaftesbury, vigorously overruled what would otherwise have been the free contractual relationships of the market, acting on behalf of the putative interests of the insane.

In the case of lunatics, the ground for intervention was simple: By reason of unreason, the insane were legally *non compos mentis,* incapable of minding their own affairs. Legally irresponsible like minors, they needed a competent body to act on their behalf. Laws licensing and regulating madhouses and preventing improper confinement would protect lunatics; in return for that protection, they were to suffer the suspension of their freedom, their civil rights. In time, the range and number of people undergoing certification increased, as the rationales for confinement were enlarged from the initial restrictive one (preventing harm being done by the lunatic to self and others), to the more expansive ideal of therapeutic cure. In other words, the state became more interventionist by moving from a negative notion of freedom (preventing harm) to a positive one (doing good). At the same time, the scope of the activities of the Lunacy Commission expanded, regulating asylum management in greater detail. The case of lunacy exemplifies the emergence of the state regulation of health at its most pure, complete, and unchallenged.[24]

The tacit ideology in the development of compulsory legislation to prevent infectious disease took a slightly different tack. Here advocates of state medicine, such as Sir John Simon and Henry Rumsey, claimed that what we might call the sovereign right of the individual to contract, die of, and spread infectious disease should be suspended for the benefit of the health of the community as a whole.[25] In this context two sets of legislation were passed during the 1850s and 1860s that made great inroads on the civil liberty of individuals to have autonomy over their health and sickness. The Compulsory Vaccination acts of 1853 and 1867 placed a legal obligation on parents to have their children vaccinated within the first year of life; fines or imprisonment were the penalties for default.[26] Compulsory smallpox vaccination constituted a remarkable infringement of the normal rights of parents over their children, especially in view of the fact that few legal restrictions on child labor existed at this time, and there was no statutory obligation on parents to educate their children; parents also still possessed an almost unlimited right to neglect or punish their offspring.

The lunacy laws had met little resistance from normally vociferous libertarians, but compulsory smallpox vaccination proved a very different kettle of fish. A powerful opposition lobby was formed, spearheaded by the Anti-Vaccination League (founded in 1867), pressing for repeal.[27] It had numerous strings to its bow, advancing statistical, technical, and medico-scientific arguments for the inefficacy—indeed, the gross danger—of vaccination itself. But it also campaigned on the platform of freedom from medical tyranny—some of its members seeing compulsory vaccination as a manifestation of the menace of medical imperialism comparable to the growing practice of vivisection.[28] At the heart of the league's campaign lay the philosophy of Mill, summarized in an epigraph at the head of each issue of its journal, the *Vaccination Inquirer:* "He who knows only his own side of the case, knows little of that."

Appealing to that cluster of populist and radical interests that paraded themselves as Davids ranged against the Goliath of the Victorian establishment, the Anti-Vaccination League was able to flex sufficient muscle to secure a substantial attenuation of the acts: The act of 1898 allowed parents to forgo vaccination if they could prove to a magistrate that they had genuine conscientious objections to the practice of injecting contaminated material into the bodies of their infants. Later, in 1907, a further amendment made exemption much easier through formal applications to a justice of the peace.[29] The new legislation merely ratified the status quo in existing antivaccinationist strongholds, such as Leicester, where the original act had proved impossible to implement against the wishes of large numbers of refractory parents, not least because the union authorities had themselves been divided on the issue.[30]

It would be inaccurate to characterize the struggle over smallpox vaccination as a simplistic division of authoritarian versus libertarian ideologies. Simon, the main architect of the 1867 act, was concerned to improve the quality of the system, making it as comprehensive as possible and ensuring the standard of lymph supply necessary for vaccination.[31] He was less concerned about the stringency of compulsion. For its part, the antivaccination lobby was not consistent in its arguments against compulsion. Although it characterized vaccination as medical despotism, it was prepared to support compulsory notification and isolation of smallpox victims in Leicester. The antivaccinationists called this the sanitarian's method, but medical officers of health, who operated notification, hailed it as the triumph of a scientific, medical approach to infectious disease and advocated its use in conjunction with vaccination, as in the 1896 Gloucester epidemic.[32]

Compulsory vaccination was one of two pieces of legislation created during the mid-Victorian period aimed at the prevention of infectious diseases. The second was the Contagious Diseases acts (1864, 1866, 1869). English legislators—all men, of course—had long since essentially accepted that prostitution was a commodity in the market economy, relating to elemental desire. So long as there were men, there would be a demand; so long as there was a market, there would be a supply. Prostitution, therefore, should essentially remain an unregulated free-market activity, subject to sporadic criminal prosecution. This "solution" (which had the additional benefit that the state was not "tainted" by giving sexual vice official recognition) was quite contrary to the system of policing employed for centuries in so many continental nations, in which prostitution came under the aegis of administrative jurisdiction through the close licensing of brothels.[33]

The consequence in England was that the chief legislation regarding prostitution was enacted ostensibly because of its threat to health. During the Crimean War it was discovered that the British army and navy were riddled with venereal disease. The euphemistically named Contagious Diseases acts (1864, 1866, 1869) attempted to counter venereal disease by enforcing the compulsory medical inspection of streetwalkers in specified garrison towns and ports. Women suspected of common prostitution could be taken into police custody, subjected to medical examination, and if found venereally infected, detained during the course of treatment.[34]

What is significant, however, is the collapse of the acts in the teeth of widespread and varied criticism (the acts were repealed in 1886). As with the antivaccination lobby, opposition to the Contagious Diseases acts formed into societies, such as the National Anti-Contagious Diseases Association (formed in 1869 and led by Josephine Butler), which won the support of a range of radical elements battling against what they saw as the improper encroachments on civil liberties.[35] Libertarian arguments against the acts were advanced: Even the *British Medical Journal* initially denounced the acts on the grounds that they infringed the "civil liberties" of prostitutes.[36] Medico-scientific arguments were added: The acts (it was alleged) were bound to prove ineffective in reducing venereal diseases. And most powerfully of all, perhaps, a moral groundswell stigmatized the acts—with their explicit avowal of the sexual double standard—as deeply offensive to women and as condoning vice by rendering such sex safe for men.[37]

There is no denying that a vocal section of the medical profession—army and navy doctors in particular—supported the acts, backing their case with an ingrained professional misogyny. Others, including no less an eminence than Sir John Simon, expressed considerable reservations, being unwilling to embroil the profession in the disreputable business of acting as moral jailers.[38] Neither can one find a simple libertarian/authoritarian polarization in the minds of the repealers. For many members of the Ladies National Association, the "liberal" campaign to spare prostitutes from the police and the "instrumental rape" of the surgeon often accompanied a revivalist "social purity" campaign (eventually organized in the National Vigilance Movement) to "protect" women by introducing legal restrictions aimed at outlawing prostitution. "Votes for women, chastity for men" soon became Christabel Pankhurst's suffragist rallying call.[39]

The argument legitimating compulsory legislation to prevent infectious disease championed the health of the community over the individual's autonomy in matters of health and sickness. The common argument of the repealing organizations objected to the gross invasion of the bodies of its subjects by an authoritarian state: "Against the body of a healthy man Parliament has no right of assault whatever under pretence of the Public Health; nor any the more against the body of a healthy infant. . . . The law is an unendurable usurpation, and creates the right of resistance."[40] The development of compulsory intervention in public health began with the bodies of those who were least able to protest. The interventionist state was then able to achieve its aim under the guise of paternalism, protecting those unable to protect themselves—lunatics and children (in the case of vaccination)—and later moved to protecting society against a section of its supposedly least responsible elements, such as prostitutes.

It is often alleged nowadays—indeed, in the case of AIDS itself—that governments, particularly those of the right, irresponsibly whip up scaremongering "moral panics," which they then exploit to introduce repressive legislation dressed up in the benign language of public health.[41] The compulsory smallpox vaccination legislation and the Contagious Diseases acts indicate a rather different scenario. For in both these cases, the legislation itself was passed sub rosa, without a noisy, public panic, because a small band of committed advocates, politicians, and civil servants diplomatically pushed a bill (in the case of the 1853 vaccination act, a private member's bill) through the House with minimal discussion. The *grande peur* was then created by *repealers,* who, in the case of smallpox, argued that vaccination was more liable to create epidemics, not prevent them, and in the case of prostitution, claimed that no woman was now safe from suspicion.

The successes of the repeal cause in both cases is a sign of the relative weakness of the alliance between government and the organized medical profession, and of deep internal divisions within both as to the propriety and prudence of health enforcement. No Victorian government was prepared to take its commitment to preventive medicine to the point of great unpopularity. Equally, the scions of the medical profession—above all the Royal Colleges of Physicians and Surgeons—were keen to preserve their independence and to keep government at arm's length.

It is significant, then, that the major instance of the successful introduction of compulsory powers over adults in the sphere of public hygiene and preventive medicine should have been on a local and case-by-case basis. This lay in the development of the idea of notifiable diseases; i.e., those socially contagious infections that had proved such a hazard in the Victorian urban environment. Under the Local Government Act of 1875, medical officers of health were granted powers to remove sufferers from such diseases out of the community and place them in isolation or fever hospitals on the ground that they were "nuisances." This procedure was taken one stage further by an adoptive Notification of Diseases Act of 1889, made compulsory under a new act in 1899. This rendered obligatory the notification to the medical officer of health (MOH) of any incidence of a listed infectious disease (including typhus, typhoid, smallpox, erysipelas, scarlet fever, diphtheria, measles, etc.) by the attending physician or head of household. The MOH was subsequently empowered to remove the patient to an isolation hospital until rendered noninfectious and to disinfect the site of infection.[42]

In some ways this legislation represents a striking infringement of the traditional freedom to be sick, and to spread one's sickness, with impunity.[43] There was no organized public opposition to this measure. But some friction was created between the different branches of the medical profession itself. Thomas Crawford, chairman of the Sanitary Institute, pointed out in 1895 that the behavior of medical officers of health regarding the operation of notification and isolation had alienated general practitioners in their districts. The procedure of secondary (bacteriological) diagnosis often undermined the general practitioner's authority, and the detection and threat of prosecution of default infuriated the MOH's clinical colleagues.[44] Crawford claimed that this hostility from general practitioners was matched by that of families who objected to the law: "The English people are not afraid of risking either their lives or their health in the interests of those whom they love and they are consequently not easily persuaded to part with any member of their family simply because he or she happens to be suffering from an infectious disease."[45] The response of medical officers of health, by contrast, was to deny the existence of hostility from family members completely, claiming that the majority was pleased to attend hospital during their sickness, and that in London, at least, the Metropolitan Asylum Board was overburdened by the demand for isolation and its costs. But they were forced to admit the open hostility of the general practitioners, and acknowledged that the success of the notification system depended on the tact and diplomacy of individual officers.[46]

It is noteworthy that Infectious Diseases acts met with so little public opposition. When comparable powers of removal had first been introduced during the 1832 cholera epidemic, the public reacted with extensive rioting[47] (partly on the ground that cholera was what the radical journalist William Cobbett called a "humbug" promulgated to distract attention from the new Poor Law).[48] This new tractability of the British public suggests that by the last quarter of the nineteenth century the public was becoming acclimated to a new medical rationality that might involve the trimming of its liberties.

For reasons initially more connected with improved nutrition and a healthier environment than with innovations in curative medicine, infectious diseases that had constituted lethal, epidemic health hazards in earlier centuries gradually ceased to pose such a threat. The Notification of Diseases Acts still remain on the statute books but, mercifully, rarely have to be invoked. It is perhaps, then, not surprising that the key debates this century upon the propriety and necessity of compulsory powers for the treatment of disease and the prevention of epidemics have centered on venereal disease (V.D.). New methods of detecting and curing syphilis, with the development of the Wasserman test in 1906 and Paul Ehrlich's development of salvarsan in 1910, revived a preoccupation with reducing the prevalence of the disease[49] (one estimate claimed that in 1913 there were half a million sufferers in London alone).[50] The advent of World War I also fueled fears that wartime morality and concentrations of soldiers would swell the disease to epidemic proportions, threatening the armed forces' fighting ability.[51]

The Royal Commission on Venereal Diseases was therefore established in 1913 and reported to Parliament in 1916. A notable shift in medical and official opinion emerged from the debate. The failures of the Contagious Diseases Acts were accepted from the outset, and the terms of the inquiry were to regard a return to these measures as a nonoption—not least because the prostitute was no longer seen as the most dangerous source of infection. Increasing social emancipation for women—especially as the result of high levels of female employment during the war—led to increased sexual freedom for "ordinary" as well as "professional" women. These so-called amateurs were held responsible for spreading venereal disease at a far greater rate than prostitutes.[52]

The commission made an important discrimination between the prevention of socially transmitted diseases and those that are transmitted sexually—the former being visible and necessitating treatment in their earliest stages, the latter lying dormant and being difficult to detect; sexually transmitted diseases remained contagious without presenting life-threatening symptoms to the carrier. The commission's report acknowledged that early detection was essential to prevent spread, and required the voluntary, active cooperation of infected persons presenting themselves for treatment. It consequently concluded that the stigma of official notification would hinder rather than help effective control, driving venereal disease underground to quack physicians and their remedies.[53]

Instead, a system of V.D. clinics, for men and for women, was to be established. Attendance would be voluntary. Anonymity and confidentiality would be preserved, and for that reason, the clinics were to have no formal connections with general practitioners and hospitals. Attenders would be encouraged, but not compelled, to inform their sexual contacts. Treatment would be free. It was a system that would "condone vice" no less than the Contagious Diseases Acts. But—a sign of the times—it condoned male and female vice equally, and involved no stigmatization of prostitutes. The underlying philosophy was to create conditions that encouraged maximum cooperation and attendance among patients.[54] These recommendations were issued as new regulations by the Local Government Board in July 1916 and became law under a 1917 act.[55] The commission had also recommended that the task of mass education be given to a voluntary organization, the National Council for Combating Venereal Disease (NCCVD), formed in 1914. The NCCVD (later to become the British Social Hygiene Council) subsequently undertook a propaganda lecture program among the troops and the civilian population, together with poster campaigns and documentary films.[56]

The medical profession's response to the commission's report was generally favorable; the doctors welcomed the free treatment centers and laboratory services provided by the state.[57] A section of the profession (mostly those who had served in the army and navy medical corps during the war) formed themselves, however, into the Society for the Prevention of Venereal Disease, which promoted the adoption of compulsory notification and the free dispensing of prophylactics, which had been so successful in reducing levels of infection among the troops. They pressed also for penalties to be imposed on defaulting patients who failed to complete, or deliberately refused, treatment.[58]

In 1923 the Trevethin Committee examined the workings of the clinics and argued that their success made notification unnecessary.[59] Those who continued to support notification, however, cited the successes of Sweden and Western Australia, which had adopted compulsory systems in 1915 and 1911. Sweden had attacked vice and venereal disease at their heart, it was claimed, by making detention compulsory, introducing prosecution for knowingly spreading infection, and making marriage illegal for a patient until he or she was cured.[60] The medical profession largely rejected these examples. *The Lancet* in 1916 suggested that the Swedish approach could be successful only for a small population, and emphasized that because it "bristles with penalties," it ran the risk that patients "may so dread this compulsory pilgrimage to health that they will refuse to seek medical help, . . . a risk which must be avoided in the working of the new legislation in this country."[61] In 1937 a delegation from the Ministry of Health was sent to Scandinavia and Holland to report on the system but concluded that "the degree of success in reducing the incidence of syphilis in the countries employing compulsory treatment and in those which rely on a voluntary system is broadly similar."[62]

As the result of a sharp rise in the incidence of venereal disease from 1939 to 1941, and a slower but steady increase in 1942,[63] the government added Regulation 33B to the Defence (General) Regulations. This regulation made compulsory the medical treatment of a person identified as a contact by two or more people. The relative merits of a voluntary system and a compulsory one were once more evaluated.[64] Advocates of compulsion, including prominent members of the Medical Society for the Study of Venereal Diseases (MSSVD) claimed that the rates of people defaulting on treatment in some parts of the country had reached 82 percent compared with only 2.5 percent in Sweden.[65] The operation of Regulation 33B was questioned by promoters of general notification, such as Dr. Edith Summerskill.[66] She claimed it operated unfavorably against women, who were more reluctant to identify contacts[67] and were, moreover, liable to imprisonment for failing to comply with treatment, while her male contacts were not: "Can the minister justify the position in which an individual informed against under Regulation 33B can be sent to prison, but the two informers, people suffering from the disease and liable to transmit it . . . are not penalised in any way?"[68] The Health Ministry dodged Dr. Summerskill's questions and her demands for a comprehensive system of compulsory notification for all patients, which she believed would restore the balance.

The *British Medical Journal* lent its support to the arguments of M. J. Laird who, at a widely reported meeting of the MSSVD in April 1942, suggested that to assert that compulsion was not consonant with the "British idea of the liberty of the subject" was outdated by the facts of rising incidence and default from treatment. The journal suggested that it was "late in the day to talk about the liberty of the subject" when the medical profession and the British public

> raise no objection to a law which may inflict a penalty upon any person who, "(a) knowing he is suffering from a notifiable disease, exposes other persons to the risk of infection". . . . Nor is any voice raised against the regulations which make it possible to "remove to hospital any person suffering from a notifiable disease if . . . [there is] a serious risk of infection being caused to other persons."[69]

The editorial believed that notification of venereal disease would operate efficiently and equitably, provided that confidentiality were maintained. By the end of the war it was clear that this line of argument was supported, as *The Lancet* pointed out, by a majority of medical officers of health but was opposed by "those in closest touch with the patient."[70]

Critics of compulsion, such as Dorothy Manchee from the British Hygiene Council, deplored the fact that notification "struck at the root of the relationship of trust and confidence between doctor and patient"; it would, moreover, open the door to blackmail. Colonel L. W. Harrison, who was the inspector at the Ministry of Health responsible for the V.D. service, believed that "private practitioners would not notify their cases." Manchee also agreed that doctors would "not comply" with such a system, which "smacked of Hitlerite Germany."[71] Physic and police should not be unwisely mingled.

The medical profession generally came out strongly in favor of the existing system of voluntary clinics, whose efficacy could best be improved by free and frank educational campaigns, removing shame and the conspiracy of silence, and putting V.D. on an equivalent footing with every other disease. The wartime Ministry for Information, the Central Council for Health Education, and the Ministry of Health combined forces to launch a new propaganda campaign through the newspapers and via the radio, giving out "Ten Plain Facts about V.D."[72] The publicity was more explicit than ever before, so much so that it only just managed to carry the support of the church (the archbishop of Canterbury demanded that the government should insist on denouncing the moral evils of promiscuity).[73] The propaganda stressed that family life was the safe, if not the sole, sexual course. For some, the campaign still fell short of what was needed. *The Lancet* suggested that "unfortunately, as the *Daily Mirror* has pointed out, the original wording of the advertisement has been watered down to meet the mistaken sense of delicacy of the proprietors of the daily press."[74]

Correspondents to *The Lancet* agreed that "prudery, hypocrisy and cant"[75] continued to dog efforts to educate the public about the plain fact that V.D. was preventable. This body of opinion held that the public should be told that "if abstinence is not possible, a condom intelligently used will give a high degree of protection."[76] John Ryle, the first professor of social medicine, was criticized, for example, for taking only a long-term view of the need for social and economic change, and not acknowledging the immediate need to inform the public that "if during the next six months every man in the British Isles wore a condom for extramarital intercourse, syphilis . . . would disappear entirely."[77] The campaign continued throughout the war, and the demobilized population was targeted by new propaganda in 1945 and 1946.[78]

MEDICAL POWER, PRIVACY, AND AIDS

The analysis offered in this chapter has charted how connections between medical practice and state power in Britain have increased. The state has made greatest inroads on the freedom of individuals in the causes of giving asylum to the mentally ill and preventing infectious disease.

The legal basis for the operation of the notification laws and the incarceration of the mentally disturbed has been a form of internment without trial. To reduce levels of infectious diseases, the state has suspended the right of habeas corpus in order to prevent an individual from infecting his or her fellow citizens. This suspension of liberty has been justified by the advocates of state medicine on the grounds that the period of "unfreedom" is limited and that hospitalization would give the best chances of cure; but, most important, it has argued the benefit to the community at large gained from the reduction of risks of epidemics.

In the case of diseases that are transmitted through ordinary social contact, the aim of "internment" was to prevent dissemination, because the very presence of the patient among the healthy spread infection to them. In the case of sexually transmitted diseases, the patient, once informed of his or her condition, could not spread infection unless he or she deliberately chose to do so. After 1916 those who supported compulsory detention of V.D. sufferers offered statistics to suggest that the high levels of default demonstrated that the efficiency of the system could not be entrusted to the voluntary cooperation of patients. Those who argued against compulsion claimed that default was no greater in voluntary than in compulsory systems—indeed default would certainly increase once confidentiality were breached. Thus, in the twentieth century the focus of the controversy surrounding prevention of venereal disease moved from disease to default.[79]

The Victorians recognized that the balance between individual liberty and the higher public good of preventing infectious disease was a delicate one. Securing the health of the community frequently depended not so much on philosophical discourse but on the balance, and imbalance, of power between preventive and curative medicine. The argument that eventually won the day in the British context for the forces of nonnotification had less to do with the importance of personal liberty than with the power of the clinical profession to maintain the private, contractual relationship with the individual patient as the jewel in the crown of medical practice. Medical officers of health and practitioners of community medicine have consistently remained the Cinderellas of the profession, in contrast to the consultants and the clinicians. These legacies of a bygone age help to explain why health enforcement has always been, and remains, a low priority for the medical profession.

The AIDS policies being pursued in Britain by the Department of Health at the time of this writing reflect this legacy. No move has been made, either by government ministers or by the department itself, to make AIDS a notifiable disease. Compulsory screening has also been rejected both by the government and by the medical profession. Instead, a forceful educational program, stepped up in December 1986, has sent information leaflets to every household in the kingdom, informing the public of the existence of AIDS and its modes of transmission, warning of the possible growth of the epidemic, making it clear that it is not a "gay" disease but presents an equal threat to the heterosexual community, and advocating safe sex: "Keep to one partner. If you can't, use a condom." Advertisements, information programs, and "light entertainment" features on the national television and radio networks have been used to publicize the Health Department's messages. There have been explicit statements from health ministers condemning social prejudices against AIDS victims and stressing that the AIDS virus cannot be transmitted through normal social contact. The Department of Employment has announced plans for distributing information leaflets to employers, emphasizing the need not to discriminate against virus carriers or sufferers.

There has been a certain response to the epidemic from pockets of far right and religious fundamentalist opinion, among whom should be included the chief constable for the Greater Manchester area, James Anderton, who has claimed that AIDS demonstrates that homosexuality is unnatural and against the will of God. There have been mutterings in the popular right-wing press to the effect that AIDS demonstrates that the legalization of homosexuality over the last generation was imprudent. The government's health campaign has also itself met with some hostility on the ground that its vernacular message is needlessly offensive to delicate minds. And a few voices from within the medical profession have called for further government powers, including the power to make screening compulsory. Until now, however, government policy has been to resist all such demands.

The Department of Health and its ministers have, in fact, achieved a considerable degree of support from responsible lay and medical opinion for its current policies. The major objections from the Opposition parties (Labour, Social Democratic, Liberal) in Parliament and from its critics in the medical profession have been over the inadequate level of funding. Michael Meacher, the Labour party spokesman for Health, in particular argued that insufficient funds have been earmarked both for research and for treatment. Money is still lacking to provide additional staff and resources for the urogenital clinics, where consultations take place. Major inadequacies are predicted to arise among hospital provision for sufferers. The Department of Health, however, has claimed the need for financial caution in view of the obscure future epidemiology of the disease. Critics, however, have been suggesting that the care and support system is already breaking down from insufficient funding and that current, not merely future, needs already outstrip the means made available to the health services for coping with the epidemic.

In July 1987 a special debate on the AIDS crisis was held at the annual meeting of the British Medical Association (BMA). A motion was proposed that it was perfectly within the bounds of ethical conduct for doctors to perform tests for AIDS without the knowledge or consent of their patients, and allowing physicians discretion to do so. Those favoring this proposal suggested, inter alia, that the fear of infection among hospital staffs, medical and lay, was now so great that such procedures would be necessary to preempt industrial action. A fierce debate among doctors resulted in the resolution being passed contrary to the advice of the association's leadership. The first British professor of venereology, Michael Adler, of Middlesex Hospital, announced to the national media networks his abhorrence of the BMA's decision. His horror was echoed by the chief medical officer to the Department of Health and numerous other leading members of the medical profession. BMA members retreated from this position at the annual meeting in 1988.

Divisions within the medical profession are thus beginning to appear. In the BMA debate, a speaker who opposed the screening of hospital patients was filmed by the news network as he was announcing a list of the reasons why it would be a serious error for the profession to begin to tread the path of compulsory health policies. He concluded his speech with an emotional appeal to his colleagues to consider the "heart of this issue," the destruction of what the profession held more sacred than anything else, "the confidence, and confidentiality, between patient and practitioners." Here we have a strong echo of the attitudes of earlier generations of physicians. He and many of his profession deplored the fact that this voluntarist ideology, which has dominated British health policy on venereal disease, was, for the first time, being undermined from within the medical profession itself.

NOTES

1. See Roy Porter, "History Says No to the Policeman's Response to AIDS," *British Medical Journal* 2 (1986): 1589–1590.

2. See the discussion of Professor Julian Peto's proposals in R. Mckie, *Panic: The Story of AIDS* (New York: Thorson's, 1986), 102–107, and of Professor Richard Doll in J. Laurance, "The Ethics of Testing for AIDS," *New Society*, 13 February 1987, 20. For other medical views see E. D. Acheson (chief medical officer to the Department of Health and Social Security), "AIDS: A Challenge to the Public Health," *The Lancet* 1 (22 March 1986): 662–666, and "British Medical Association's Evidence on AIDS to Parliament," *British Medical Journal* 1 (1987): 61. For further general histories and medical background, see Graham Hancock and Enver Carim, *AIDS: The Deadly Epidemic* (London: Victor Gollancz, 1986); Nicholas Wells, *The AIDS Virus: Forecasting Its Impact* (London: Office of Health Economics, 1986).

3. M. Fitzpatrick and D. Milligan, *The Truth about the AIDS Panic* (London: Junius, 1987); M. D. Kirby, "AIDS Legislation—Turning Up the Heat?" *Journal of Medical Ethics* 12 (1986): 187–194; Raanan Gillon (editor of the *Journal of Medical Ethics*), quoted in Laurance, "The Ethics of Testing for AIDS," 20; Nigel Pugh, "Civil Rights under Threat," *Community Care: The Independent Voice of Social Work*, 22 January 1987, 13–15.

4. See R. Lambert, *Sir John Simon, 1816–1904, and English Social Administration* (London: Macgibbon and Kee, 1963); and A. Wohl, *Endangered Lives: Public Health in Victorian Britain* (London: Methuen, 1984).

5. See W. M. Frazer, *History of English Public Health, 1834–1939* (London: Ballière, Tindall & Cox, 1950); George Rosen, *A History of Public Health* (New York: M. D. Publications, 1958); C. F. Brockington, *The History of Public Health in the Nineteenth Century* (Edinburgh: Livingstone, 1965); R. H. Shryock, *The Development of Modern Medicine* (1937; Madison: University of Wisconsin Press, 1979).

6. For discussion see *Medical Fringe and Medical Orthodoxy*, ed. W. F. Bynum and Roy Porter (London: Croom Helm, 1986).

7. Don Locke, *William Godwin: A Fantasy of Reason* (London: Routledge & Kegan Paul, 1983).

8. George Rosen, *From Medical Police to Social Medicine* (New York: Sci-

ence History Publications, 1974), 120–157, and for a much earlier instance, R. Palmer, "The Control of Plague in Venice and Northern Italy, 1348–1600" (Ph.D. diss., University of Kent, 1978). The concept of medical police had been more readily taken up in Scotland by Andrew Duncan and his successors; see B. White, "Training Medical Policemen," paper presented at the conference on the History of Legal Medicine, University of Lancaster, 1987. In England the most aggressive policing had been used during the seventeenth-century plague years. See P. Slack, *The Impact of Plague in Tudor and Stuart England* (London: Routledge & Kegan Paul, 1985).

9. John Stuart Mill, *On Liberty* (1859; Harmmondsworth: Penguin Classics, 1986).

10. R. P. Anschutz, *The Philosophy of J. S. Mill* (Oxford: Oxford University Press, 1969); Isaiah Berlin, *Four Essays on Liberty* (Oxford: Oxford University Press, 1969); Gertrude Himmelfarb, *On Liberty and Liberalism: The Case of John Stuart Mill* (New York: Knopf, 1974).

11. S. E. Finer, *The Life and Times of Edwin Chadwick* (London: Methuen, 1952), 319–474.

12. Lambert, *Sir John Simon,* 261–560; R. M. Macleod, "The Anatomy of State Medicine," in *Medicine and Science in the 1860s,* ed. F. N. L. Poynter (London: Wellcome Institute, 1968), 201–227.

13. Wohl, *Endangered Lives,* 199, 308–319.

14. Lambert, *Sir John Simon,* 250–258.

15. Quoted by David Roberts, *Paternalism in Early Victorian England* (London: Croom Helm, 1979), 200.

16. Paul McHugh, *Prostitution and Victorian Social Reform* (London: Croom Helm, 1982), 35–43; Judith Walkowitz, *Prostitution and Victorian Society: Women, Class and the State* (Cambridge: Cambridge University Press, 1980), 69–89.

17. Sir Arthur Whitlegge and Sir George Newman, *Hygiene and Public Health* (London: Cassell, 1917), 526–543; D. E. Watkins, "The English Revolution in Social Medicine" (Ph.D. diss., University of London, 1984), 214–239.

18. Sir John Simon, *Report of the Medical Officer to the Local Government Board,* vol. 9 (London: His Majesty's Stationery Office, 1869), 11.

19. Finer, *Edwin Chadwick,* 12–37; see also R. A. Lewis, *Edwin Chadwick and the Public Health Movement* (London: Longmans, Green, 1952).

20. For a review of the debate see R. M. Macleod, "Statesmen Undisguised," *American Historical Review* 78 (1973): 1386–1405.

21. Michel Foucault, *Madness and Civilization: A History of Insanity in the Age of Reason,* trans. Richard Howard (New York: Random House, 1985).

22. W. L. Parry-Jones, *The Trade in Lunacy* (London: Routledge & Kegan Paul, 1971), 14.

23. N. Hervey, "The Lunacy Commission, 1845–60, with Special Reference to the Implementation of Policy in Kent and Surrey" (Ph.D. diss., University of Bristol, 1987).

24. D. J. Mellett, *The Prerogative of Asylumdom* (New York: Garland, 1982).

25. See Henry Rumsey, *Essay on State Medicine* (London: Churchill, 1856),

and *Essays and Papers on Some Fallacies of Statistics* (London: Smith, Elder & Co., 1875), 30–36; John Simon, *English Sanitary Institutions* (London: Cassell, 1890), 433–487.

26. B. J. Stern, *Should We Be Vaccinated? A Survey of the Controversy in Its Historical and Scientific Aspects* (London: Harper, 1927), 58–61.

27. William White, *The Story of a Great Delusion* (London: Allen, 1885), is the best account of the history of the antivaccination movement told by a historian from within the movement's own ranks. In this vein, see also William Scott Tebb, *A Century of Vaccination and What It Teaches Us* (London: Swan Sonnenschein, 1899).

28. Dorothy Porter and Roy Porter, "The Politics of Compulsory Smallpox Vaccination and the Gloucester Epidemic 1895–96," *Medical History,* forthcoming.

29. Porter and Porter, ibid.; R. M. Macleod, "Law, Medicine and Public Opinion: The Resistance to Compulsory Health Legislation, 1870–1907," *Public Law* 107 (1967): 189–211.

30. Stuart M. F. Fraser, "Leicester and Smallpox: The Leicester Method," *Medical History* 24 (1980): 315–332.

31. Lambert, *Sir John Simon,* 391–394, 437–447.

32. Porter and Porter, "The Politics of Smallpox Vaccination."

33. Alain Corbin, *Les Filles de Noce* (Paris, 1978), and "Commercial Sexuality in Nineteenth-Century France: A System of Images and Regulations," in *The Making of the Modern Body: Sexuality and Society in the Nineteenth Century,* ed. C. Gallagher and T. Laqueur (Berkeley and Los Angeles: University of California Press, 1987), 209–219.

34. McHugh, *Prostitution,* 35–53; Walkowitz, *Prostitution and Victorian Society,* 69–89.

35. McHugh, *Prostitution,* 55–70.

36. Walkowitz, *Prostitution,* 77.

37. Keith Thomas, "The Double Standard," *Journal of the History of Ideas* 20 (1959): 195–210.

38. McHugh, *Prostitution*, 48; Lambert, *Simon,* 405–406.

39. Walkowitz, *Prostitution,* 108–136.

40. This was a quotation from Francis W. Newman, professor at University College London, which the *Vaccination Inquirer* frequently used, together with the quotation from Mill, as an epigraph to each issue. See, for example, April–July 1894.

41. Fitzpatrick and Milligan, *AIDS Panic,* 1–4. There are historical parallels of scaremongering during the cholera epidemics of the nineteenth century leading to a variety of social responses, from "choleraphobia" to riot. See Michael Durey, *The Return of the Plague: British Society and Cholera 1831–32* (London: Gill and Macmillan Humanities Press, 1979), 131–140, and R. J. Morris, *Cholera 1832: The Social Response to an Epidemic* (London: Croom Helm, 1976), 95–127; Roy Porter, "Plague and Panic," *New Society* (12 December 1986): 11–13.

42. Watkins, "English Revolution in Social Medicine"; Whitlegge and Newman, *Hygiene,* 526–543; A. Newsholme, *Hygiene and Public Health* (London:

Gill, 1902), 317–334; B. Burnett Ham, *Handbook of Sanitary Law* (1899; London: Lewis, 1938), 69–94.

43. This is true with the exception of emergency powers for medical policing introduced during periods of widespread epidemics such as cholera in 1832–1833. See Durey, *Return of the Plague*, and Morris, *Cholera 1832*.

44. Watkins, "English Revolution," 299–302.

45. Thomas Crawford, "The Position of Medical Officers of Health in Regard to the Administration and Working of the Infectious Diseases and Notification Act," *Journal of the Sanitary Institute* 16 (1895–96): 353–361.

46. Watkins, "English Revolution," 215–216, 301–302.

47. Morris, *Cholera 1832*, 109–114.

48. Ibid., 97.

49. "The Control of Venereal Diseases," *Public Health* 26 (1913): 51–52; "The History of the Fight against Venereal Disease," *British Medical Journal* 2 (1916): 230–231.

50. *Public Health* 26, ibid., 51. The editorial in *Public Health* is quoting from an official inquiry into venereal disease, undertaken for the Local Government Board by Dr. R. W. Johnstone in 1912 and published as part of the *Annual Report of the Medical Officer of the Local Government Board, 1913–14*.

51. "Final Report of the Royal Commission on Venereal Diseases," *The Lancet* 1 (1916): 575–576; "The Treatment of Venereal Diseases by the State," *The Lancet* 2 (1916): 869–870.

52. See quotations from Johnstone's report and Arthur Newsholme's introduction in the *Annual Report of the Medical Officer to the Local Government Board, 1913–14* in Frazer, *History of English Public Health*, 338. See also Arthur Newsholme, *Medicine and the State* (London: Allen and Unwin, 1932), 212.

53. *Final Report of the Royal Commission on Venereal Diseases* [cd.8189] (London: His Majesty's Stationery Office, 1916).

54. Ibid., 60–62; *The Lancet* 1 (1916): 575–576.

55. The Venereal Diseases Act, 1917.

56. *Final Report . . . on Venereal Diseases*, 64. For a history of some of the controversies that surrounded the education policy, see Bridget A. Towers, "Health Education Policy 1916–1926: Venereal Disease and the Prophylaxis Dilemma," *Medical History* 24 (1980): 70–87.

57. "The Prevention and Treatment of Venereal Diseases: The Intervention of the State," *The Lancet* 1 (1916): 153–154; "The Fight against Venereal Disease," *The Lancet* 1 (1916): 682; "The State Treatment of Venereal Diseases," *The Lancet* 2 (1916): 283–284.

58. Towers, "Health Education," 75–77, 80–83.

59. "Control of Venereal Disease," *British Medical Journal* 2 (1942): 611–612.

60. "Medical Society for the Study of Venereal Diseases," *The Lancet* 1 (1942): 561–562.

61. *The Lancet* 2 (1916): 284.

62. *British Medical Journal* 2 (1942): 611.

63. "Venereal Disease in War-Time," *The Lancet* 2 (1942): 21.

64. "New Compulsory Powers in Control of Venereal Disease," *The Lancet* 2 (1942): 589; N. P. Shannon, "The Compulsory Treatment of Venereal Diseases under Regulation 33B," *British Journal of Venereal Diseases* 19 (1943): 22–25.

65. *British Medical Journal* 2 (1942): 611.

66. *The Lancet* 1 (1943): 691–692.

67. *The Lancet* 1 (1944): 167.

68. *The Lancet* 1 (1943): 723.

69. *British Medical Journal* 2 (1942): 612.

70. *The Lancet* 1 (1946): 615–616.

71. Ibid., 615.

72. "Control of Venereal Disease," *The Lancet* 2 (1942): 577–578; the Ministry of Health and The Central Council for Health Education, "Ten Plain Facts About V.D.," newspaper advertisement issued in 1942.

73. *The Lancet* 2 (1942): 738.

74. *The Lancet* 1 (1943): 317 (27 February).

75. R. A. Lyster, "Prevention of Venereal Disease," *The Lancet* 1 (1943): 476. Lyster was then president of the National Society for the Prevention of Venereal Disease.

76. Shakespeare Cooke, "Prevention of Venereal Disease," *The Lancet* 1 (1943): 350–351. See also correspondence of James Sequeira in *The Lancet* throughout 1943.

77. Ibid., 511.

78. *The Lancet* 1 (1945): 324; "Venereal Diseases: Educational Campaign," *Ministry of Health Circulars 42/45 and 92/45,* 1945.

79. Frank Mort has suggested that the British state opted for a basically noninterventionist policy with regard to STDs largely because the "personal life of mass society" remained outside the traditional boundaries of its broader political culture. See Frank Mort, *Dangerous Sexualities: Medico-Moral Politics in England since 1830* (London: Routledge & Kegan Paul, 1987). For a history of American policy, including the current issues surrounding the AIDS epidemic, see Allan M. Brandt, *No Magic Bullet: A Social History of Venereal Disease in the United States since 1880—With a New Chapter on AIDS* (Oxford: Oxford University Press, 1987).

Sin versus Science: Venereal Disease in Twentieth-Century Baltimore

Elizabeth Fee

Ways of perceiving and understanding disease are historically constructed. Our social, political, religious, and moral conceptions influence our perceptions of disease, just as do different scientific and medical theories. Indeed, these different elements often cannot be easily separated, as scientists and physicians bring their own cultural ideas to bear in the construction of scientific theories. Because these cultural ideas may be widely shared, their presence within medical and scientific theory may not be readily apparent. Often, such cultural conceptions are more obvious when reviewing medical and scientific theories of the past than they are in contemporary medical practice.[1]

Just as cultural conceptions of disease may be embodied in the framing of scientific theories, so these theories also influence popular perceptions of disease. At times, such scientific theories may reinforce, or contradict, other cultural conceptions; for example, religious and moral ideas, or racial stereotypes. The aspects of disease that we call "social" and "biological" are parts of a single social reality in which disease is produced, experienced, and reproduced, and in which the cultural meanings of the experience are defined, acted upon, and struggled over. The germ theory of disease tends to remove disease from its social context and to define disease as a biological phenomenon best studied in the laboratory. But a more complete understanding of disease must deal with its social as well as its biological aspects, with its cultural meanings as well as its statistical incidence.

In the case of the venereal diseases, it is clear that our attitudes embody a fundamental cultural ambivalence: Are venereal diseases to be studied and treated from a purely biomedical point of view—as the result of infection by a microorganism—or as social, moral, or spiritual afflictions?[2] As the name implies, venereal diseases are inevitably associated with sexuality, and therefore our perceptions of these diseases tend to be entangled with our ideas about the social meanings and moral evaluations of sexual behaviors. In the case of syphilis, a major killer in the first half of the twentieth century, health officials could decide that the true "cause" of syphilis was the microorganism *Treponema pallidum,* or they could define the "underlying cause" as "promiscuous sexual behavior." Each claim focuses on a different part of social reality, and each carries different messages of responsibility and blame. Each is part of a different language in which the disease may be described and defined. The first suggests the primacy of the clinic for treating disease; the second, the primacy of moral exhortation.

The parallel between syphilis and AIDS lends a special relevance to the study of that earlier epidemic. Both diseases, in laboratory terms, are caused by a microorganism—in the case of AIDS, by the HIV retrovirus. Both diseases can be transmitted by sexual contact; both can also be transmitted nonsexually. The social perception of each disease has been heavily influenced by the possibility of sexual transmission and the attendant notions of responsibility, guilt, and blame. In each case, those suffering from the disease have often been regarded as both the cause and embodiment of the disease, and have been feared and blamed by others who define themselves as more virtuous.

Until the advent of AIDS, syphilis was the most feared of the venereal diseases. Syphilis can be transmitted by body fluids during sexual contact, and by blood transfusions during the early stages of infection. It can be contracted by health workers after clinical examination of infectious lesions, and can occasionally be transmitted by contact with contaminated articles. It can be passed from mother to fetus during pregnancy.

Syphilis has an incubation period of several weeks. Initial infection is marked by a primary lesion on the skin or mucous membranes at the site of infection. This may then be followed by a latency period of several weeks or several years. The secondary stage of syphilis is marked by secondary lesions on the skin and mucous membranes. Syphilis is most communicable during the primary and secondary stages and the latent period. There is no natural immunity to syphilis; approximately 10 percent of exposures result in infection. Late syphilis, five to twenty years after initial infection, is marked by disabling lesions of the skin, viscera, cardiovascular system, and central nervous system, and may cause death.

Nonvenereal syphilis is spread by the same spirochete, *Treponema pallidum,* and is a common childhood disease in some Asian and African countries characterized by poor socioeconomic conditions and primitive sanitary arrangements. It is spread by direct contact with infectious skin lesions and by poor sanitation. The terms "venereal" and "nonvenereal" syphilis are, of course, problematic, because "venereal" syphilis may sometimes be transmitted by nonsexual contacts, but the term "venereal syphilis" does remind us of the inextricable identification of syphilis with sexual behavior in Western societies.

Throughout the twentieth century struggles have been waged over the meaning and definition of the venereal diseases. At times these diseases have been blanketed in silence, as though they belonged to a "private" realm not open to public discussion. Wars, however, have tended to make venereal diseases visible. The need to mobilize a large and healthy armed force brings venereal disease out of the private sphere and into the center of public policy discussions, highlighting the struggle over the proper definition and treatment of disease. During World War I, for example, the American Social Hygiene Association consistently equated venereal disease with immorality, vice, and prostitution.[3] Its members thus tried to close down brothels and taverns, to arrest prostitutes, and to advocate continence and sexual abstinence for the soldiers. The Commission on Training Camp Activities tried to suppress vice and liquor, and also to organize "good, clean fun": sports events, theatrical entertainments, and educational programs.[4] Meanwhile, the army quietly issued prophylactic kits to the soldiers and made early treatment after possible exposure compulsory. Any soldier who failed to get treatment could face court martial and imprisonment for "neglect of duty." These different approaches illustrate alternative conceptions of disease: the first viewing infection as the consequence of "vice," the second as a medical problem requiring prevention and treatment.

When dealing with major disease problems, we often try to find some social group to blame for the infection. During World War I, educational materials clearly presented the fighting men as the innocent victims of disease; prostitutes were the guilty spreaders of infection, implicitly working for the enemy against patriotic American soldiers.[5] In many communities prostitutes were the focus, and often the victims and scapegoats, of the new attention to venereal infections. Prostitutes—the women responsible for the defilement of the heroic American soldier—

would be regularly rounded up, arrested, and jailed in the campaign against vice.

The end of World War I brought a waning of interest in venereal disease and a return to "normal life," freed of the restrictions and regulations of military necessity. The once-energetic public discussion of venereal disease fell silent. Prostitutes and their customers were again permitted to operate without much official harassment; health departments quietly collected statistics on venereal disease but avoided publicity on the subject.[6]

Here we will examine the subsequent history of venereal disease, and especially syphilis, by focusing on a major industrial city, Baltimore, where a struggle between the moral and biomedical views of disease was played out in the context of city politics in the 1930s and 1940s. Although syphilis is no longer such a significant public health problem, this account should be useful in helping us reflect on the contemporary problem of AIDS. The politics and policies surrounding AIDS are characterized by a remarkably similar set of tensions between the moral and biomedical conceptions of disease.

TREATMENT FOR VENEREAL DISEASE: THE PUBLIC HEALTH CLINICS

In Baltimore, in the 1920s, a great social silence surrounded the problem of syphilis. The negative social stigma associated with venereal diseases caused extensive underreporting. Physicians endeavored to save patients and their families from possible embarrassment by attributing syphilis deaths to other causes. A tacit social conspiracy of silence resulted: Patients did not talk about their diseases, physicians did not report them, the health department did not publicize them, and the newspapers never mentioned them. The diseases were thus largely invisible. Many hospitals and physicians refused to treat patients with venereal diseases; physicians who specialized in these diseases could make a great deal of money from private patients.[7] Many patients, however, could not afford private medical care.

In the aftermath of World War I, the city health department began quietly to treat venereal diseases in its public clinics. The first such clinic, which opened in 1922, had thirteen thousand patient visits in its first year of operation. The clinic population grew so fast that the city soon opened a second clinic, and then a third. These patients, brought to the public clinics through poverty, were recorded in health department files as venereal disease cases. Like all the diseases of the poor, they attracted little public attention. Syphilis among the wealthy was covered with the silence of discretion; syphilis among the poor was covered with a silence of public disinterest.

The venereal disease problem in Baltimore was, however, turned into news by a survey conducted by the U.S. Public Health Service in 1931.[8] The Public Health Service described syphilis as a major problem in Baltimore, and defined it as a problem of the black population. The "colored" rate was especially high at 22/1000 for males and 10/1000 for females; this contrasted with a reported white rate of 4/1000 for males and 1.3/1000 for females. Of course, whites were more likely to be seeing private physicians and were therefore less likely to have their disease reported to the health department. Syphilis, which had originally been perceived as a disease of vice and prostitution, was thus redefined as a black disease.

The treatment of syphilis might well have been considered a punishment for sin. The recommended treatment required sixty or more weekly clinic visits, with painful injections in alternating courses of arsenicals and heavy metals. The minimum effective treatment required forty weekly visits. To the distress of health officials, many patients drifted away from the clinics as soon as their symptoms had been relieved; only half the white patients and a third of the black patients stayed to receive the minimum necessary treatment.[9] Fewer black patients continued in treatment because many of the white physicians and nurses were said to have an unsympathetic attitude to black patients. In 1932 the health department employed black physicians and nurses, hoping to increase the rate of successful treatments:

> Indeed, after several years of experience along these lines, it can safely be concluded that the best results are obtained by encouraging the colored race to take care of its own people. . . . The success of these clinics is unquestionably due to the fact that colored physicians have a more sympathetic approach and a better understanding of the psychology of the Negro race.[10]

As the depression deepened, patients who previously would have been able to pay were increasingly forced to depend on the free public clinics. In 1932 the public clinics were becoming more crowded than ever before, now with more than 84,000 annual visits. The city health department, already burdened with tight budgets and increasing health problems of every kind, complained that the hospitals in town were dumping poor patients on the city clinics.[11] The city health department wanted to distribute the then current chemotherapy—neoarsphenamine, sulpharsphenamine, and salvarsan—free of charge to physicians and hospitals for the treatment of indigent patients; but with cuts in their own budgets, they could do little beyond helplessly watching while the clinic population continued to grow.

In 1933 the problem of overcrowding became so acute that the city health department was faced with a real crisis. The department decided to concentrate on patients at the infectious stage of syphilis. They discontinued treatment to any patients who had already received four courses of arsphenamine—that is, patients who had received sufficient drugs to render them noninfectious to others, even though they had not themselves been cured.[12] The reason for the change in policy was reduced health department funding; its justification, that health departments should primarily be concerned with rates of infection, and not with individual cures.

The new operating rules instituted in 1933 effectively changed the character of the health department clinics. Previously, the clinics had been operated as treatment facilities for patients who could not afford the fees of private physicians; however crowded, however inadequate the medical attention, they had at least intended to cure their patients. Now the clinics no longer pretended to cure but simply to render people noninfectious. For the poor, it became impossible to receive full treatment. The unemployed could not afford the expensive series of weekly treatments given by private physicians, but they could not get jobs if they tested positively for infection.

VENEREAL DISEASE AND RACISM

In the 1930s, as today, health statistics were gathered by race but not by income. The statistics on venereal diseases confirmed the definition of syphilis as predominantly a black or "colored" problem. It is difficult to know the extent to which these statistics reflected a bias in reporting, as blacks were more likely to attend the public health clinics where cases of syphilis were reported for health department records. The bias in reporting presumably emphasized and exaggerated racial differences in rates of infection, and fed the belief that syphilis was a "colored" disease. In fact, almost all infectious diseases were far more prevalent among blacks than whites, reflecting the effects of poverty, poor housing, and overcrowding. The distribution of syphilis, for example, was virtually identical with the distribution of tuberculosis, and both were heavily concentrated in the slums and ghettos. Ferdinand Reinhard, the head of the bureau of venereal diseases, blamed both diseases on economic conditions, noting that the black population "suffered severely under the depression . . . actually existing near the bread line."[13] Reinhard deplored the poor quality of public clinic facilities and expressed the forlorn hope that "at some future time, when the social conscience of the community becomes more highly developed, something may be done to rectify these conditions."[14]

Although Reinhard described the venereal disease problem among blacks as an effect of economics and social conditions, most whites saw venereal disease as a question of sexual immorality. Blacks were popularly perceived as highly sexual, uninhibited, and promiscuous. The historian James Jones, writing about the "notoriously syphilis-soaked race," has graphically described the sexual perceptions and attitudes underlying syphilis programs in the southern states. Briefly stated, white doctors saw blacks as "diseased, debilitated and debauched," the victims of their own uncontrolled or uncontrollable sexual instincts and impulses.[15] Baltimore, lying on the border between north and south, was little different: If, as nobody doubted, venereal diseases were more prevalent among blacks, this fact was seen as both consequence and evidence of their promiscuity, sexual indulgence, and immorality.

Because the problem was perceived as one of sexual behavior, it seemed appropriate for the city health department to begin an energetic public education project, aimed at changing sexual attitudes—by persuasion or by fear. In 1934, for example, a new program of "sex hygiene" was directed at the black population. Talks were given at the Colored Vocational School and the Frederick Douglass High School; exhibits were held for Negro Health Week and for the National Association of Teachers in Colored Schools. Nearly fourteen thousand pamphlets on venereal diseases were distributed. A "social hygiene motion picture" with the discouraging title, *Damaged Lives,* played in twenty-three theaters, thus reaching more than 65,000 people, one-tenth of Baltimore's adult population.[16]

The main aim of this health propaganda was to stress the dangers of sexual promiscuity, but it also emphasized the need for early detection and treatment of disease. Apparently unaware that the public clinics no longer offered full treatment to their patients, the famous and controversial Baltimore journalist H. L. Mencken thundered in local newspaper columns that "we must either teach and advocate the use of prophylactic measures [condoms] or force patients to take adequate treatment until they are cured."[17] Although the first suggestion was perfectly sensible as a method of prevention, it flew in the face of public morality as seeming to encourage "sexual irregularity"—only Mencken seemed to have the courage to publicly advocate such an approach. Pamphlets distributed by the national Social Hygiene Association and the city health department continued to urge chastity before marriage and sexual fidelity within marriage as the only solution to syphilis.

In 1935 syphilis was by far the most prevalent communicable disease in the city, with 5,754 reported cases; the next most prevalent disease was chickenpox—not a disease considered of much importance—with 3,816 reported cases.[18] The same year, the staff of the bureau of venereal diseases gave twenty-one public talks on syphilis, published five articles in the local press, produced a radio talk for Negro Health Week, and distributed sixteen thousand pamphlets. The facilities for actually treating syphilis were still completely inadequate.

As head of the bureau of venereal diseases, Ferdinand Reinhard continued to argue that venereal disease patients needed adequate treatment. Syphilis deaths were now running at between 110 and 150 per year. Reinhard complained: "Any other group of diseases scattered throughout the community to this extent would be considered to have taken on epidemic proportions and would be cause for alarm on the part of health authorities."[19] Perhaps despairing of the efficacy of moral arguments, Reinhard began to stress the economic costs of the refusal to treat syphilis. At least 12 percent of the patients refused treatment would probably end their days in insane asylums; 10 percent more would be charges on the public purse because of cardiovascular complications—conservatively estimated at a direct charge to the city of $180,000 annually, without counting the economic costs of lost individual and family earnings, or of medical treatment prior to complete physical or mental collapse.[20]

Reinhard continued for several years to struggle against the partial treatment plan and to advocate extended clinic facilities, sufficient for all syphilis patients, and staffed with black physicians, nurses, and social workers. It seemed, at the time, to be a one-man campaign. Most physicians approved of the fact that the health department was not offering treatment, the proper domain of fee-for-service medicine. Particularly during the depression years, when many physicians found it difficult to make a living on patient fees, the medical profession was antagonistic to efforts by public health officers to offer free treatments to any patients, whatever their illness.

SYPHILIS BECOMES EVERYONE'S DISEASE: THE NATIONAL CAMPAIGN

In 1936 Reinhard's "one-man campaign" against syphilis in Baltimore suddenly became part of a major national effort. Thomas Parran, surgeon general of the U.S. Public Health Service, now lent the full weight of his energy and authority to a campaign against venereal diseases. A forceful and dynamic man, Parran decided to break through the wall of silence and make the public confront the scope and magnitude of the problem. He thus redefined syphilis as a disease that struck "innocent" victims: the educated, respectable, white population. Although his books, *Shadow on the Land* and *Plain Words about Venereal Disease* are best remembered in public health circles, Parran's short popular article, "Why Don't We Stamp Out Syphilis?" published in *Survey Graphic* and the *Reader's Digest* in 1936, reached a much larger popular audience.[21] In this article, Parran called syphilis "the great American Disease" and declared: "We might virtually stamp out this disease were we not hampered by the widespread belief that nice people don't talk about syphilis, that nice people don't have syphilis, and that nice people shouldn't do anything about those who *do* have syphilis."[22] Parran's point was that nice people *did* have syphilis, and he never tired of pointing out that respectable physicians, innocent children, and heads of industry were among those infected.[23] If people could only free their minds of "the medieval concept that syphilis is the just reward of sin," he said, they could "deal with it as we would any other highly communicable disease, dangerous to the individual and burdensome to the public at large."[24]

In order to separate syphilis from its well-worn associations with sin, black immorality, vice, and prostitution, Parran peppered his talks and articles with a series of little anecdotes such as the following: "Remember that a kiss may carry the germ. In an eastern state recently one of our health officers traced 17 cases of syphilis to a party at which kissing games were played."[25]

Parran declared that half the victims of syphilis were "innocently infected": "Many cases come from such casual contacts as the use of a recently soiled drinking cup, a pipe or cigarette, in receiving services from diseased nursemaids, barber or beauty shop operators, etc., and in giving services such as those of a dentist, doctor, or nurse to a diseased person."[26] Syphilis was just another contagious disease, although a highly threatening and dangerous one. The point was to find syphilis cases and to treat them; the state should be obliged to provide treatment, said Parran, and the patient should be obliged to endure it. Syphilis would be the next great plague to go—as soon as the public broke with the old-fashioned and prescientific notion that syphilis was "the wages of sin." From a financial point of view, the state and the individual would profit from early identification and treatment before the disease had a chance to produce "human wrecks, the incompetents, the criminals."

In Baltimore, Huntington Williams, the young commissioner of health, took up the campaign as articulated by Parran. He termed syphilis "the greatest unmet problem of public health" but declared that "medical science has all the weapons it needs to defeat this tiny but ferocious enemy, once the defenses thrown up by society itself are beaten down."[27]

Beginning in 1936 the new syphilis campaign began to have an impact on the local press. The *Baltimore Health News,* a popular health magazine published by the city, began the process with two issues devoted to syphilis. The American Public Health Association broadcast a radio message on syphilis from its annual meeting in New Orleans; the Baltimore health department reprinted Parran's *Reader's Digest* article and showed a "talking-slide film" entitled "For All Our Sakes" to large and apparently enthusiastic audiences; the local press and radio stations picked up the campaign.[28]

But while the city health department was consolidating the new biomedical approach to syphilis, it was suddenly challenged with a new moral crusade against vice and prostitution—led by none other than the redoubtable J. Edgar Hoover and the FBI.

MEDICAL TREATMENT OR CRUSADE AGAINST VICE?

"Captives Taken in Weekend Drive against City's White Slave Traffic" declared the headlines of the *Baltimore Sun* on May 17, 1937. The newspaper reported:

> Striking at Baltimore's white slave traffic, thirty-five Federal agents, commanded by J. Edgar Hoover, chief of the Federal Bureau of Investigation, Department of Justice, swept down on ten alleged haunts of vice here late Saturday night and early yesterday morning, taking forty-seven persons into custody. . . . Mr. Hoover said the crusade will continue "until Baltimore is completely cleaned up."[29]

The raids generated great excitement and controversy in Baltimore, magnified when local prostitutes implicated a number of high-level police officers and at least one state senator in Baltimore's "white slave trade."[30] The local newspapers delighted in the revelations of an organized racket, reporting on Baltimore as a now-famous center of vice and iniquity. As a result of a succession of titillating revelations, the Baltimore police force was discredited and Hoover was admired for his resolute action.

State Senator Raymond E. Kennedy seized the political opportunity and accused the city health department and the police department of implicitly condoning vice. He demanded that all prostitutes being treated in city clinics be immediately incarcerated. Meanwhile, a grand jury investigation of Baltimore's "haunts of vice" had been organized, and Parran was called to appear as a witness. On his arrival in Baltimore, however, Parran pulled a public relations coup for the health department. He managed to turn the public fervor away from prostitution, and toward a medical program for venereal disease control. He announced a state survey of venereal diseases, suggested that Baltimore follow the successful Swedish model of disease control, including the provision of free drugs, and he declared to enthusiastic mass meetings that Maryland would take the lead in the fight against "social diseases."[31]

Public interest in Parran's speeches was so great that when city budget officials refused a health department request for an extra $21,000 to combat syphilis, their action was publicly denounced as "incredible." Even Senator Raymond Kennedy now joined in the popular demand for adequate medical services, and Mayor Howard Jackson was forced to agree to an increased health department budget. As Kennedy declared: "There has been more discussion of syphilis in the last ninety days than in the twenty years before."[32]

In 1938, when the American Society for Social Hygiene complained that prostitution still flourished in Baltimore, the local press had lost interest in exposés of vice, and no local politician emerged to carry a crusade. When "National Social Hygiene Day" was announced for February 2, 1938, Commissioner Williams decided to celebrate it in Baltimore, but changed its name to "Syphilis Control Day." Obviously, the change in name was significant: Not only did the new name recognize the word "syphilis" as acceptable public discourse, it also associated Baltimore's program with the biomedical approach to disease, and distanced it from the traditional focus of the social hygienists on vice, prostitution, and morality.[33] Thanks to citywide publicity and political pressure on Mayor Jackson, Williams was able greatly to expand his budget and open the Druid Hill Health Center for black patients in west Baltimore—the first time that adequate public health facilities had been available in that area of the city.[34]

The city health department now tackled the problem of syphilis in industry. At the time, industrial workers were being fired (or never hired in the first place) if they were found to have positive blood tests for syphilis. Employers fired infected workers on the grounds that they were more likely to be involved in industrial accidents and would thus increase the costs of workmen's compensation and insurance premiums. The health department started to provide free laboratory blood tests for industrial workers; they kept the test results confidential and referred those infected for appropriate treatment. The health department followed individual workers to make sure they were receiving treatment but—at least in theory—no worker who accepted treatment could be fired. The fact that no guarantee of confidentiality was made for workers refusing treatment meant that syphilis treatment was essentially made compulsory for industrial workers participating in the plan.[35]

Baltimore's industrial employers were gradually persuaded of the plan's value; by 1940 eight industries with eighty-five hundred workers were participating. Some industries, however, still insisted on their right to fire infected workers—and many of the physicians to whom workers were referred had little idea how to treat syphilis. Despite these problems, the "Baltimore Plan" for industry was said to be relatively successful in treating syphilis while protecting workers' jobs.[36]

THE IMPACT OF WAR

In the late 1930s there was considerable optimism that the campaign against the venereal diseases was beginning to show results. The more open public health attitude toward syphilis as a problem of disease rather than of morality seemed to be successful. The industrial screening plan was convincing reluctant employers, the city was supporting the health department with larger budget appropriations, and the new Druid Hill Health Center was treating patients.[37] The numbers of reported cases of syphilis were decreasing each year despite increased screening efforts and probably more effective reporting mechanisms. In 1938, 8,236 new cases were reported; in 1939, 7,509; and in 1940, only 6,213. Spot surveys of selected populations, such as that of the black Dunbar High School in 1939, suggested that syphilis was indeed declining and was less prevalent than the more pessimistic reports had suspected. These records of syphilis incidence and prevalence may have been quite unreliable from an epidemiological point of view, but this was the first time that syphilis rates had even seemed to be declining, and it was a natural conclusion that health department efforts were finally showing demonstrable results.

Amid such optimism, however, came the prospect of war and, with it, the fear that war mobilization and an influx of sixty thousand soldiers would upset all previous gains.[38] By 1941, with the institution of selective service examinations, reported venereal disease rates had already started to climb. In Baltimore in that year, 1.7 percent of the white enlistees had positive blood tests for syphilis, as had 24 percent of the black recruits.[39] Mirroring the racial separations of civil society, black and white troops were segregated, and even black and white blood donations continued to be segregated throughout the war.

Baltimore City now had the dubious distinction of having the second-highest syphilis rate in the country, second only to Washington, D.C. Of 6,081 Baltimore draftees examined, 616 had tested positively for syphilis. Baltimore's rate was therefore 101.3 cases per 1,000 men examined, more than twice the national rate.[40] In an effort to justify these statistics, the city health department blamed the situation on the nonwhite population: The relatively high proportion of blacks to whites "explained" why Baltimore had the second-highest venereal disease rate among the country's largest cities (the same way it "explained" the city's soaring tuberculosis rate).[41]

Such justifications were hardly sufficient for a country at war. With the war mobilization had come renewed national attention to protecting the health and fighting efficiency of the soldiers. As during World War I, the first concern was with the control or suppression of prostitution in the vicinity of army camps, and with "social hygiene" rather than treatment programs. The May Act passed by Congress made prostitution in the vicinity of military camps a federal offense.

In Baltimore, as in several other cities, the FBI called a conference of local law enforcement agencies to discuss the problem of prostitution.[42] Almost immediately, wrangling and mutual accusations broke out between the military officials and different local authorities involved. Major General Milton Reckord of the U.S. Army accused the police department of having failed to control prostitution or the liquor trade.[43] Police Captain Joseph Itzel, in turn, accused the military officials, the liquor board, and the courts of hampering the police in their fight against prostitution and venereal diseases: The military officials had refused to ban the nightclubs and taverns believed to be sources of venereal infections; the liquor board had not revoked their licenses; and the courts had either dismissed charges of prostitution or levied such trivial fines as to be completely ineffective.[44] As if there were not problems enough, Itzel also charged that Baltimore congressmen were protecting some of the establishments that his police officers had tried to close.

Perhaps mindful of J. Edgar Hoover's attack on the police department in 1935, the Baltimore police seemed determined to prove their dedication in the battle against prostitution. By early 1943 they claimed to have closed most of Baltimore's brothels and to have driven prostitutes from the streets.[45] Police Commissioner Stanton demanded statewide legislation to allow police officers to arrest prostitutes, force them to submit to medical examination, and, if infected, to take medical treatment.[46]

Jumping into the controversy, Dr. Nels A. Nelson, head of the state venereal-disease-control program, declared that arrests of prostitutes and compulsory medical examinations were completely ineffective: Only a few prostitutes could be arrested at any one time, and as soon as they were treated and released, they would immediately return to the streets to become reinfected and to continue to spread the infection. The only real control of venereal disease, concluded Nelson, depended on the complete "repression of sexual promiscuity." Nelson advocated closing all houses of prostitution, jailing all those who derived profit from prostitution and all "confirmed prostitutes," institutional rehabilitation of "girls who are simply on the wrong road," employment of policewomen to take charge of "girls who seem headed for trouble" and closing all dance halls, taverns, and nightclubs to unescorted women.[47] Nelson also accused physicians of failing to cooperate with the effort and of not wanting to be associated with venereal diseases.[48]

Alarmed by the growing conflict between local health and law enforcement agencies, the Maryland State Senate now set up a vice inquiry, and invited Nelson and Robert H. Riley, the state director of health, for a "full and frank" discussion behind closed doors.[49] At this meeting Police Commissioner Stanton repeated his demand for the compulsory examination and treatment of prostitutes, while the state and city health departments reiterated their opposition to the Stanton plan, which would, in their view, only be a way for the police to harass prostitutes.[50] Meanwhile, the city health commissioner stated that reported cases of syphilis were rapidly increasing. Between 1940 and 1942 new cases of syphilis had almost doubled, from 6,213 to 11,293. In 1942 selective service records showed that almost 3 percent of the white draftees and more than 32 percent of the black soldiers had syphilis.[51] Thousands of worker hours were also being lost in the war industries from hospitalization of workers with venereal diseases.

In an effort to develop some kind of cooperative effort between the feuding agencies, the city organized the Baltimore Venereal Disease Council in December 1942. The council members represented the Medical and Chirurgical Faculty of Maryland, the Baltimore Retail Druggists Association, the Venereal Disease Control Office of the Third Service Command, the Baltimore Criminal Justice Commission, the Board of Liquor License Commissioners, the Emergency Medical Services for Maryland, the Johns Hopkins University, the Maryland State Health Department, the State Supreme Court, the police commissioner of Baltimore, the Maryland Medical Association, and the city health department.[52] Three committees were created: the Committee on Rehabilitation; the Committee on Legislation; and the Committee on Medicine, Public Health, and Pharmacy. The rehabilitation committee offered a social, rather than moral, analysis of prostitution: "Prostitution exists because of the urge for sexual gratification in numerous males, on the one hand, and the inadequacies of conventional social arrangements to meet these demands." For women, prostitution was bound up with "inadequate income, bad housing, insufficient diet, lack of recreation and other facets of total life," although a small number were thought to enter prostitution because of "an overwhelming craving for sex stimulation."[53] The committee carefully divided all prostitutes into three main types and thirteen subtypes, ranging from "bats, or superannuated prostitutes rendered unattractive by drink and drugs and by the least particular of bums and homeless men," to "potential prostitutes who are willing to accept money for sex relations which, however, may also be on a volunteer or free basis."[54] The committee recommended that older "hardened" prostitutes be jailed, that "mental cases" be institutionalized, and that "young and potential" prostitutes be offered rehabilitation services, care, and assistance.

Nels Nelson of the state Health Department had abandoned the fight against prostitution. He was busily distributing free drugs for the control of syphilis to private physicians; the city had wanted such a program but had been unable to afford it. Nelson publicly declared the city venereal disease clinics "little more than drug pumping stations in dirty, unattractive quarters."[55] He told the press he was tired of hearing the V.D. rate discussed as though it were only a black problem: "Negroes are plagued by venereal diseases because of their economic and social position. . . . They have had the benefits of only two or three generations of Western civilization."[56]

The army was also under attack for failing to organize an effective V.D. program.[57] Its programs and policies were plagued by contradictions; publicly it advocated chastity while privately providing prophylactics for the men. Those in charge of the army's venereal disease program were caught between those advocating the suppression of prostitution and sexual continence for the soldiers, and many army officers who felt that "any man who won't f———, won't fight."[58] The army finally adopted a pragmatic approach and simply attempted to reduce the sources of infection. The pragmatic approach lacked the fervor of a purity crusade, but tried to steer some middle course between laissez-faire attitudes and moral absolutism.

In Baltimore the new acting directors of the city's venereal disease program, Ralph Sikes and Alexander Novey, shared this pragmatic view. Noting that syphilis cases were continuing their sharp increase during the war, they philosophically began their annual report for 1943 by remarking that "the close association between Mars and Venus has existed since historians first recorded human annals."[59] Under their leadership, the bureau concentrated on rendering patients noninfectious as rapidly as possible; health officers cooperated with the armed services in distributing prophylactic kits throughout the city—in police stations, firehouses, transportation terminals, hospitals, and clinics.[60] The V.D. control officers had thus implicitly accepted the idea that this was a campaign *against* disease, not a campaign *for* sexual morality; they concentrated on a fairly mechanical, albeit effective, approach to prevention, while leaving the struggle around prostitution to social hygiene reformers, the police, and the courts.

SEX EDUCATION DURING THE WAR

During the war the city health department and a research group at the Johns Hopkins School of Hygiene and Public Health undertook a daring task—to teach "sex hygiene" in the public schools. They gave talks to groups of high school students (separated by sex), showed plaster models of the male and female reproductive systems, and gave simple explanations of "menstruation, conception, pregnancy, nocturnal emissions and masturbation, but omitting intercourse and childbirth."[61] The project organizers found that "the boys frequently asked for further information about masturbation, and often about prophylaxis which had purposely been omitted from the talk."[62]

The talk presented to the students offers an interesting glimpse of sex education in 1944 and of a project regarded with much interest, and some nervousness, by the city health department. Sex was introduced with military metaphors; sex, the students were told, was like "the fast, tricky fighter planes of the Army"—very difficult to handle. "Sex is just as difficult a problem to handle as any airplane. . . . It is no wonder then that there are so many crashes in the field of sex. When a plane crashes, a person may not walk away from such an accident, or if he does he may carry injury that will last his lifetime. Similar results occur from crashes in the field of sex."[63]

Having been assured that sex was both exciting and dangerous, students were then given a brief description of male reproductive physiology, ending with a caution against masturbation. Masturbation was not dangerous, students were told, merely unnecessary and possibly habit-forming: "It is true that having formed the habit a person may devote too much time and thought to that sort of thing which will hurt the other things in life, such as studies, athletics, and normal friendships."[64] A brief description of the female reproductive system was followed by a discussion of morals and ethics, warning of the need for judgment, but avoiding any definite conclusion: "Since this problem differs for each one, because of different religions, different stages of financial independence and varied ethical standards, we cannot answer anyone's special problem here."[65] Students were urged to discuss their questions with parents and teachers and to read a social hygiene pamphlet entitled "Growing Up in the World Today."[66]

The third part of the presentation, on venereal diseases, emphasized the dangers of sex. Intimacy brought the germs of syphilis—sexual intercourse was the most threatening, but even kisses could carry disease. Early treatment could help before much damage was done, but the best strategy was to avoid any possible contact with these sexual germs: "They can be caught only from an infected person and therefore, we should avoid intimate contact with an infected person. But we cannot tell by *looking* at a person whether he or she is infected or not; the answer is to avoid intimate contact with all persons except in marriage. This is the only sure way of avoiding these diseases."[67]

At least for these high school students, the link between sexual morality and venereal disease was clear—sexual intimacy led to syphilis and was therefore to be avoided except in marriage (why marital sex should be "safe" was never explained, nor was congenital syphilis ever mentioned).

AFTER THE WAR: THE NEW PENICILLIN THERAPY

By the end of World War II the problem of syphilis was beginning to recede, both in public consciousness and in terms of statistical measures. Part of this was the normal relaxation in the immediate aftermath of war, the return to home and family, the desire for stability, and a reluctance to confront social and sexual problems or to dwell on their existence. Even more important, however, was the success of the new drug, penicillin: At last, it appeared that venereal diseases could be quickly and effectively treated. It seemed to be only a matter of time before the venereal diseases would finally be eliminated with the aid of modern medicine's "miracle cures."

By 1940 the new "miracle drug" penicillin had been discovered and purified. In 1943 it was used for the first time to treat syphilis but was not yet generally available; supplies were still strictly rationed.[68] Soon it would completely transform the old methods of treating venereal diseases. Penicillin treatments for syphilis were given over a period of eight days; because supplies of the drug were then very limited, only cases judged to be highly infectious were sent for "an eight-day cure, or what is for the present considered to be a cure."[69] On December 31, 1944, the Baltimore City Hospitals opened the first rapid treatment center for treating syphilis with penicillin. From all initial reports, the new experimental treatment was remarkably effective.

On June 20, 1945, Mayor Theodore R. McKeldin approved a new city ordinance, making treatment for venereal diseases compulsory for the first time. Those suspected of having syphilis or gonorrhea were required to take penicillin therapy at the Rapid Treatment Center.[70] Those refusing treatment could be isolated in the venereal disease division of the Baltimore City Hospitals; members of the Church of Christ Scientist, who could not be forced to take treatment, could still be quarantined. This new ordinance was much stricter than previous health regulations but was passed with little controversy. The new penicillin therapy was, apparently, safe and effective, requiring, at most, a few days' treatment. Legislators who might have hesitated in requiring a prolonged or possibly dangerous therapy—such as the older treatment with arsenic and heavy metals—had few qualms about mandating the new penicillin treatment.

The ordinance was, however, rarely invoked. Most patients were eager to go to the Rapid Treatment Center when diagnosed. In 1946 nearly two thousand people with infectious syphilis received treatment: Most were reported as completely cured. (Before penicillin, only an estimated 25 percent of patients completed the lengthy treatments considered necessary for a full cure.)[71] In 1947 the *Baltimore Sun* reviewed the city's experience with the new ordinance: "On the basis of this experience [over the last 16 months], it is clear that the protection of the public against persons carrying the disease and refusing to be treated more than outweighs the sacrifice of individual rights by so small a number. . . . Under the circumstances, the enactment of a permanent ordinance seems fully justified."[72]

In 1947 the State Health Department announced that "for the first time in history any resident of Maryland who contracts syphilis can obtain treatment resulting in prompt and almost certain cure."[73] For the first time, there were sufficient supplies of penicillin to treat everyone—not just the veterans, not just the infectious cases, but every patient with syphilis or gonorrhea. By 1948 gonorrhea could be cured with a single injection, and syphilis with a short series of treatments.

CONCLUSION: THE END OF THE STRUGGLE?

The biomedical approach to venereal diseases had been stunningly successful. Diseases that only ten years before had been described as the most serious of all the infectious diseases had now been tamed by chemotherapy with a simple, safe, and effective cure. Diseases that twenty years previously had been guilty secrets, virtually unmentionable in the press and quietly ignored by health departments, now became glorious examples of the triumph of modern medicine in overcoming ancient plagues. The ideological struggle between those who had seen the fight against venereal disease as a battle for sexual morality and those who had seen it as simply another form of bacteriological warfare was over. The social hygiene reformers had to concede defeat to the public health officers, epidemiologists, and laboratory researchers. Or did they?

In 1947 the Maryland State Department of Health, announcing the success of the rapid treatment program, concluded its press bulletin with the warning: "To decrease the number of repeat patients and prevent venereal diseases it will be necessary to reduce sexual promiscuity. If fear of disease is a less powerful restraining factor the problem must be attacked more strongly through moral training and suppression of prostitution."[74] Baltimore's health department sounded even more pessimistic: "It may be stated that so far there is little or no evidence that the apparently miraculous one and eight day cures of gonorrhea and infectious syphilis (respectively) with penicillin have accomplished much toward the control of these diseases. . . . Certainly this new therapy has done nothing to correct the promiscuous sexual behavior which is the ultimate cause of the spread of venereal disease."[75]

In 1948 Thomas B. Turner, the prominent bacteriologist at Johns Hopkins, gave a talk to the American Social Hygiene Association entitled, "Penicillin: Help or Hindrance?" His title alone expressed a curious ambivalence about the new "miracle drug." As head of the Hopkins research group on syphilis, Turner was in a better position than most to understand the extraordinary difference the new chemotherapy had made to patients. He catalogued the successes of penicillin "on the credit side of the ledger" but cautioned that nobody should be "dazzled by the apparent potentialities of this fine new drug." On "the debit side of the ledger" was the loss of fear as a deterrent to exposure and the possibility of multiple reinfections; Turner assured his audience that the real concern of venereal disease prevention programs was "the moral, spiritual and economic health of a community" and urged them to "strengthen those forces in the community which help to preserve not only our physical well being, but our spiritual health as well."[76]

Official admiration for the new chemotherapy was thus linked to warnings that the "real" causes of disease were unsolved. Even those most committed to the bacteriological view of disease seemed uneasy about the decoupling of venereal disease from sin and promiscuity: How would sexual morality be controlled if not by the fear of disease? Would "rampant promiscuity" defeat the best efforts of medical treatment?

A brief review of health statistics in the years since the discovery of penicillin suggests that syphilis has, in the main, been effectively controlled. New cases of syphilis are reported each year, and doubtless others are unreported, but the rates are relatively low. In 1986 a total of 373 cases of primary, secondary, and early latent cases were reported in Baltimore; in 1987, a total of 364 cases. Although these cases are of continuing concern to health department officials, at least from the perspective of the 1930s and 1940s, the miracle of control really has occurred. Gonorrhea, however, is another story. Gonorrhea continues to be the most frequently reported infectious disease in the United States, in Maryland, and in Baltimore City; as press reports like to say, in numbers of cases, it is second only to the common cold.[77] But gonorrhea, too, is declining. In 1980 there were eighteen thousand cases in Baltimore, in 1986, sixteen thousand cases, and in 1987, thirteen thousand cases. In 1986, Baltimore ranked second in numbers of cases of gonorrhea among cities with populations of more than 200,000.

Although gonorrhea is of epidemic proportions, it creates little popular concern. A remarkable effort in 1976 to form a coalition in Baltimore against venereal disease—composed of the Boy Scouts, the National Organization for Women, the League of Women Voters, the Benevolent Order of Elks, and the Baltimore Gay Alliance—was unable to fire public interest.[78] Parents were more concerned about drug use than sex; those infected, or potentially infected, knew the cure was simple, available, and cheap. As Turner had noted, the vital element of *fear* was missing: Gonorrhea was perceived as an uncomplicated infection, easily treated and readily cured.

As we have since discovered, the fear, and the underlying attitudes toward sexuality, were only lying dormant. The recent public concern, horror, and fear of AIDS have reignited the older social hygiene movement, albeit in a new form. Attitudes once expressed toward the black population as sexually promiscuous, sexually threatening, and a reservoir of disease have now been, in revived form, turned against the gay male population. AIDS is popularly seen as caused by gay promiscuity and, even more broadly, as a punishment for unconventional or unapproved sexual behavior, rather than simply as the result of infection by a microorganism. Just as in the case of syphilis, AIDS is often perceived as the "wages of sin" or, as Jerry Falwell says: "A man reaps what he sows. If he sows seed in the field of his lower nature, he will reap from it a harvest of corruption." Again, the argument pits a new generation of biomedical researchers—eager, in the main, to dissociate a medical problem from a moral crusade—against a new generation of moral reformers, eager to use the new AIDS threat to reform sexual behavior.

The "moral" and "scientific" attitudes toward venereal disease are not, of course, completely separate. As we have seen in the ambivalent responses to the success of penicillin therapy, even the most dedicated scientists tend to share the social and sexual values of their culture—in this case, expressing some regret or misgiving, lest effective and safe chemotherapy act as an encouragement to disapproved sexual activity by removing the fear of disease. Moral reformers know that scientific successes, especially in the form of new "miracle drugs," will weaken, but not destroy, their case. If a new "miracle drug" is discovered to be effective against AIDS, it will weaken, but certainly not destroy, their social, moral, and cultural objections to homosexuality.

Both the biomedical and moral perspectives or attitudes toward venereal disease select out specific aspects of a complex social reality. As the history of public health demonstrates, venereal diseases—as all other diseases—occur in a social context within which disease is perceived, experienced, and reproduced. One realm comprises both "biological" and "social" aspects of disease. We may separate out one or the other for purposes of analysis, but any complete understanding of a disease problem must involve both as interrelated parts of a single social reality.

Social and cultural ideas or ideologies provide a variety of ways in which diseases can be perceived and interpreted. The germ theory provides an explanation of disease that largely, but not completely, isolates it from this social context, robbing it of some of its social (in this case, moral) meaning. But the purely "scientific" interpretation is never wholly victorious, for social and cultural meanings of disease reassert themselves in the interstices of science and prove their power whenever the biomedical sciences fail to completely cure or solve the problem. Only when a disease condition is completely abolished do social and cultural meanings cease to be relevant to the experience and perception of human illness.

NOTES

Another version of this paper appeared in the *Journal of the History of Medicine and Allied Sciences* 43 (1988): 141–164.

1. For a fascinating analysis of the history of cultural and scientific conceptions of syphilis, see Ludwig Fleck, *Genesis and Development of a Scientific Fact* (1935; rpt. Chicago: University of Chicago Press, 1979).
2. For an excellent recent history of the controversies around venereal diseases in the United States, see Allan M. Brandt, *No Magic Bullet: A Social History of Venereal Diseases in the United States since 1880* (New York: Oxford University Press, 1985).
3. *Scientific and Technical Societies of the United States and Canada,* 8th ed. (Washington, D.C.: National Academy of Sciences, 1968), 62.
4. Edward H. Beardsley, "Allied against Sin: American and British Responses to Venereal Disease in World War I," *Medical History* 20 (1976): 194.

5. As one widely reprinted article, said to have reached 8 million readers, described "The Enemy at Home": "The name of this invisible enemy is Venereal Disease—and there you have in two words the epitome of all that is unclean, malignant and menacing. . . . Gonorrhoea and syphilis are 'camp followers' where prostitution and alcohol are permitted. They form almost as great an enemy behind the lines as do the Huns in front." "V.D.: The Enemy at Home," cited by William H. Zinsser, "Social Hygiene and the War: Fighting Venereal Diseases a Public Trust," *Social Hygiene* 4 (1918): 519–520.

6. In 1920 William Travis Howard, a member of the city health department, complained: "The Baltimore health department has never inaugurated a single administrative measure directed at the control of the venereal diseases. . . . The Baltimore health department has contented itself with receiving such reports as were made and with lending its power, when called upon, to force a few recalcitrant patients to appear at the venereal disease clinic established by the United States Government." William Travis Howard, *Public Health Administration and the Natural History of Disease in Baltimore, Maryland, 1797–1920* (Washington, D.C.: Carnegie Institution, 1924), 154–155.

7. *Baltimore City Health Department Annual Report* (Baltimore, 1930).

8. Taliaferro Clark and Lida Usilton, "Survey of the Venereal Diseases in the City of Baltimore, Baltimore County, and the Four Contiguous Counties," *Venereal Disease Information* 12 (Washington, D.C.: U.S. Public Health Service, 20 October 1931), 437–456.

9. Ferdinand O. Reinhard, director, Bureau of Vital Statistics, Baltimore, "Delinquent Patients in Venereal Disease Clinics: Result of a Study in Baltimore City Health Department," *Journal of the American Medical Association* 106 (1936): 1377–1390.

10. *Baltimore City Health Department Annual Report* (Baltimore, 1932), 63.

11. Ibid., 62.

12. *Baltimore City Health Department Annual Report* (Baltimore, 1933), 93.

13. Ibid., 97.

14. Ibid., 99.

15. James H. Jones, *Bad Blood: The Tuskegee Syphilis Experiment* (New York: Free Press, 1981), 16–29. The Tuskegee experiment was conducted by the U.S. Public Health Service between 1932 and 1972. Four hundred black Alabama sharecroppers and day laborers were followed to determine the effects of untreated syphilis; treatment was deliberately withheld from the subjects of the study, even after effective penicillin therapy became available.

16. *Baltimore City Health Department Annual Report* (Baltimore, 1934), 107.

17. "Plague," *Baltimore Evening Sun,* 13 August 1934.

18. *Baltimore City Health Department Annual Report* (Baltimore, 1935), 115.

19. Ferdinand O. Reinhard, "The Venereal Disease Problem in the Colored Population of Baltimore City," *American Journal of Syphilis and Neurology* 19 (1935): 183–195.

20. Ferdinand O. Reinhard, "Late Latent Syphilis—A Problem and a Challenge," *Journal of Social Hygiene* 22 (1936): 360–363.

21. Thomas Parran, *Shadow on the Land: Syphilis* (New York: Reynal and Hitchcock, 1937); Thomas Parran and R. A. Vonderlehr, *Plain Words about Venereal Disease* (New York: Reynal and Hitchcock, 1941); also see n. 20.

22. Thomas Parran, "Why Don't We Stamp out Syphilis?" rpt. from *Reader's Digest,* July 1936, in *Baltimore Health News* 13 (August 1936): 3.

23. E.g., Parran, *Shadow on the Land,* 207, 230.

24. Thomas Parran, "Why Don't We Stamp out Syphilis?" rpt. *Baltimore Health News* 13 (August 1936): 8.

25. Ibid., 3.

26. Thomas Parran, "Why Don't We Stamp out Syphilis?" *Reader's Digest,* July 1936, 65–73.

27. "Open Attack on Age-Old Curse," *Baltimore Sun,* 9 August 1936.

28. "War on Venereal Disease Impends," *Baltimore Sun,* 24 December 1936.

29. "G-Men's Haul in Vice Raids Totals 47," *Baltimore Sun,* 17 May 1937.

30. "Vice Witness Names Police Lieutenant," *Baltimore Sun,* 18 May 1937; "Vice Arrests May Total 100; Bierman Named," *Baltimore Sunday Sun,* 19 May 1937.

31. "Starts to Survey Venereal Disease," *Baltimore Sun,* 29 July 1937; "Venereal Disease Fight Is Planned," *Baltimore Sun,* 22 August 1937; "Fight Opens Here on Social Disease," *Baltimore Sun,* 25 August 1937; "Syphilis Control Unit Begins Work," *Baltimore Sun,* 21 October 1937; "Over 2,000 Attend Talks on Syphilis," *Baltimore Sun,* 26 October 1937.

32. "Failure to Assist Syphilis Fight Hit," *Baltimore Sun,* 6 December 1937; "Jackson Pledges Aid in War on Syphilis," *Baltimore Sun,* 7 December 1937.

33. "Attention Called to Syphilis Here," *Baltimore Sun,* 1 February 1938.

34. *Baltimore City Health Department Annual Report* (Baltimore, 1938), 159, and (Baltimore, 1939), 159.

35. Ibid. (1938), 16; "21 Employers Asked in Drive on Syphilis," *Baltimore Sun,* 27 March 1938; "Syphilis Control Is Under Way Here," *Baltimore Sun,* 22 May 1938; W.M.P. "We Join the Anti-Syphilis Crusade," *The Kalends* (periodical of the Williams and Wilkins Company), June 1938, rpt. *Baltimore Health News* 15 (July 1938): 53–54; "Syphilis in Industry" (Baltimore City Health Department, n.d.).

36. Huntington Williams, "Discussion on the Symposium on Syphilis in Industry," 15 January 1940. Second Annual Conference on Industrial Health, sponsored by the Council on Industrial Health of the American Medical Association, Chicago, 15–16 January 1940; editorial, "Syphilis and Unemployment," *Journal of Industrial Hygiene and Toxicology* 19 (1937): 189–192; *Baltimore Health News* 15 (July 1938): 50–57.

37. *Baltimore City Health Department Annual Report* (Baltimore, 1938), 159–163, and (Baltimore, 1939), 159–163.

38. Ibid. (1940), 149–151.

39. Ibid. (1941), 139.

40. "City Shown Second in Syphilis Survey," *Baltimore Sun,* 22 October 1941.

41. "High Syphilis Rate Laid to Race Ratio," *Baltimore Sun,* 26 October 1941.

42. "FBI and City Agencies Schedule Parley on Vice," *Evening Sun,* 15 July 1942.

43. "Reckord Tells O'Conor of Vice," *Baltimore Sun,* 17 July 1942.

44. "Itzel Charges War on Vice Hampered," *Baltimore Sun,* 26 January 1943.

45. "Says Vice Control Has Improved Here," *Baltimore Sun,* 27 January 1943.

46. "State Law Held Needed in War on Vice," *Baltimore Sun,* 28 January 1943.

47. Nels A. Nelson, "The Repression of Prostitution for Venereal Disease Control," *Baltimore Health News* 20 (January 1943): 107–108.

48. "High Venereal Disease Rate Cited in Maryland," *Baltimore Sun,* 4 December 1942.

49. "Vice Inquiry Transferred to Annapolis," *Baltimore Sun,* 29 January 1943.

50. "Stanton Idea for Examination of Prostitutes Is Denounced," *Baltimore Sun,* 29 January 1943.

51. "Venereal Picture Dark: Dr. Huntington Williams Says No Improvement Is Expected for Some Time," *Baltimore Sun,* 21 January 1943.

52. "Baltimore Disease Council Is Organized," *Baltimore Health News* 20 (February 1943): 109–110.

53. "Three Venereal Disease Council Committee Reports," *Baltimore Health News* 20 (March 1943): 119–120.

54. Ibid., 118–119.

55. "Clinics Here under Fire," *Baltimore Sun,* 30 March 1943.

56. "Venereal Disease Rate High in State," *Baltimore Sun,* 15 June 1943.

57. Parran and Vonderlehr, *Plain Words about Venereal Disease,* esp. 96–120.

58. Ibid., 77.

59. *Baltimore City Health Department Annual Report* (Baltimore, 1943), 147.

60. Ibid., 148.

61. C. Howe Eller, "A Sex Education Project and Serologic Survey in a Baltimore High School," *Baltimore Health News* 21 (1944): 81–87.

62. Ibid., 84.

63. J. D. Porterfield, Baltimore City Health Department, "A Talk on Sex Hygiene for High School Students," April 1944, Rockefeller Foundation Archives, RG 1.1, ser. 200, 1.

64. Ibid., 4.

65. Ibid., 7.

66. Emily V. Clapp, *Growing Up in the World Today* (Boston: Massachusetts Society for Social Hygiene, n.d.).

67. Ibid., 14.

68. For the development of penicillin therapy, see Harry F. Dowling, *Fighting Infection: Conquests of the Twentieth Century* (Cambridge: Harvard University Press, 1977), 125–157.

69. *Baltimore City Health Department Annual Report* (Baltimore, 1945), 29.

70. Ibid., 145–146; "Venereal Law Made Specific," *Baltimore Sun,* 26 August 1945.

71. "End of VD—Cure Center Seen as Calamity," *Evening Sun,* 12 June 1946.

72. "A Temporary Power Made Permanent," *Baltimore Sun,* 9 January 1947.

73. "Rapid Treatment: Maryland State Department of Health," Press Bulletin No. 1043, 27 January 1947, Enoch Pratt Public Library of Baltimore, Maryland Room.

74. Ibid.

75. *Baltimore City Health Department Annual Report* (Baltimore, 1946), 28.

76. Thomas B. Turner, "Syphilis: Help or Hindrance?" Talk to American Social Hygiene Association, 2 February 1948, Rockefeller Foundation Archives, RG 1.1, ser. 200, 4.

77. "Baltimore City STD Fact Sheet" (Baltimore City Health Department, November 1981).

78. "City Assembles Coalition to Battle Venereal Disease," *Baltimore Sun,* 10 June 1976.

AIDS: From Social History to Social Policy

Allan M. Brandt

Despite the philosopher George Santayana's famous injunction that those who do not remember the past are condemned to repeat it, history holds no simple truths. Nevertheless, there are a number of significant historical questions relating to the AIDS epidemic. What does the history of medicine and public health have to tell us about contemporary approaches to the dilemmas raised by AIDS? Is AIDS something totally new, or are there instances in the past that are usefully comparable? Are there some lessons in the way science and society have responded to epidemic disease in the past that could inform our understanding of and response to the current health crisis?

There are obviously no simple answers to such questions. History is not a fable with the moral spelled out at the end. Even if we could agree on a particular construction of past events, it would not necessarily lead to consensus on what is to be done. Yet history provides us with one means of approaching the present. In this regard, the history of responses to particular diseases can inform and deepen our understanding of the AIDS crisis and the medical, social, and public health interventions available.

The way a society responds to problems of disease reveals its deepest cultural, social, and moral values. These core values—patterns of judgment about what is good or bad—shape and guide human perception and action. This, we know, has most certainly been the case with AIDS; the epidemic has been shaped not only by powerful biological forces, but by behavioral, social, and cultural factors as well. This essay analyzes the process by which social and cultural forces affect our understanding of disease—the "social construction of disease"—and examines several analogues to the current health crisis. But disease is more than a metaphor. These "social constructions" are more than merely metaphors. They have very real sociopolitical implications.[1]

SEXUALLY TRANSMITTED DISEASES IN HISTORICAL CONTEXT

An examination of the first decades of the twentieth century—a time of intense concern and interest in sexually transmitted diseases not unlike those today—may demonstrate how this process has worked. Indeed, the first two decades of the twentieth century witnessed a general hysteria about venereal infections. The historical analogues are striking; they relate to public health, science, and, especially, social and cultural values.

This period, often referred to as the Progressive era, combined two powerful strains in American social thought: the search for new technical, scientific answers to social problems, and the search for a set of unified moral ideals. The problem of sexually transmitted diseases (STDs) appealed to both sets of interests. The campaign against these infections—the "social hygiene" movement—was predicated on a series of major scientific breakthroughs. The specific organism that causes gonorrhea, the *gonococcus* bacterium, and the causative agent for syphilis, the spirochete, were identified. By the end of the first decade of the twentieth century diagnostic exams had been established.[2] In 1910 German Nobel laureate Paul Ehrlich discovered the first major chemotherapy effective against the spirochete—salvasan. Science thus had the effect of reframing the way in which these diseases were seen.

The enormous social, cultural, and economic costs of venereal disease were revealed when doctors defined what they called "venereal insontium," or venereal disease of the innocent. In the early twentieth century physicians traced the tragic repercussions of syphilis within the family. Perhaps the best-known example of venereal insontium is ophthalmia neonatorum, gonorrheal blindness of the newborn, and as late as 1910 as many as 25 percent of all the blind in the United States had lost their sight in this way, despite the earlier discovery that silver nitrate solution could prevent infection. Soon many states began to require the use of this prophylactic treatment by law.[3]

But doctors stressed the impact of venereal disease on women even more than on children. In 1906 the American Medical Association (AMA) held a symposium on "The Duty of the Profession to Womanhood." As one physician at the conference explained:

> These vipers of venery which are called clap and pox, lurking as they often do, under the floral tributes of the honeymoon, may so inhibit conception or blight its products that motherhood becomes either an utter impossibility or a veritable curse. The ban placed by venereal disease on fetal life outrivals the criminal interference with the products of conception as a cause of race suicide.[4]

Family tragedy was a frequent cultural theme in these years. In 1913 a hit Broadway play by French playwright Eugene Brieux, *Damaged Goods,* told the story of young George Dupont, who, although warned by his physician not to marry because he has syphilis, disregards this advice only to spread the infection to his wife and, later, to their child. This story was told and retold, revealing deep cultural values about science, social responsibility, and the limited ability of medicine to cure the moral ailments of humankind.[5]

But physicians expressed concerns that went beyond the confines of the family; they also examined the wider social repercussions of sexually transmitted diseases. The turn of the century witnessed the most intensive periods of immigration to the United States in its entire history; more than 650,000 immigrants came to these shores each year between 1885 and 1910. Many doctors and social critics suggested that these individuals were bringing venereal disease into the country. As Howard Kelly, a leading gynecologist at the Johns Hopkins School of Medicine, explained: "The tide [of venereal disease] has been raising [*sic*] owing to the inpouring of a large foreign population with lower ideals." Kelly elaborated, warning: "Think of these countless currents flowing daily from the houses of the poorest into those of the richest, and forming a sort of civic circulatory system expressive of the body politic, a circulation which continually tends to equalize the distribution of morality and disease."[6]

Examinations at ports of entry failed to reveal a high incidence of disease; nevertheless, nativists called for the restriction of immigration. How were these immigrants thought to be spreading sexually transmitted diseases to native, middle-class, Anglo-Saxon Americans? First, it was suggested that immigrants constituted the great bulk of the prostitutes inhabiting American cities; virtually every major American metropolis of the early twentieth century had clearly defined red-light districts where prostitution flourished. These women, it was suggested, were typically foreign-born.[7]

But even more important, physicians asserted that syphilis and gonorrhea could be transmitted in any number of ways. Doctors catalogued the various modes of transmission: Pens, pencils, toothbrushes, towels and bedding, and medical procedures were all identified as potential means of communication.[8] As one woman explained in an anonymous essay in 1912:

> At first it was unbelievable. I knew of the disease only through newspaper advertisements [for patent medicines]. I had understood that it was the result of sin and that it originated and was contracted only in the underworld of the city. I felt sure that my friend was mistaken in diagnosis when he exclaimed, "Another tragedy of the common drinking cup!" I eagerly met his remark with the assurance that I did not use public drinking cups, that I had used my own cup for years. He led me to review my summer. After recalling a number of times when my thirst had forced me to go to the public fountain, I came at last to realize that what he had told me was true.[9]

The doctor, of course, had diagnosed syphilis. One indication of how seriously these casual modes of transmission were taken is the fact that the U.S. Navy removed doorknobs from its battleships during World War I, claiming they had been a source of infection for many of its sailors (a breathtaking act of denial). We now know, of course, that syphilis and gonorrhea typically are not contracted in these ways. This poses a difficult historical problem: Why did physicians believe they could be?

Theories of casual transmission reflected deep cultural fears about disease and sexuality in the early twentieth century. In these approaches to venereal disease, concerns about hygiene, contamination, and contagion were expressed, anxieties that revealed a great deal about the contemporary society and culture. Venereal disease was viewed as a threat to the entire late Victorian social and sexual system, which placed great value on discipline, restraint, and homogeneity. The sexual code of this era held that only marital sex should receive social sanction. But the concerns about venereal disease also reflected a pervasive fear of the urban masses, the growth of the cities, and the changing nature of familial relationships. Finally, the distinction between venereal disease and venereal insontium had the effect of dividing victims; some deserved attention, sympathy, and medical support, others did not, depending on how the infection was obtained. Victims were separated into the innocent and the guilty.

In short, venereal disease became a metaphor for late Victorian anxieties about sexuality, contagion, and social organization. But these metaphors are not simply innocuous linguistic constructions. They have powerful sociopolitical implications, many of which have been remarkably persistent throughout the century.

Concerns about sexually transmitted diseases led to a major public health campaign to stop their spread. In fact, many of the public health approaches we apply today to communicable infections were developed early in this century. Educational programs formed a major component of the campaign, although to speak of education is far too vague. The question, of course, is the precise content of the education offered. During the first decades of the twentieth century, when schools first instituted sex-education programs, their basic goal was to encourage premarital continence by inculcating a fear of sex. Indeed, these programs could more accurately be termed "antisexual education."

The newly acquired ability to diagnose syphilis and gonorrhea led to the development of other important public health interventions. Reporting, screening, testing, and the isolation of carriers were all initiated in the early years of the twentieth century as venereal-disease-control measures, and American cities began to require the reporting of venereal diseases around 1915. Some states used reports to follow contacts and bring individuals in for treatment, and by the 1930s many had come to require premarital and prenatal screening. Some municipalities mandated compulsory screening of food-handlers and barbers, even though it was by then understood that syphilis and gonorrhea could not be spread through casual contact. The rationale offered was that these individuals were at risk for infection anyway and that screening might reveal new cases for treatment.

Perhaps the most dramatic public health intervention devised to combat sexually transmitted diseases was the campaign to close red-light districts. In the first two decades of the twentieth century, vice commissions in almost all American cities had identified prostitutes as a major risk for American health and morals, and decided that the time had come to remove the "sources of infection." Comparing the red-light districts to malaria-producing swamps, they attempted to "drain" them; during World War I more than a hundred red-light districts were closed.

The crackdown on prostitutes constituted the most concerted attack on civil liberties in the name of public health in American history. Not surprisingly, in the atmosphere of crisis engendered by the war, public health officials employed radical techniques in their battle against venereal disease. State laws held that anyone "reasonably suspected" of harboring a venereal infection could be compulsorily tested, and prostitutes were now subject to quarantine, detention, and internment.[10] United States Attorney General T. W. Gregory explained: "The constitutional right of the community, in the interest of the public health, to ascertain the existence of infections and communicable diseases in its midst and to isolate and quarantine such cases or take steps necessary to prevent the spread of disease is clear."[11] In July 1918 Congress allocated more than $1 million for the detention and isolation of venereal carriers. During the war more than thirty thousand prostitutes were incarcerated in institutions supported by the federal government. As one federal official noted:

> Conditions required the immediate isolation of as many venereally infected persons acting as spreaders of disease as could be quickly apprehended and quarantined. It was not a measure instituted for the punishment of prostitutes on account of infraction of the civil or moral law, but was strictly a public health measure to prevent the spread of dangerous, communicable diseases.[12]

Fear of venereal disease during the war had led to substantial inroads against traditional civil liberties. Although many of these interventions were challenged in the courts, most were upheld; the police powers of the state were deemed sufficient to override any constitutional concerns. The program of detention and isolation, it should be noted, had no impact on rates of venereal disease, which increased dramatically during the war. Although this story is not well known, the parallels to the internment of Japanese Americans during World War II are unavoidable.

THE AIDS EPIDEMIC

In light of the history of sexually transmitted diseases in the last century, it is almost impossible to watch the AIDS epidemic without a sense of *déjà vu*. AIDS raises a host of concerns traditional to the debates about venereal infection—from morality to medicine, sexuality and deviance, and prevention and intervention. In many instances the situation with AIDS is similar to that of syphilis in the early twentieth century, described in the previous chapter by Elizabeth Fee. Like syphilis then, AIDS can cause death; there is currently no curative treatment; it is being addressed in the meantime via education and social engineering; and it arouses fears that reveal deeper social and cultural anxieties about the disease, its transmissibility, and its victims. Yet AIDS is different, too.

AIDS threatens our sense of medical security. After all, the age of transmissible, lethal infections was deemed long past in the Western world. Ours was the age of chronic disease—heart diseases and cancers that principally strike late in life; epidemics of infectious diseases had receded in the public memory. Not since the polio epidemics of the early 1950s has fear of infection reached such a high pitch as it has in the 1980s. Indeed, no epidemic since the swine flu pandemic of 1918 has had such a dramatic impact on patterns of mortality, and, ironically, the concerns in 1976 about a new epidemic of swine flu, which never materialized, seemed to confirm that fear of epidemic infection was unfounded in this modern age of antibiotics. AIDS has fractured this false sense of confidence. Effective responses to such a problem are further complicated by its "social construction," those attitudes and values that shape the public view of the disease. The social construction of AIDS will in turn have a powerful impact on the choices made in responding to the disease.

SOCIAL ATTITUDES AND STIGMA

Though AIDS is an enormous public health problem, public perceptions of the epidemic have not always been accurate. Despite considerable evidence that AIDS is not easily communicated, widespread fears persist, reminiscent of the belief that syphilis could be transmitted by drinking cups, toilet seats, and doorknobs. Such late Victorian concerns are now cast in a contemporary light. In the fall of 1985 a *New York Times*/CBS poll found that 47 percent of Americans believed that AIDS could be transmitted via a shared drinking glass, while 28 percent believed that toilet seats could be the source of contamination.[13] Another survey found that 34 percent of those polled believed it unsafe to "associate" with an AIDS victim even when no physical contact was involved. The California Association of Realtors instructed its members to inform prospective buyers whether or not a house on the market had been owned by an AIDS patient.[14]

Because of the considerable fear the AIDS epidemic has engendered, and the fact that the disease has principally affected two already marginal social groups (gays and intravenous drug users), its victims have been further victimized by stigmatization and discrimination. AIDS patients have lost jobs, housing, and social support. At risk not just from a serious, terminal disease, AIDS sufferers also have to deal with a series of social perceptions and attitudes that encourage further discrimination and isolation. Even the medical profession has not been free from the fear of AIDS: Early in the epidemic some physicians refused to treat AIDS patients, despite assurances that the virus was not easily transmitted.[15]

The hysteria and stigma have even led to attempts to segregate victims. The first major skirmish in this battle arose over whether children with AIDS should be permitted to attend school. Ryan White, a thirteen-year-old AIDS victim, was banned from his Indiana school. This issue has attracted a vehement, ongoing debate, but most jurisdictions have permitted children with the disease to attend when they posed no risk to other students. In Queens, New York, angry parents kept their children home in two school districts because a child with AIDS was permitted to go to school. The boycott reflected a pervasive mistrust of scientific authority, as well as a lack of understanding about the nature of uncertainty in science. Could officials assure—absolutely—that the disease could *not* be passed in the classroom? Medical science, which deals in probabilities, could not offer the definitive guarantees that many demanded.[16]

Stigma goes beyond AIDS patients to anyone considered at risk of carrying the infection. Indeed, not only have AIDS patients been subject to discrimination, but the public response to the disease has also been accompanied by a rise in attacks on homosexuals. Fire officials have refused to resuscitate men they suspected might be homosexual, and police have worn gloves in apprehending suspects in some municipalities.[17]

Our understanding of AIDS and its meaning has been powerfully shaped by the media in what has been a complex process. AIDS has generated outstanding science writing as well as scurrilous reports bent on raising irrational fears and public hysteria. The death of movie idol Rock Hudson in October 1985 demonstrates the paradoxical relationship of AIDS and the media. Hudson's death became the occasion for recognizing that AIDS was a vast problem that merited more attention; his death put a human face on the epidemic for many Americans. It also became the occasion for speculation about Hudson's sexuality and for a prurient interest in the gay subculture. Hudson's plight was heavy with irony. This macho screen star, the press now speculated, had lived a secret life. AIDS brought a pale, thin, dying Hudson out of the closet, and President Ronald Reagan finally uttered the dangerous monosyllable, "AIDS."

But Hudson's death also led to heightened fears of hidden disease.

Who knew who was gay? Who knew who might have the disease? Hudson's death created alarm among Hollywood actors that they might contract the disease in the course of making movies and television shows. Some critics suggested that Hudson had acted irresponsibly by not informing his fellow cast members of the television serial "Dynasty" and by kissing his costar, Linda Evans, in one episode. In this respect, Hudson's death again raised concerns that AIDS victims and those who carry the virus could place others at risk. Shortly after Hudson's death, his estate was sued by a lover, who claimed that Hudson had never informed him he had AIDS.[18]

The fact that the two principal high-risk groups are already highly stigmatized in American society has had a powerful impact on responses to the epidemic. Some have seen the AIDS epidemic in a purely "moral" light: AIDS is a disease that occurs among those who violate the moral order. As one journalist concluded: "Suddenly a lot of people fear that they and their families might suddenly catch some mysterious, fatal illness which until now has been confined to society's social outcasts." AIDS, like other sexually transmitted diseases, has been viewed as a fateful link between social deviance and the morally correct. Such fears have been exacerbated by an expectant media. "NO ONE IS SAFE FROM AIDS," announced *Life* magazine in bold red letters on its cover.[19] Implicit was the notion that "no one is safe" from gays and intravenous drug users. The disease had come to be equated with those who are at highest risk of suffering its terrible consequences.

Underlying the fears of transmission were deeper concerns about homosexuality. Just as "innocent syphilis" in the first decades of the twentieth century was thought to bring the "respectable middle class" in contact with a deviant ethnic, working-class "sexual underworld," now AIDS threatened heterosexuals with homosexual contamination. In this context, homosexuality—not a virus—causes AIDS. Therefore, homosexuality itself is feared as if it were a communicable, lethal disease. After a generation of work to strike homosexuality from the psychiatric diagnostic manuals, it had suddenly reappeared as an infectious, terminal disease.[20]

The AIDS epidemic thus offered new opportunities for expressions of moral opprobrium. Patrick Buchanan, conservative columnist and former Reagan speechwriter, explained, "The poor homosexuals—they have declared war upon Nature, and now Nature is exacting an awful retribution."[21] Criticizing government expenditures on research to produce a vaccine, *Commentary* editor Norman Podhoretz asked: "Are they aware that in the name of compassion they are giving social sanction to what can only be described as brutish degradation?" Podhoretz's position—that gays get what they deserve, that to investigate treatments would merely encourage unhealthy behaviors—is a classic position in the history of sexually transmitted diseases. It also demonstrates a remarkably uninformed view of the epidemic, as well as a complete disregard for the public health.[22]

In a now classic work, *Stigma: Notes on the Management of Spoiled Identity,* sociologist Erving Goffman defined what he considered to be three types of stigma. The first is an abomination of the body; clearly AIDS could be so categorized. The second is a blemish of individual character; again victims of AIDS and other sexually transmitted diseases have traditionally been seen as lacking control, as immoral and promiscuous. And third, Goffman identified the tribal stigmas of race, nation, or religion. This, too, has been a recurring theme in considerations of venereal disease—the notion that particular groups were especially prone to infection. Perhaps the sexually transmitted diseases carry a particularly weighty stigma because they cut through each of these categories; an undesired *difference,* of a sexual nature, that sets its victims apart. Victims of AIDS thus suffer the biological consequences of a terrifying, fatal disease as well as a deep social stigma.[23]

Fear of disease and the homophobia it has generated have forced the gay-rights movement into defensive action in order to fight a rising tide of discrimination. In fact, the epidemic threatens to undo a generation of progress toward gay rights. Not only does AIDS threaten the lives of many members of the gay community, it has unleashed a considerable political and legal threat. In June 1986 the Justice Department issued a decision that held it permissible for employers to bar AIDS patients or those infected with the virus from work. The ruling held that federal law did not protect the civil rights of those who *might* be considered dangerous to others; moreover, the ruling left the evaluation of such "real or perceived" risks to the employer. The decision was issued despite government scientists' repeated statements, on the basis of considerable epidemiological and biological evidence, that the disease was not casually transmitted.[24]

Public health officials openly expressed their dismay with the ruling, which threatened to encourage the irrational fears of the disease that they had worked so diligently to alleviate. Calling the ruling a "license to hound AIDS victims," the *New York Times* wrote in an editorial that "no one should want to curb the powers of public health officials to control a disease as deadly as AIDS. But to throw AIDS victims out of their jobs is a capitulation to unwarranted fear that protects no one."[25] As journalist Charles Krauthammer noted, the ruling undercut all antidiscrimination legislation: "The whole point of such laws is to say this: It may indeed cause you psychological distress to mix with others who you irrationally dislike or fear. Too bad. The state has decided that these particular prejudices are destructive and irrational. Therefore the state will prohibit you . . . from acting upon your groundless prejudices." As Krauthammer concluded, "It should not matter if people think you can get AIDS in the Xerox room. You can't. Ignorance is a cause of discrimination. It is not a justification for it."[26]

Such a ruling may not be upheld in court. But the courts have not supported recent attempts to provide basic civil liberties for homosexuals. Soon after the Justice Department ruling in 1986, the Supreme Court upheld, in a five to four decision, the constitutionality of a state's sodomy law in a case that was considered a major setback to the gay-rights movement.[27] This ruling, which conflicted with the court's recent affirmations of the right to privacy, can be fully understood only in the context of the AIDS epidemic. Nevertheless, in 1987 and 1988 the court ruled that people with infectious disease are protected by the statute prohibiting discrimination against the handicapped.

SCREENING FOR HIV

Although scientific knowledge about AIDS has grown at an exponential rate, much remains unknown. At the same time, AIDS presents a series of highly problematic social policy questions that demand answers even in the face of incomplete medical knowledge and widespread fear. AIDS makes explicit a central tension in our polity: the premium we place on the rights of the individual to fundamental civil liberties versus the notion of the public good and the role of the state in assuring public welfare. Both sets of values, highly prized in our culture, have necessarily been brought to bear in the AIDS crisis. In the course of the twentieth century civil liberties were expanded and strengthened in the courts, making the conflicts posed by AIDS even more contentious.

Nowhere is this more clearly seen than in the current debate about testing and screening for human immunodeficiency virus (HIV) antibody. The discovery of the enzyme-linked immunosorbent assay (ELISA test) not only made possible the screening of blood to preserve the quality of the blood supply, it also made it technically possible to identify individuals with HIV. Although many, especially in the gay community, have viewed the test with grave concern because of the potential for misuse in identifying and segregating, or even quarantining, individuals testing positive, others have viewed the test as the critical element in a campaign to stem the epidemic. The debate currently rages about the appropriate use of this test.

Beginning in late 1985 the U.S. Department of Defense announced that all new recruits for military service would be screened for HIV antibody and rejected if found to test positive. One justification of the screening program was that military personnel receive a wide variety of live-virus vaccinations that might cause serious disease in individuals whose immune systems were compromised. Military officials also contended that combat would provide a high risk for transmission of HIV, given that soldiers routinely serve as blood donors in the field. As Dorothy Porter and Roy Porter note in their chapter, the armed forces are typically the first to undergo massive screening for transmissible diseases. Although the military suggested that the screening program would maintain absolute confidentiality, in practice this may be difficult to achieve inasmuch as rejected candidates may suffer the stigma of HIV infection. Critics of the military screening program also argued that the test was being used to identify and remove gays from service.[28]

The military screening program was merely the first; many others have been proposed, from the mandatory screening of high-risk groups to premarital testing, testing in prisons, and universal screening. Some proposals have called for mandatory testing of high-risk individuals, but they fail to recognize the implicit impossibility of identifying such groups and requiring them to be tested.[29] How would officials implement legislation that mandated testing for only certain, ill-defined social groups? Because such proposals are impossible to enforce, only universal screening programs could be mandated. But such programs would have obvious problems.

Conservative columnist William F. Buckley, Jr., has recommended mandatory universal screening, with all seropositive individuals being tattooed on their forearms and buttocks. This, he suggests, would serve to stem the epidemic by warning those who might share needles or have sex with such individuals. The sorriness of Buckley's logic, however, is more than apparent. First, he fails to differentiate between those with AIDS and those who are positive for the antibody. Second, he fails to note the possibility of false positives, which, with mandatory testing, would become much more likely. As epidemiologists recognize, the incidence of false positive tests increases when the prevalence of infection in the population being tested is low. "We face a utilitarian imperative," wrote Buckley.[30] But there is no evidence whatsoever that such an invasive and stigmatizing program would slow the spread of this epidemic. Buckley's proposal is all the more remarkable in light of his consistent attacks on intrusive government. A powerfully moralistic homophobia is only thinly veiled by such proposals.

When the epidemic worsens, as it most certainly will, society's desire to identify and segregate infected individuals will probably become more intense, even though massive, compulsory screening would offer little in the interests of public health. The public will cease clamoring for such measures only if the full costs and negligible benefits are clearly explained and understood. Otherwise, the irrational desire to segregate may be overwhelming.

Finally, it is worth questioning the purpose of testing, especially in light of the fact that, at this writing, there is no effective treatment for AIDS. In the 1930s, when states began to mandate premarital blood testing for syphilis, individuals found to be infected could seek treatment, become noninfectious, and go on with their lives; their contacts could be found, tested, and, if infected, treated. Such programs obviously served the interests of the individuals who were infected as well as the public interest. Such a program is not possible in the case of AIDS, for which there is currently no cure and no means of rendering noninfectious those individuals who carry HIV.

Some have argued that testing is advisable because knowing one's antibody status will encourage individuals to act responsibly, to avoid spreading the infection, and perhaps to avoid further risks that could contribute to the development of disease. This may be true for some, but it has yet to be determined; individuals may have quite variable psychological and behavioral responses to learning of their infection status. Many individuals, especially in the gay community, have altered their behavior without knowing their antibody status. The test has risks in that it is difficult, even in the best of circumstances, to guarantee that the results will be held strictly confidential. Fears that a positive test could lead to discrimination seem realistic in light of Justice Department rulings and the highly stigmatized view of the disease.[31]

All this, of course, is not to argue that testing is useless. Many individuals, especially those likely to have come in contact with the virus, may want to learn their antibody status. Obviously, they should be able to do so under the strictest standards of confidentiality. Moreover, as treatments become available, it is likely that they will be most effective if initiated before the development of symptoms. It would thus become important for infected individuals to find out on a timely basis—while they are still asymptomatic—so they may seek treatment.

It is crucial to maintain the distinction between voluntary use of the test and mandatory screening. The test could be used as a "marker" to license discrimination in employment, housing, and the availability of health and life insurance. Mandatory screening could therefore have the effect of creating an underground epidemic in which infected individuals, fearing discrimination, isolation, or quarantine, refuse to cooperate with public health officials. Hidden infection is the nemesis of any effective campaign to halt an epidemic disease.

Among those asserting their right to require individuals to take the ELISA test are insurance companies, which argue that individuals who have been exposed to HIV are likely to have higher health-care costs than the population in general; therefore, they contend, such individuals should pay higher premiums. "If America's private voluntary-insurance system is to remain workable, AIDS tests must be allowed so the disease can be underwritten in the same manner as heart disease, cancer, or alcohol and drug abuse," explained Claire Wolkoff of the American Academy of Actuaries. "The alternative is to spread the risk factor over the whole population, thus raising the price of insurance for everyone."[32] Several states have taken legislative action to bar insurers from requiring the test, or to assure its absolute confidentiality. When the District of Columbia passed such a resolution, Senator Jesse Helms, the conservative Republican from North Carolina, said "the truth is the so-called homosexual rights crowd has snookered the entire District of Columbia into footing the bill to provide special treatment for those who are at health risk because of AIDS." At least four life and health insurance companies announced a decision to stop doing business in Washington, D.C., rather than comply with the legislation.[33]

The question at the heart of the debate over insurance testing is, who will bear the cost of AIDS? Should the costs of the epidemic be spread over the whole society, or should they be borne by those who have been and will be infected by HIV? Early studies estimated the average health-care costs for AIDS patients to be about $150,000, although later investigations soon determined that this figure might be overestimated by as much as 100 percent. Total direct and indirect costs of the epidemic—the losses from medical care and income—rose to $3.3 billion by mid-1986. An added problem was that hospitals often had to pick up the tab for AIDS patients. This has been particularly true in New York City, where close to 30 percent of all AIDS victims are intravenous drug users, whose health care costs tend to be higher and who are less likely to be insured.[34] In this respect, AIDS again reveals deep and persistent social problems, in this instance, the problem of financing health care. How should the risks of catastrophic disease be spread? Should we apply an individualist ethic, or look to social programs to distribute the costs of disease more equitably? These questions have been on the national agenda for more than a generation. AIDS forces them out of the shadows.

At issue on who should bear the costs of the epidemic is the critical question: Who is responsible? This has been especially significant in the history of sexually transmitted diseases, traditionally viewed as diseases of individual moral failing.

The debate over screening for HIV antibody is ultimately part and parcel of a larger debate in American society over testing in general. New biotechnologies make it possible for tests to reveal a great deal about any individual: his or her health status, behaviors, medical risks, and genetic makeup. This is information that not only insurers but also employers and the state might want to have. The right to require tests, and the question of whose interests such tests are to serve, promise to be bitter and controversial issues in the years ahead. Indeed, they raise the question of whose interest medical science will serve. The issue of compulsory testing reflects the most fundamental tensions between civil liberties and social control.

AIDS AND PUBLIC HEALTH

Although Edward Brandt, then assistant secretary of health and human services, called AIDS the nation's "number-one priority" in public health in mid-1983, the federal government's response has been poorly coordinated and haphazard. In 1985 the Office of Technology Assessment (OTA) issued a report analyzing the federal government's response to AIDS; the report revealed a number of significant shortcomings. First, the government had been slow to respond: Although the Centers for Disease Control (CDC) had identified AIDS in 1981, research at the National Institutes of Health (NIH) did not begin in earnest until 1983; bureaucratic procedures appear to have prevented a more timely response to this public health emergency. Second, when NIH did take up the AIDS problem, research funding was inadequate. In 1982 and 1983 the administration did not budget any money for AIDS research; nevertheless, Congress allocated $33 million. The following year, the administration asked for $39 million. Congress appropriated $61 million. In 1986 Congress allocated $234 million, but the Reagan administration proposed cutting this to $213.2 million; this, despite the fact that cases had been doubling every year.[35] Underlying this debate over funding was the controversial nature of AIDS itself and its close association with homosexuality. Funding for the research and treatment of sexually transmitted diseases has always been suspect in the federal health budget.

The OTA report also pointed out the inattention paid to social and psychological factors associated with the disease—especially noteworthy in that preventive measures offered the only immediate hope of slowing the epidemic. Nevertheless, funds for education have been meager. In 1986 the CDC had $25 million available for education, although a full program would have required three times that amount. As Harvey V. Fineberg, dean of the Harvard School of Public Health, noted, "We understand enough about the cause and spread of the AIDS virus to give people the knowledge they need to protect themselves."[36] And yet, outside the gay community, this is not being done.

Sex education has typically been an area of significant controversy, and this has proved especially true with respect to education programs about the AIDS epidemic for schoolchildren of various ages. As Walter Dowdle of the CDC explained: "The sense of urgency is somewhat different here. It's not a matter of philosophy and religious taboos. We are talking about prevention in life and death situations."[37] The federal government, however, refused to issue educational materials explicitly advising "safe sex" practices, apparently fearing they would be construed as an "endorsement" of homosexuality. In this respect, federal officials were as fearful as the Victorian legislators (discussed by the Porters in the last chapter) that public health education might seem to "condone" vice.

Although behavioral means are the only current hope for preventing the further spread of the disease, as the history of the sexually transmitted diseases makes clear, altering behavior is no simple matter. Sexuality is a powerful force, certainly subject to individual will, but not completely so. Such problems as intravenous drug use highlight the issue of addiction, which clearly points to the fact that behavior is not always subject to control. Behavioral practices, though clearly related to patterns of disease, are poorly understood in contemporary biomedicine. Indeed, the underlying assumption about behavior, and one deeply ingrained in our culture, is that it is entirely voluntary. According to this logic, individuals "should" modify their behavior once appropriately informed about risks. Moreover, we know too little about how to assist individuals who seek to make and maintain difficult behavioral alterations. This is as true for sexual behavior as it is for drug addiction, the two principal mechanisms for the transmission of the AIDS virus. Preventive medicine and health promotion have had inadequate attention in modern medicine, where the emphasis has been on treatment, cure, and technology—the search for "magic bullets."

AIDS IN A CULTURAL CONTEXT

AIDS makes explicit, as few diseases could, the complex interaction of social, cultural, and biological forces. Given the social history of venereal disease in the United States, this is hardly surprising. But, as disease is shaped by its particular social and historical context, so will the response. Nevertheless, the analogues that AIDS poses to the broader history of sexually transmitted diseases in the United States are striking: the pervasive fear of contagion, concerns about casual transmission, the stigmatization of victims, the conflicts between public health and civil liberties, and the search for magic bullets. How these issues will be resolved as the AIDS epidemic continues to unfold in the years ahead is far from certain.

History is not a predictive science. AIDS is not syphilis, and the historical moment has shifted. But one thing is certain: The response to AIDS, as can already be seen, will not be determined strictly by the disease's biological character; rather, that response will be deeply influenced by our social and cultural understanding of disease and its victims. And, indeed, even our scientific understanding of the disease will be refracted through our cultural values and attitudes. History provides us with a way of understanding and approaching the present. The recognition of the process by which AIDS has been culturally defined provides us with an opportunity to guide and influence responses to the epidemic in ways that will be constructive, effective, and humane.

A series of difficult dilemmas are just offstage. Can we protect the rights of AIDS victims while avoiding the victimization of the public? How will the conflict between individual liberties and public welfare be resolved?[38] In the months and years ahead the problem of constructing cost-benefit ratios for various policies will be confronted. Who will bear the burdens of any particular intervention? What are the potential unintended consequences of any particular policy? Traditional public health policies have been advocated: screening, testing, reporting, contact tracing, isolation, and quarantine. Will these measures be effective in the case of AIDS, which is complicated by the large number of healthy carriers perhaps infectious for life?

There are two criteria by which any proposal must be evaluated. First, *effectiveness:* There must be considerable evidence that any particular policy offers substantial benefit. The second criterion for public interventions should be *justice:* Is it the least restrictive of all possible positive measures?

Although we know a good deal about AIDS, much still lies outside current scientific understanding. Policies relating to AIDS will, of course, be created in this atmosphere of uncertainty, complicated by the decline of the authority of scientific experts—from Three Mile Island, to Love Canal, to the space shuttle, to Chernobyl—which has had the effect of creating significant public distrust.[39] Our fortunate inexperience, as a society, with major epidemics (since polio) accounts for our relative lack of social and political savvy in dealing with such problems. In fact, we would probably have to go back to the influenza pandemic of 1918 to identify a pathogen as dangerous as the AIDS virus. That is, we have few models for dealing with public health issues of this magnitude and complexity.

Our notions of cost-benefit analyses and social policy are characterized by a naïve belief in policies without costs. All social policies carry certain costs, but in our political culture we tend to reject policies when the costs become explicit, even if they promise significant benefits. This has been seen in two proposals to slow the spread of the infection. As in the early twentieth century, education has been proffered as one of the few strategies capable of slowing the spread of disease. But discussions must assess the meaning and content of such education. Explicit sexual education has been rejected by some officials because it is viewed as encouraging homosexuality; the costs are thus evaluated as too high. Another recent proposal has met a similar fate—the idea of providing sterile needles to intravenous drug users to slow down the rapid spread of the disease among that community. This idea has proved unpopular thus far because it is seen as contributing to the drug problem. Underlying such assessments, of course, is the idea that AIDS is a "self-inflicted" disease.

As was the case in the early twentieth century, public health measures that require dramatic infringements of civil liberties are again being proposed. As we saw in the Porters' chapter on the enforcement of health measures in Britain, such steps have had little if any impact on the public health. In the United States, similar harsh measures have been ineffective: For example, rates of venereal disease climbed rapidly during World War I, despite radical government measures regarding the incarceration of prostitutes. This is not to suggest the purely pragmatic notion that if an intervention works it is right. Rather, if an intervention does not produce results, and yet is supported by officials and the public, one must look for secondary reasons to explain that support. The issue thus becomes not the desire to protect the public from hazard—an idea so basic to modern governments that few would question it in principle; our most fundamental notions of social welfare are based upon it. Rather, these activities indicate a transformation from protection to punishment; a clear signal that the disease and those who get it are socially disvalued.

In view of the fear and aversion that surround AIDS, there is a clear danger that policies with little or no potential for slowing the epidemic could nevertheless have considerable legal, social, and cultural appeal. What can be done to separate realistic concerns from irrational fears? How can victim-blaming and stigmatization of high-risk, already marginal, groups be avoided? This process of dividing victims into blameless and blameful categories is analogous to early twentieth-century notions of venereal disease insontium, and is evident, for example, in assessments such as the following 1983 article appearing in the *New York Times Magazine:*

> The groups most recently found to be at risk for AIDS present a particularly poignant problem. Innocent bystanders caught in the path of a new disease, they can make no behavioral decisions to minimize their risk: hemophiliacs cannot stop taking bloodclotting medication; surgery patients cannot stop getting transfusions; women cannot control the drug habits of their mates; babies cannot choose their mothers.[40]

This passage illustrates a number of problems. First, it suggests that the disease is somehow more "poignant" when it attacks nonhomosexuals. Second, if these groups are "innocent bystanders," then those at highest risk of contracting AIDS are "guilty." This discussion implies that the entire community is at risk from the sexual practices of homosexuals. In some quarters the misapprehension persists: AIDS is caused by homosexuality, not by a retrovirus. According to this confused logic, the answer to the problem is simple: Repress these behaviors. Implicit in this approach to the problem are powerful assumptions about culpability and guilt.

Indeed, assessments of AIDS—as of most sexually transmitted diseases in the twentieth century—rest on the essentially simplistic view that the problem can be solved if individuals conduct their sexual life more responsibly, a view that rests on the explicit assumption that an individual's behavior is free from external forces—that a "life-style" is strictly voluntary. These persistent assumptions about health-related behavior rest on an essentially naïve view of human nature. If anything has become clear in the course of the twentieth century it is that behavior is subject to complex forces, internal psychologies, and external pressures, all of which are not subject to immediate modification or, arguably, to modification at all. Sexuality is subject to a number of powerful influences, social and economic, conscious and unconscious, many more powerful than even the fear of disease and death. In this view, sexuality is equated with other risk-taking behaviors—smoking, drinking, poor eating habits, driving too fast. Individuals can, of course, be held partly accountable for these behaviors, but the questions of to what extent and whether they should be are not as simple.

The persistence of such values and attitudes calls into question the received view of the sexual revolution in whose aftermath we are living. Serious and important changes in sexual mores and practices have undoubtedly taken place—the gay-liberation movement is but one example. But this makes certain continuities all the more striking. Social values continue to define sexually transmitted diseases as uniquely sinful and, indeed, to transform them into evidence of moral decay; some still believe that fear of disease encourages a higher morality. It thus seems naïve and wishful to assert that we have conquered moral puritanism within ourselves, because underlying tensions in American sexual values persist, tensions that are brought forward in our approach to AIDS as well as to venereal diseases. To conservative foes of the sexual revolution, the message is clear: The way to control sexually transmitted disease is not through medical means but through moral rectitude. A disease such as AIDS is controlled by controlling individual conduct.

The final chapter by Daniel Fox demonstrates that one current trend in health care policy is to accept this model of disease and to apply it to a myriad of other illnesses, to reduce the emphasis on social or external determinants of disease and health, and to stress individual responsibility.[41] This model, however, has failed venereal disease, and the historical record renders it a dubious precedent. The presumption nevertheless remains. Behavior—bad behavior at that—is seen as the cause of disease. These assumptions may be powerful psychologically, and in some cases they may influence behavior, but so long as they are dominant—so long as disease is equated with sin—there can be no "magic bullet."

In this sense the old scare tactics have failed; denial and repression of sexuality have failed; victim-blaming and moralizing have failed as effective public health mechanisms. Although biomedical solutions offer much hope, they, too, have been unable to free us from infectious disease. More creative and sophisticated approaches to this set of diseases are necessary. Behavioral changes may indeed be a significant factor in disease, and new techniques to assist those who seek to change are needed. But we need to recognize that "behavioral change" does not have to mean celibacy, heterosexuality, or morality; rather, it means avoiding contact with a pathogen.

AIDS makes painfully explicit the limits of our ability to intervene against the course of the biological world. Sexual contact is one of a number of ways in which microorganisms are transmitted from human to human. New or altered infectious agents are passed this way; no single medical treatment has proved effective for these infectious organisms. This, then, reveals the fundamental flaw in the biomedical model; that is, the search for magic bullets. Venereal diseases, indeed, all infectious diseases, constitute complex bioecological problems in which host, parasite, and a number of social and environmental forces interact. No *single* medical or social intervention can thus adequately address the problem. Just as social mores and practices change, so, too, does the biological system. New infections such as AIDS may appear, or older, once-controlled infectious diseases, such as gonorrhea, may become intransigent in the face of agents whose effectiveness is attenuated as the organism itself changes. As one observer recently remarked, the battle against infectious disease is an ongoing "leap-frog war."[42]

Caught in the complex web of social and scientific questions surrounding AIDS, we easily forget the dimensions of the tragedy. While disease tells us much about the nature of our society, it also reveals the nature of illness, suffering, and death and dying. The high mortality associated with AIDS and the growing number of cases could become the justification for drastic measures. "Better safe than sorry" could well become a catch phrase to justify dramatic abuses of basic human rights in the context of an uncertain science. Moreover, the social construction of this disease, its close association in much of the public's eye with violations of the moral code, could contribute to spiraling hysteria and anger. This cycle has already led to further victimization of patients, the double jeopardy of lethal disease and social oppression.

The social costs of ineffective, draconian public health measures would only augment the crisis we know as AIDS. But such measures can be avoided only if we are adept in both our medical and cultural understanding of this disease. For we need to perform a difficult task, that of separating deeply irrational fears from scientific understanding. Only when we recognize the ways in which social and cultural values shape this disease will we be able to begin to deal effectively and humanely with a problem as serious and complex as AIDS.

AIDS is an unfinished chapter in our medical and social history, demonstrating the nature of contemporary biomedical science and research; our beliefs about health, disease, and contagion; and our ideas about sexuality and social responsibility. AIDS demonstrates how economics and politics cannot be separated from disease; indeed, these forces shape our response in powerful ways. In the years ahead we will, no doubt, learn a great deal more about AIDS and how to control it. We will also learn a great deal about the nature of our society from the manner in which we address the disease: AIDS will be a standard by which we may measure not only our medical and scientific skill but also our capacity for justice and compassion.

NOTES

This essay first appeared in somewhat different form in *Law, Medicine, and Health Care* 14 (1986): 231–241.

1. One model has already been proposed in Susan Sontag's brilliant polemic, *Illness as Metaphor*. In this work, Sontag assessed the important ways in which tuberculosis and cancer have been used as metaphors. Using techniques of literary analysis, she demonstrated prevailing cultural views of these diseases and their victims. See Sontag, *Illness as Metaphor* (New York: Vintage, 1978).
2. The following discussion is abbreviated from my book, *No Magic Bullet: A Social History of Venereal Disease in the United States since 1880*, rev. ed. (New York: Oxford University Press, 1987).
3. On the problem of ophthalmia neonatorum, see Abraham L. Wolbarst, "On the Occurrence of Syphilis and Gonorrhea in Children by Direct Infection," *American Medicine* 7 (1912): 494; Carolyn Von Blarcum, "The Harm Done in Ascribing All Babies' Sore Eyes to Gonorrhea," *American Journal of Public Health* 6 (1916): 926–931; and J. W. Kerr, "Ophthalmia Neonatorum: An Analysis of the Laws and Regulations in Relation thereto in Force in the United States," *Public Health Service Bulletin* no. 49 (Washington, D.C.: U.S. Government Printing Office, 1914).
4. Albert H. Burr, "The Guarantee of Safety in the Marriage Contract," *Journal of the American Medical Association* 47 (1906): 1887–1888.
5. See Eugene Brieux, *Damaged Goods*, trans. John Pollack (New York:

Brentano's, 1913). On the critical reception of the play see "Demoralizing Plays," *Outlook* 150 (1913): 110; John D. Rockefeller, "The Awakening of a New Social Conscience," *Medical Reviews of Reviews* 19 (1913): 281; "Damaged Goods," *Hearst's Magazine* 23 (1913): 806; "Brieux's New Sociological Sermon in Three Acts," *Current Opinion* 54 (1913): 296–297. See also, Barbara Gutmann Rosenkrantz, "Damaged Goods: Dilemmas of Responsibility for Risk," *Milbank Memorial Fund Quarterly* 57 (1979): 1–37.

6. Howard Kelly, "Social Diseases and Their Prevention," *Social Diseases* 1 (1910): 17, and "The Protection of the Innocent," *American Journal of Obstetrics* 55 (1907): 477–481.

7. On prostitution during the Progressive era in America, see Paul S. Boyer, *Urban Masses and Moral Order* (Cambridge: Harvard University Press, 1978); Ruth Rosen, *The Lost Sisterhood: Prostitution in America, 1900–1918* (Baltimore: Johns Hopkins University Press, 1982); and Mark Thomas Connely, *The Response to Prostitution in the Progressive Era* (Chapel Hill: University of North Carolina Press, 1980).

8. On nonvenereal transmission, see especially L. Duncan Bulkey, *Syphilis of the Innocent* (New York: Bailey and Fairchild, 1894).

9. "What One Woman Has Had to Bear," *Forum* 68 (1912): 451–454. See also "New Laws About Drinking Cups," *Life* 58 (1911): 1152.

10. The wartime policy for the attack on the red-light districts and the testing and incarceration of prostitutes is described in greater detail in Brandt, *No Magic Bullet*, 80–95.

11. T. W. Gregory, "Memorandum on Legal Aspects of the Proposed System of Medical Examination of Women Convicted Under Section 13, Selective Service Act," National Archives, Washington, D.C., Record Group 90, Box 223. See also Mary Macey Dietzler, *Detention Houses and Reformatories as Protective Social Agencies in the Campaign of the United States Government Against Venereal Diseases*, United States Interdepartmental Social Hygiene Board (Washington, D.C.: Government Printing Office, 1922).

12. C. C. Pierce, "The Value of Detention as a Reconstruction Measure," *American Journal of Obstetrics* 80 (1919): 629.

13. "AFRAIDS," *New Republic*, 14 October 1985, 7–9. See also Charles Krauthammer, "The Politics of a Plague," *New Republic*, 1 August 1983, 18–21.

14. *New York Times*, 26 June 1985.

15. Jay A. Winsten, "Fighting Panic on AIDS," *New York Times*, 26 July 1983.

16. "The Fear of AIDS," *Newsweek*, 23 September 1985, 18–25. On the school controversy see *New York Times*, 13, 24 October 1985, and 8 December 1985. Also David J. Rothman, "Public Policy and Risk Assessment in the Case of AIDS," in *AIDS: Public Policy Dimensions* (New York: United Hospital Fund, 1986).

17. Leon Eisenberg, "Private Trust/Public Confidence in Science and Medicine: The Genesis of Fear," *Law, Medicine and Health Care* 14 (1986): 243–249; Robert Balzell, "The History of an Epidemic," *New Republic*, 1 August 1983, 14–18; Richard Goldstein, "The Uses of AIDS," *Village Voice*, 5 November 1985, 25–27.

18. "Fear and AIDS in Hollywood," *People*, 23 September 1985, 28–33; *New York Times*, 7 November 1985; *Washington Post*, 28 July 1985.

19. *Life*, July 1985, 12–21.

20. See Ronald Bayer, *Homosexuality and American Psychiatry: The Politics of Diagnosis* (New York: Basic Books, 1981).

21. *New York Post*, 24 May 1983.

22. Quoted in *New York Times*, 18 March 1986.

23. Erving Goffman, *Stigma: Notes on the Management of Spoiled Identity* (Englewood Cliffs, N.J.: Prentice-Hall, 1963).

24. On the Justice Department ruling, see *New York Times*, 23, 27 June 1986; *Wall Street Journal*, 27 June 1986.

25. *New York Times*, 26 June 1986.

26. Charles Krauthammer, "Fear Him and Fire Him," *Washington Post*, 27 June 1986.

27. *New York Times*, 1 July 1986.

28. On military testing, see *New York Times*, 13 October 1985, 31 January, and 2 February 1986; *Science* 232 (16 May 1986): 818–820. The results of military screening have shown relatively high rates of infection. In Manhattan 2 percent of individuals applying to enter the service have been found to be infected; these numbers are fifteen to twenty times higher than the estimated national prevalence.

29. Among those who have recommended mandatory screening for those at high risk are Lewis Kuller, professor of epidemiology at the University of Pittsburgh, and Paul Starr, professor of sociology at Princeton. See *Chronicle of Higher Education*, 4 June 1986.

30. William F. Buckley, Jr., "Identify All the Carriers," *New York Times*, 18 March 1986.

31. See, for example, Mark Senak, "Ban AIDS Blood Tests," *New York Times*, 27 May 1986.

32. *New York Times*, 11 June 1986. See also the full-page advertisement of the American Council of Life Insurance and the Health Insurance Association of America, *Washington Post*, 11 May 1986.

33. Quoted in *Washington Post*, 20 June 1986, and 28 June 1986.

34. *New York Times*, 8 June and 10 January 1986, 3 November 1986; on the problem of financing AIDS see also George R. Seage, "The Medical Cost of Treatment of AIDS/ARC Patients," unpublished paper, Boston Department of Health and Hospitals, 12 May 1985; Philip R. Lee, "AIDS: Allocating Resources for Patient Care," *Issues in Science and Technology* 2 (1986): 66–73; and especially Rashi Fein, "AIDS and Economics," unpublished paper, AIDS Institute of the New York State Department of Health, 29 May 1986.

35. *Washington Post*, 25 May 1983, 23 July 1985; *New York Times*, 15 June 1983, and 29 July, 24 October 1985; and especially, U.S. Congress, Office of Technology Assessment, *Review of the Public Health Service's Response to AIDS: A Technical Memorandum*, February 1985.

36. Harvey V. Fineberg, "A Way to Tackle AIDS Education," *New York Times*, 13 July 1986; also Paul Cleary et al., "Health Education about AIDS," *Health Education Quarterly* 13 (Winter 1986): 317–330.

37. *New York Times*, 6 July 1986.

38. For an analysis of the difficult social policy questions raised by AIDS, see Ronald Bayer, "AIDS, Power, and Reason," *Milbank Quarterly* 64 (1986): 168–182. On legal issues see Harlon Dalton and Scott Burris, eds., *AIDS and the Law* (New Haven: Yale University Press, 1987).

39. See Leon Eisenberg, "Private Trust/Public Confidence in Science and Medicine: The Genesis of Fear," *Law, Medicine, and Health Care* 14 (1986): 243–249.

40. Robin Marantz Henig, "AIDS: A New Disease's Deadly Odyssey," *New York Times Magazine,* 6 February 1983, 36.

41. See, for example, John H. Knowles, "The Responsibility of the Individual," *Daedalus* 106 (1977): 68; and Robert Carlen, "Against Free Clinics for Sexually Transmitted Diseases," *New England Journal of Medicine* 307 (1982): 1350.

42. Harry Dowling, *Fighting Infection: Conquests of the Twentieth Century* (Cambridge: Harvard University Press, 1977), 228–250; *New York Times,* 23 January 1977.

Images of Plague: Infectious Disease in the Visual Arts

Daniel M. Fox and Diane R. Karp

The word *plague* is of ancient origin. For thousands of years people have used it to describe events that provoked fear and suffering. The modern concept of infectious disease has, however, profoundly changed the way people think about plagues, both in the past and in our own time.

Artists have represented the impact of plagues throughout recorded history. They have necessarily employed the conventions of their time and their medium: the ways they and their audiences agreed to see and represent people and objects. The images on the following pages exemplify some of the ways artists have depicted the experience of plague during the past four centuries. We selected those images from an exhibition we assembled in 1987, "In Time of Plague: Five Centuries of Infectious Disease in the Visual Arts." This exhibition was mounted at the American Museum of Natural History in New York City between January and March of 1988 with support from the Rockefeller Foundation and the museum. The Smithsonian Institution Travelling Exhibition Service is sponsoring a two-year national tour for it, beginning in 1989.

The exhibition included about 120 objects on paper—prints, posters, and photographs—selected to tell two stories. One story is about changing conventions among artists for depicting the effects of physical afflictions that have causes not visible to the unaided eye. The other is about the impact on artists of the gradual emergence of the concept of infectious disease. During the past several centuries, most people in Western nations have come to believe that most illnesses with a sudden onset and a rapid course have distinctive natural histories that, if understood, could lead to their containment, prevention, and even cure. Our two stories embrace the history both of art and of medicine. We have each addressed elsewhere some of the complexities we can only suggest here.[1] The purpose of this group of prints and photographs is to introduce readers to some of the imagery that has been created where art and illness intersect.

The concept of conventions is central to viewing these or any other visual representations. Conventions are the rules by which artists array their subjects, configure space, and use light. Artists of any age choose from the available conventions when they depict the course and consequence of illness, or any other subject. Pictures usually ratify the way contemporaries see. But artists can also use conventions to direct their audiences to new ways of seeing, for example, to new theories of the causes of infectious disease and ways of preventing or treating them.

The artists who made each of the works we present used pictorial languages of conventions that made sense to their contemporaries. Such languages must often be translated for people of other places and times. The final image in our series (fig. 15), for example, will be familiar to most late twentieth-century viewers. Many readers of this book may already have seen Alon Reininger's prize-winning photograph, taken in 1986, of Ken Meeks, a person with AIDS, being cared for by a friend. We recognize the conventions of photojournalism. This is a close-up photograph that encourages us to make up stories about particular human beings and their relationships with other people. Ken Meeks is in the foreground, looking intently at the camera. The composition directs viewers to the lesions of Kaposi's sarcoma on Meeks's arm. Many viewers would note the similarity between the pattern of the lesions and of the dots on his shirt. At the right, in the rear of the room, his friend sits in subdued light, apparently looking at Meeks and the photographer. We have all seen similar photographs of a thousand different subjects. The familiar conventions help us to interpret this one, as the photographer intended, as being about intimacy and caring for a person who is desperately ill.

Another image in the group is also about intimacy and caring (fig. 2), but it was made at a time and place that are so distant that the picture requires more explanation. This engraving by Galle depicts treatment in the sixteenth century for what we now call syphilis. The image would have been as accessible to contemporaries as Reininger's photograph is to us. They would quickly have distinguished the patient's physicians and their helpers from his domestic servants by their dress and activities. The caption would have been as redundant to them as Reininger's is to us. They would have known that the engraving depicted the preparation of a dose of hyacum, a medicine made from a log imported from the Americas and used to treat venereal disease until the twentieth century. Moreover, they would not have needed prompting to interpret the picture on the wall of the patient's room as suggesting the sexual transmission of his disease. Unlike the twentieth-century photograph, this scene is presented in conventions that emphasize both physical and emotional distance. The point of view of Reininger's camera conveys to the viewer a sense of physical proximity and emotional immediacy. His image is about a particular person and his care. Galle's sixteenth-century engraving, in contrast, generalizes about care.

We encourage readers to make similar analyses of the other images we present. For each of them, we provide a caption that identifies its origin and offers some data that will assist in interpretation.

NOTE

1. Diane R. Karp et al., *Ars Medica: Art, Medicine and the Human Condition* (Philadelphia: Philadelphia Museum of Art, 1985); Daniel M. Fox and Christopher Lawrence, *Photographing Medicine: Images and Power in Britain and America since 1840* (Westport, Conn.: Greenwood Press, 1988).

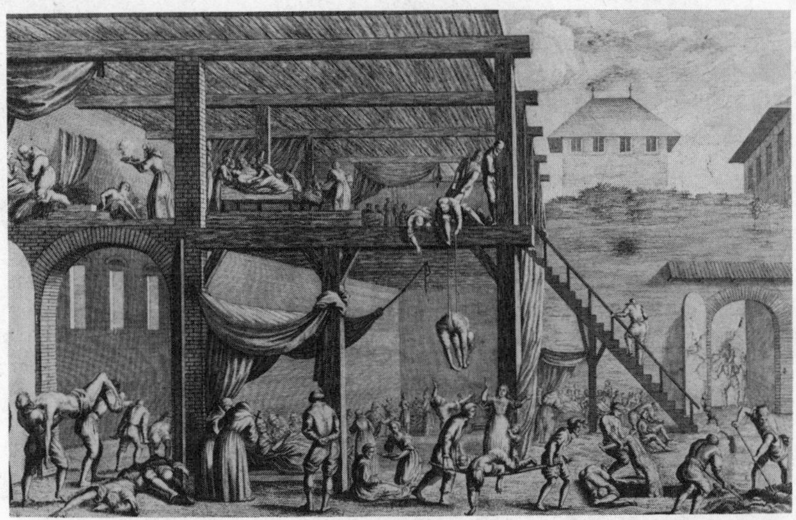

1. Plague Hospital. Sixteenth-century German engraving by Jeremiah Wolff. The New York Public Library, Print Collection.

The original meaning of *hospital* was "place of rest." By the late Middle Ages, hospitals in Western Europe had become institutions for the care of the infirm and dying. During epidemics, buildings of various origins were transformed into hospitals in order to isolate the sick from the healthy, care for the patients, and ease their passage from life into the hereafter. A hospital was a place to rest and die, not to be cured. In this engraving, a building at the edge of town has been designated as a plague hospital. The sick are carried in through the gates at lower right, and at various points in the print we can see patients being fed, cared for, given last rites, and removed to the grave in the foreground before the same gate through which they entered.

HYACVM, ET LVES VENEREA.
Grauata morbo ab hocce membra mollia
Leuabit ista sorpta coctio arboris.

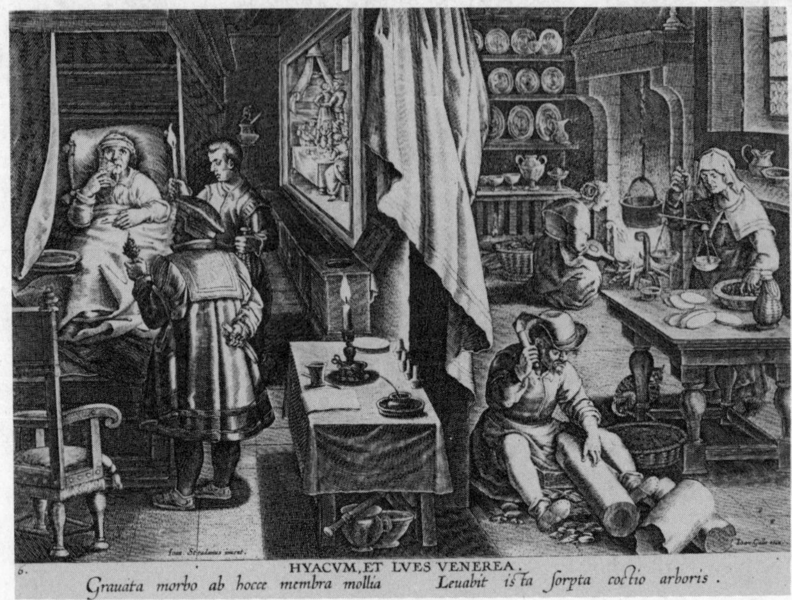

2. Hyacum et Lues Venera. French engraving, c. 1570, by Theodor Galle, after Strada. The New York Public Library, Print Collection.

See the description of this engraving in the introduction to this article.

3. *Opposite:* Examining a Leper. Early sixteenth-century German colored woodcut, possibly Johannes Wechtlin. From *Feldtbuch der Wundartzney* (Strasbourg, 1540). Philadelphia Museum of Art, Ars Medica Collection.

This woodcut appeared in a field manual used primarily by military surgeons and frequently reprinted. Didactic rather than illustrative, the woodcuts were pictorial reports of medical procedures presented in Renaissance style. The use of space is ordered and rational. The figures were simplified and idealized to demonstrate proper medical practice. The quatrains above each drawing summarized the medical knowledge appropriate for the procedure being illustrated. This picture emphasized the medical obligation to treat lepers while it demonstrated the symptoms of the disease. Four doctors examine a patient: One touches the patient's head while describing the symptoms of leprosy in the quatrain (notably distension, stinking breath, and obvious lesions), and the surgeon at the right holds a flask in order to demonstrate the traditional diagnostic technique of uroscopy.

Blůt/harn/knoll/drůßen/glyder fül/
Des athems gſtanck/vnd zeychen vil/
Fürwar red ich/die zöigen an/
Das diſer ſey ein Maltzig man.

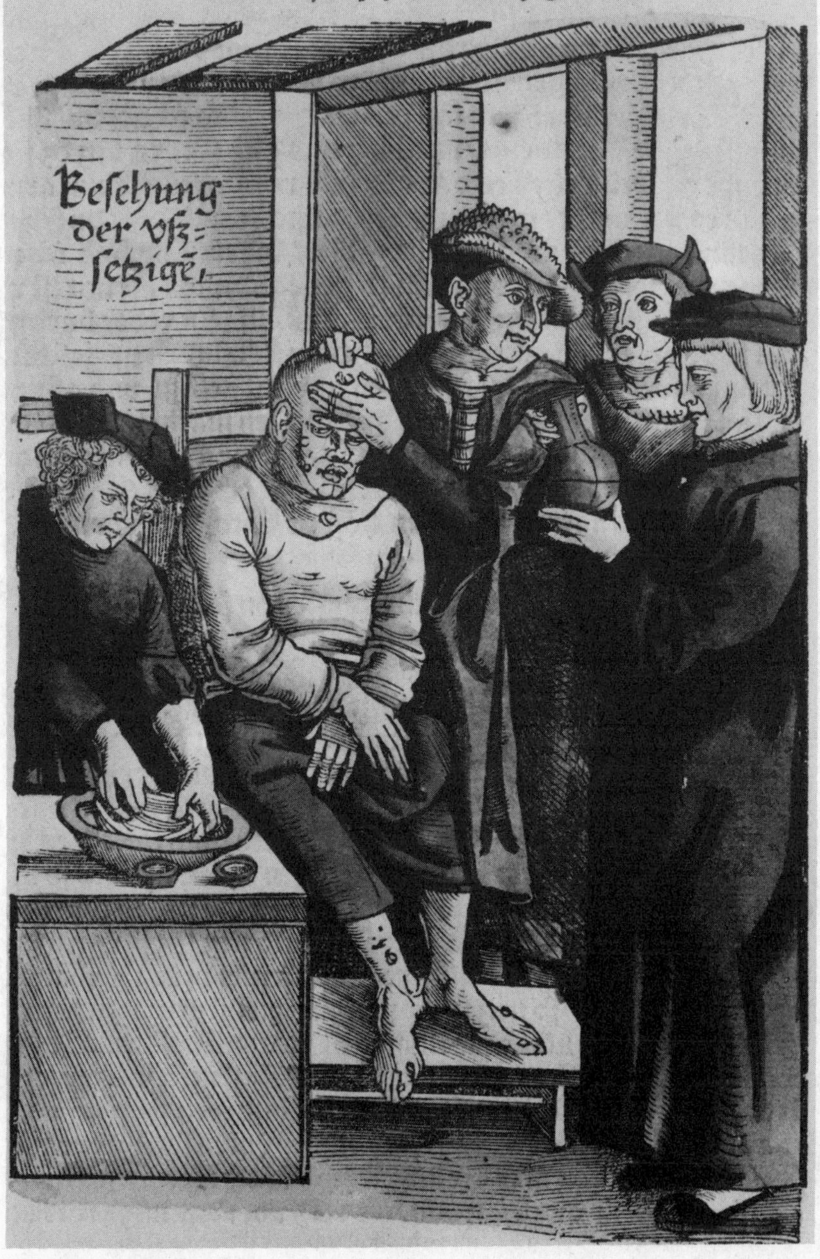

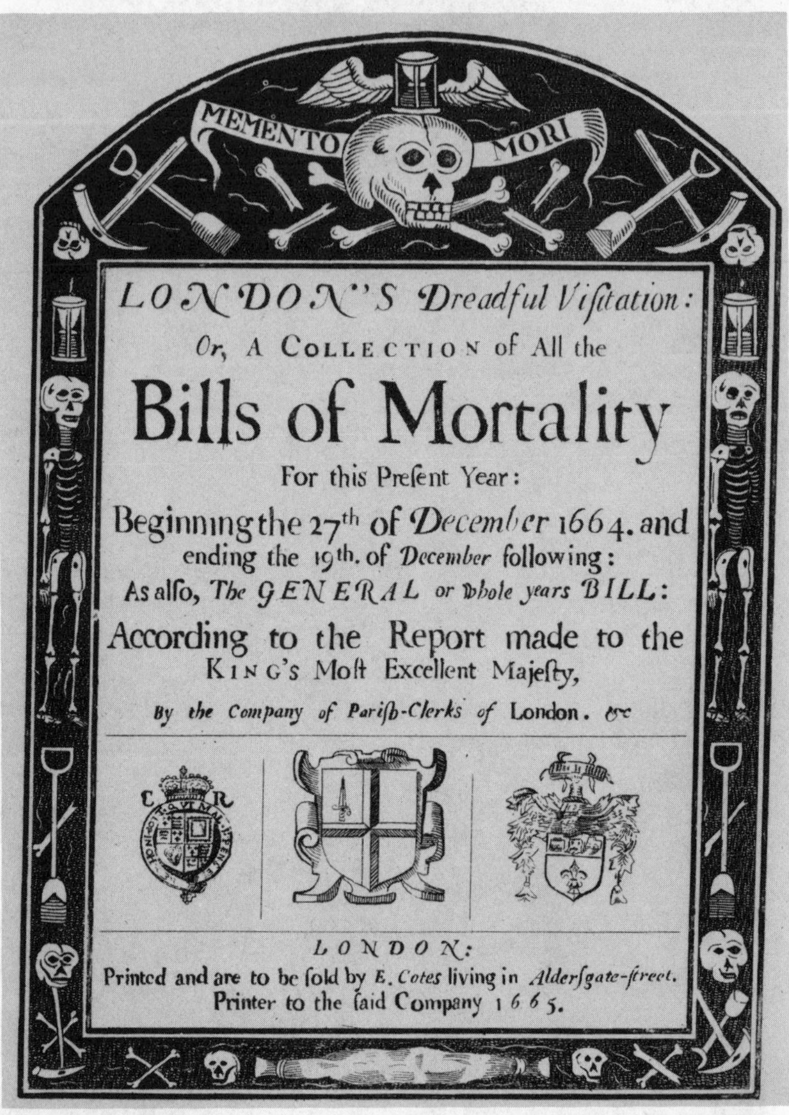

MEMENTO MORI

LONDON'S Dreadful Viſitation:

Or, A COLLECTION of All the

Bills of Mortality

For this Preſent Year:

Beginning the 27th of December 1664. and ending the 19th. of December following:

As alſo, The GENERAL or whole years BILL:

According to the Report made to the KING's Moſt Excellent Majeſty,

By the Company of Pariſh-Clerks of London. &c

C R

LONDON:

Printed and are to be ſold by E. Cotes living in Alderſgate-ſtreet. Printer to the ſaid Company 1665.

4. Frontispiece engraving for *Bills of Mortality* (London, 1665). Wellcome Institute for the History of Medicine, London.

By the seventeenth century some cities published records of the numbers of deaths and their presumed causes. This volume dates from the Great Plague of London in 1664. The *memento mori* embellishments on the border—skulls, winged hourglasses, skeletons, picks and shovels—are allegories. These conventional symbols allow viewers to contemplate death while maintaining emotional distance from the gruesome realities of their everyday lives. They also serve as reminders of the transience of life.

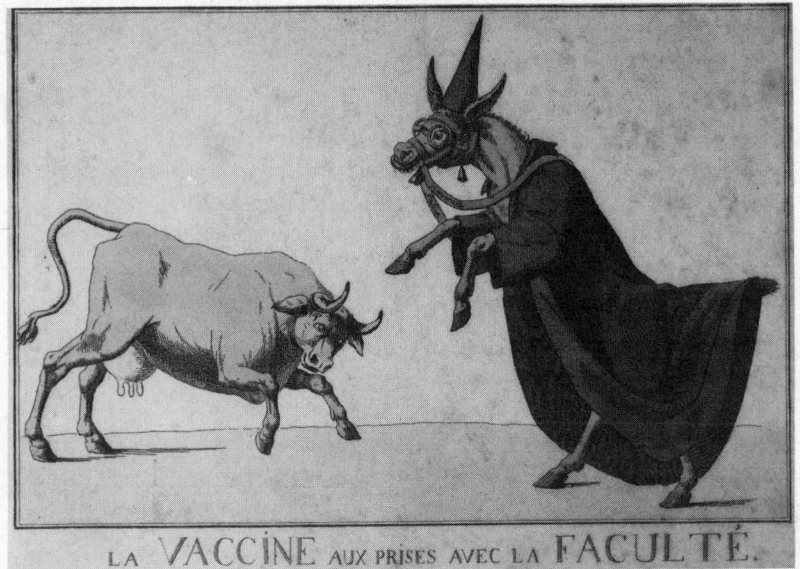

5. La VACCINE aux prises avec la FACULTÉ (Vaccine in Conflict with Academic Medicine). Late eighteenth-century colored etching of the French school. Philadelphia Museum of Art, Ars Medica Collection.

This etching satirizes the controversy over the merits of vaccination against smallpox. The cow, defiantly poised for conflict, symbolizes the medical practitioners and their lay supporters who embraced the potential of mass vaccination. The donkey, dressed in academic robes and bearing the venerable names of Hippocrates and Galen on its reins, represents the leaders of academic medicine who attacked vaccination as a mad deviation from properly informed medical practice. The conventions of the cartoon framed the issues of this debate in concise terms for the public.

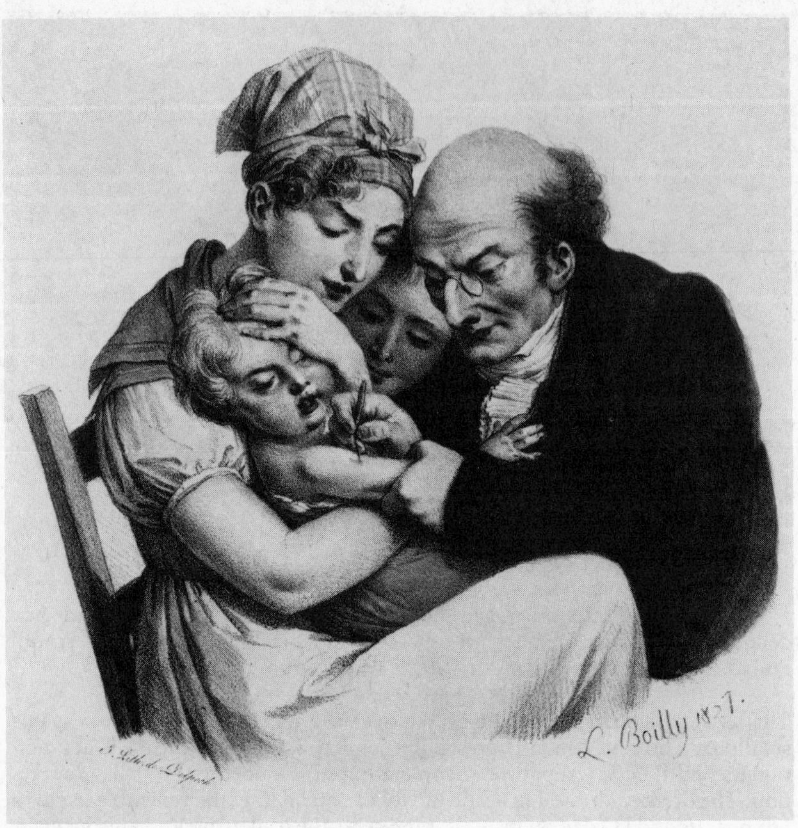

6. La Vaccine. French color lithograph, 1827, by Louis Leopold Boilly. Philadelphia Museum of Art, Ars Medica Collection.

Boilly was well known for his genre portraits of people in all ranks of French life. Here he depicts a household interior where vaccination is taking place. The procedure is now a part of everyday life, rather than a source of controversy as it was then.

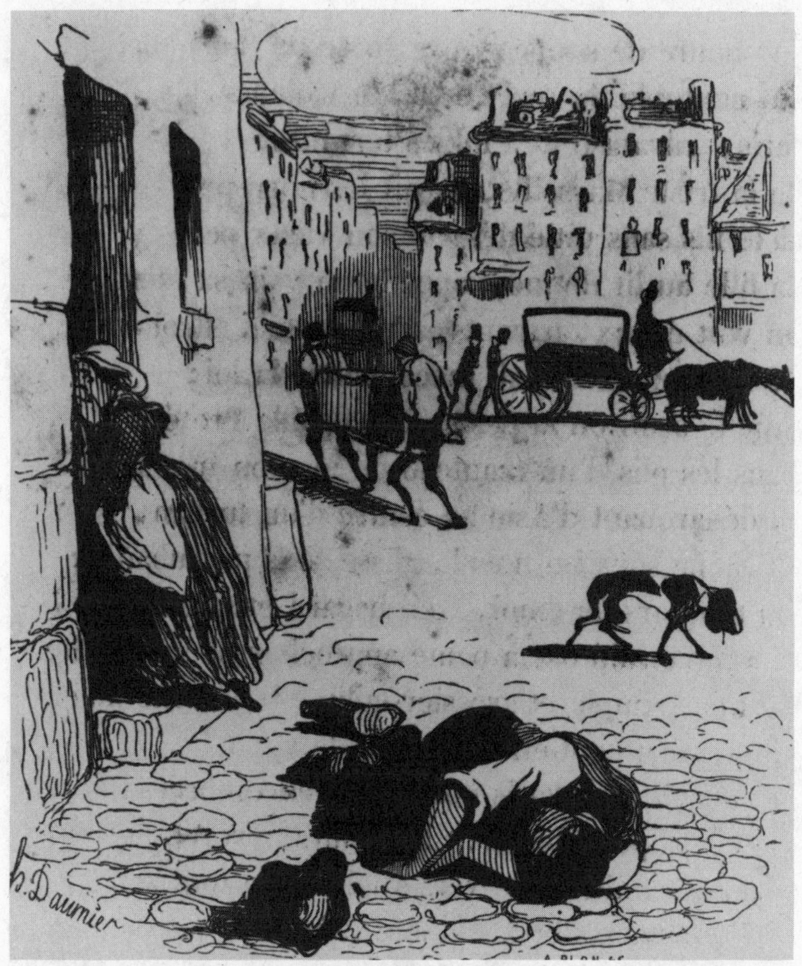

7. Cholera victim. Woodcut from *Némésis médicale illustrée, recueil de satires* (Brussels, 1841) by Antoine François Hippolyte Fabre, after a drawing by Honoré Daumier. National Library of Medicine, History of Medicine Division.

This wood engraving translates a drawing by Daumier, the great chronicler of Parisian life in the pictorial arts, into a printed image presenting the harshness of urban experience in the mid-nineteenth century. During an epidemic, another cholera victim has collapsed in the street and attracts no attention from other people, not even from a dog. The speed and energy of Daumier's lines, which were maintained in Fabre's engraving, present a powerful image of a familiar event.

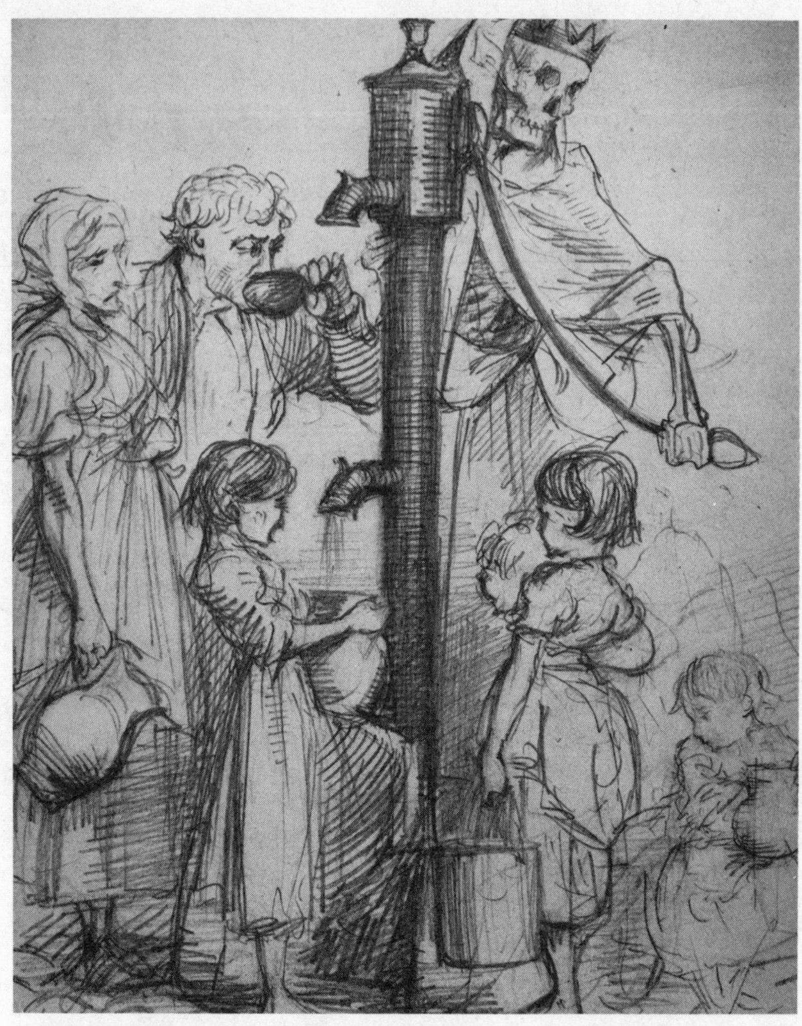

8. Death's Dispensary. English graphite on paper, c. 1866, by George John Pinwell. Philadelphia Museum of Art, Ars Medica Collection.

This powerful drawing by a noted wood engraver and water colorist was a preparatory sketch for an illustration published in the English magazine *Fun* during the outbreak of cholera in London in 1866. By 1866 most physicians and public health officials were convinced that cholera was communicated through the water supply. Pinwell's image, which shows a skeleton figure of cholera working the handle of a pump, dispensing disease to all who imbibe the contaminated water, conveys the horror of the public realization that the population in 1866 might still unwittingly be exposing themselves to disease.

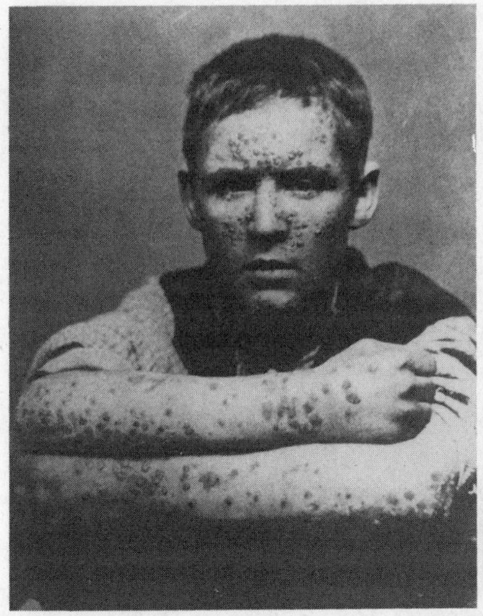
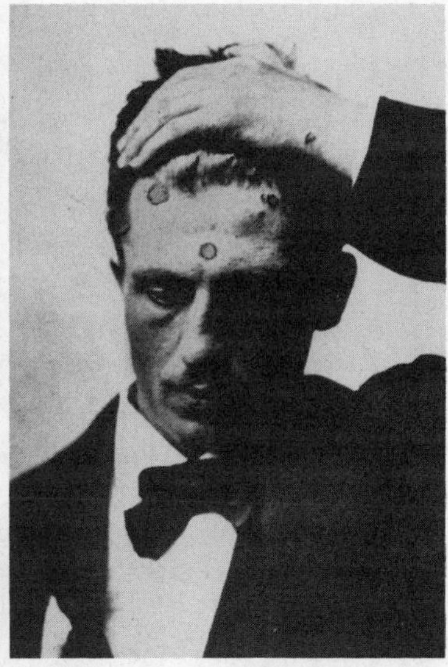

9. Photographic portraits of patients with syphilis. From George Henry Fox, *Photographic Illustration of Cutaneous Syphilis* (1891). Stanley B. Burns, M.D., and the Burns Archive.

In the late nineteenth century many physicians embraced the new technology of photography to document pathological anatomies. They appropriated for this purpose the conventions of contemporary portraiture in drawing and painting. These contrasting portraits depict the scourge of syphilis from two points of view. The boy, photographed with his arms folded to show his lesions and looking directly at the camera, is an innocent victim of heredity. The man, depicted in formal clothes with his upraised arm calling attention to the lesions on his forehead, his eyes averted from the camera, would have been recognized by contemporaries as a rake.

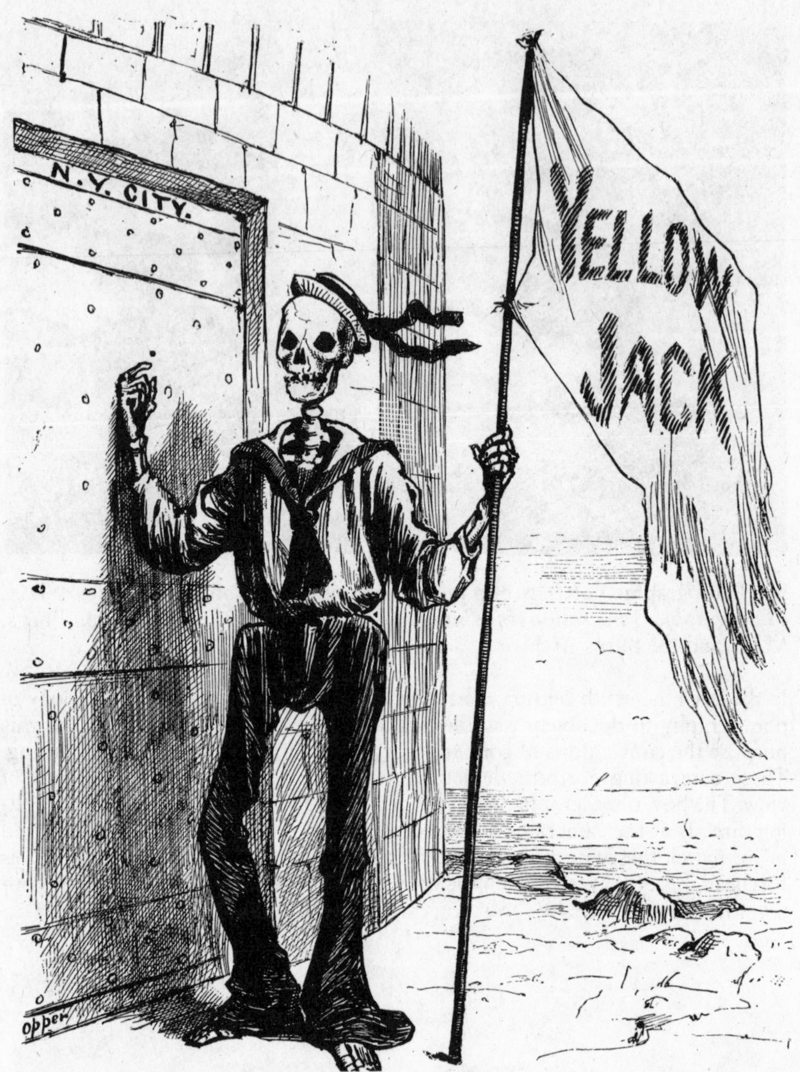

10. Yellow Jack. Engraving from *Frank Leslie's Illustrated Newspaper,* 21 September 1883. New York Academy of Medicine.

In this cartoon, Death, dressed in the uniform of an Italian sailor, brings yellow fever—popularly called Yellow Jack—to New York's door. The cartoon's social and political implications during a decade when millions of immigrants arrived in American ports needed no caption. A century later, when the authors exhibited this cartoon in New York City, it was widely reprinted, presumably because of its direct analogy with the AIDS epidemic.

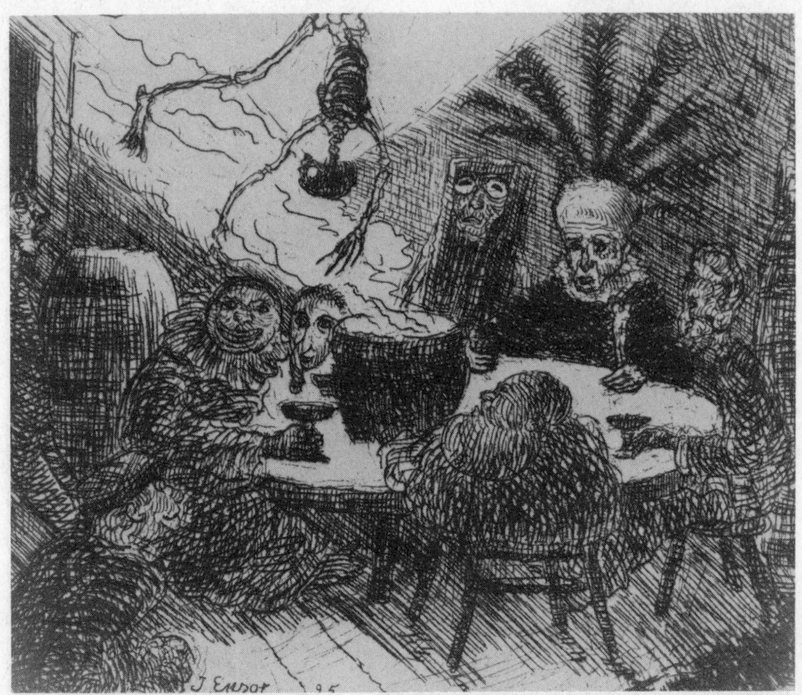

11. Le Roi Peste (King Plague). Belgian etching, 1895, by James Ensor. National Library of Medicine, History of Medicine Division.

James Ensor, painter and printmaker, combined an understanding of the tragic mystery of nature with malevolent humor. For most of his creative life he was obsessed with the specter of death, depicting it in myriad social and personal situations. In this etching, he was inspired by "King Pest," a story written by Edgar Allan Poe, whose work fueled the Symbolist-Expressionist movement in Europe. In an undertaker's room where a skeleton hangs from the ceiling, King Pest the First carouses with his ghoulish council. In literature and the fine arts, plague remained a powerful theme in the late nineteenth century, even as its epidemiological significance diminished.

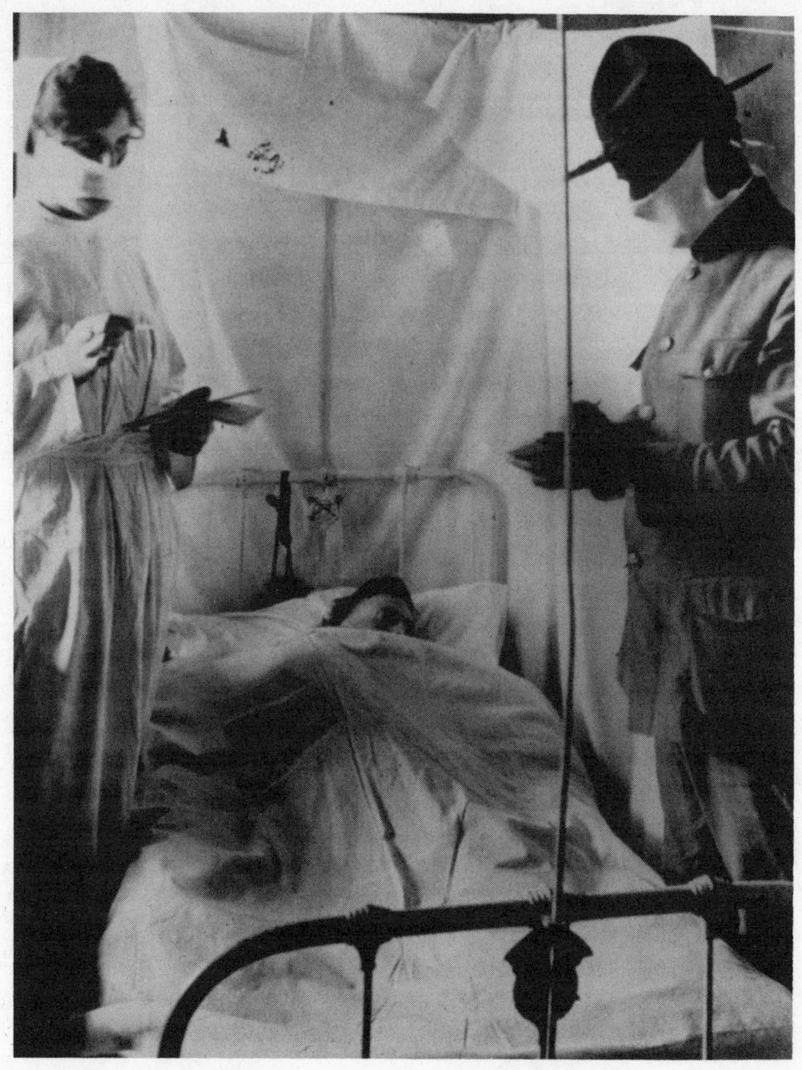

12. Army camp, New York State. By an unknown photographer, 1918. American Red Cross.

An influenza epidemic claimed more than half a million lives in Europe and America in 1918–1919. Photographers depicted medical care during the epidemic with conventions that had been changing rapidly for two decades—change that was accelerated during World War I. According to these newer conventions, photographers moved closer to their subjects in order to communicate stories about human relationships. Unlike the figures in the portraits in fig. 9, the patient here is shown with a physician and a nurse who are working—protected from contagion, they hoped—by face masks.

LIGUE NATIONALE FRANÇAISE CONTRE LE PÉRIL VÉNÉRIEN
LA COURSE A LA MORT
TUBERCULOSE
SYPHILIS
CANCER
TUBERCULOSE : 150.000 MORTS PAR AN
SYPHILIS : 140.000 " "
CANCER : 40.000 "
AFFICHE ADOPTÉE PAR LA COMMISSION GÉNÉRALE DE PROPAGANDE DE L'OFFICE NATIONAL D'HYGIÈNE SOCIALE

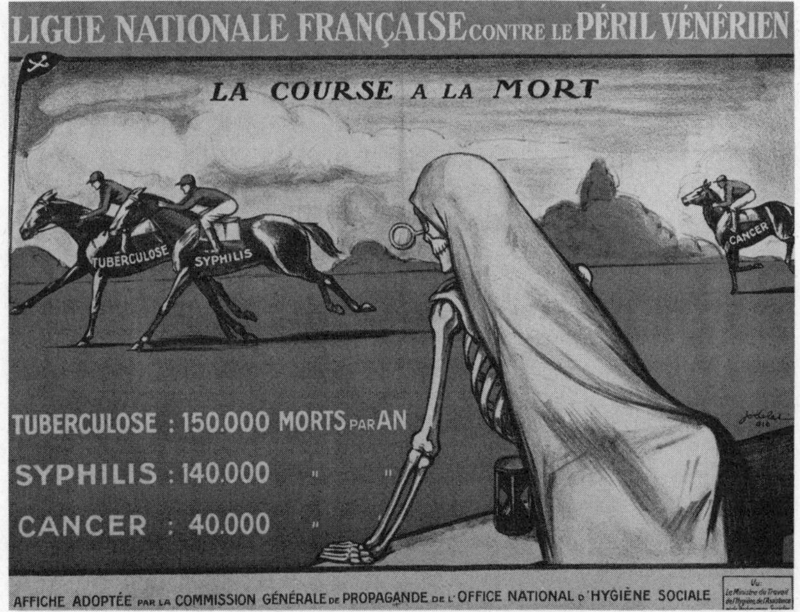

13. La Course à la Mort (The Race to Death). French colored lithograph, c. 1926, by Jodalet. Philadelphia Museum of Art, Gift of William H. Helfand.

This powerful propagandistic lithograph was published by the National Office of Social Hygiene as part of the public campaign of the National French League against Venereal Disease. Using popular imagery rather than conventions of high art, Jodalet places us at the rail along with a macabre personification of death, draped in a shroud, watching the progress of this modern apocalyptic race through a magnifying glass. We are reminded of the Four Horsemen of the Apocalypse, who trample the rich and the poor alike. The three horsemen here—tuberculosis, syphilis, and cancer—are, it would seem, about to be joined by a mysterious fourth before the hourglass (a *memento mori* image, as in fig. 4) runs down.

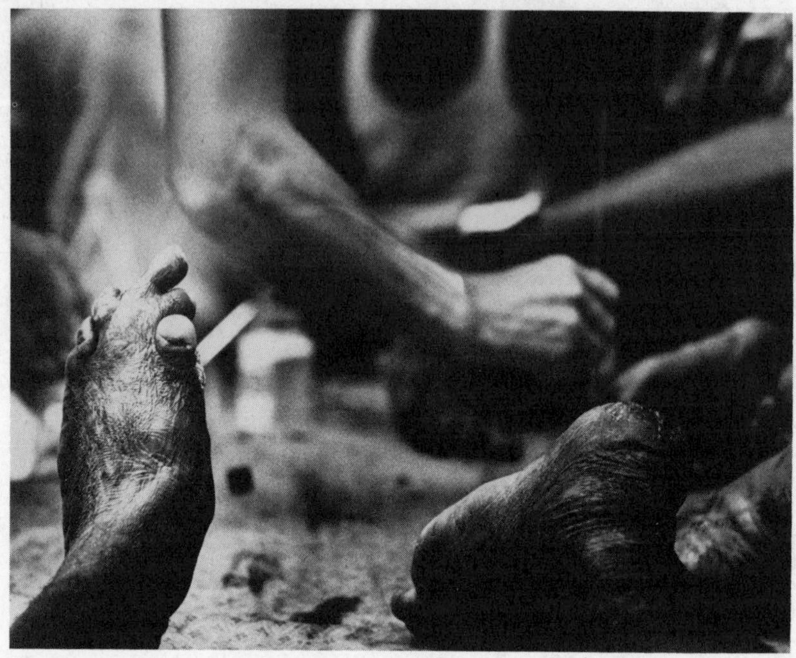

14. Leprosy from "A Man of Mercy." Photograph, 1954, by W. Eugene Smith. Black Star.

This photograph of a man suffering from leprosy presents with clarity and directness the harsh reality of a disease that, although associated with the Middle Ages, remains widespread today. Rather than focusing on the patient, Smith depicts the disease and the deformity in a way that initially appears to be clinical. Smith was one of the foremost photojournalists of his generation, however, and he took this photograph to illustrate a *Life* magazine essay on the work of Dr. Albert Schweitzer. Thus, the interplay of the leper's feet and the arm of the unknown person above him creates a story that suggests truth, power, and humanity. The image is beautiful and haunting, despite its subject matter.

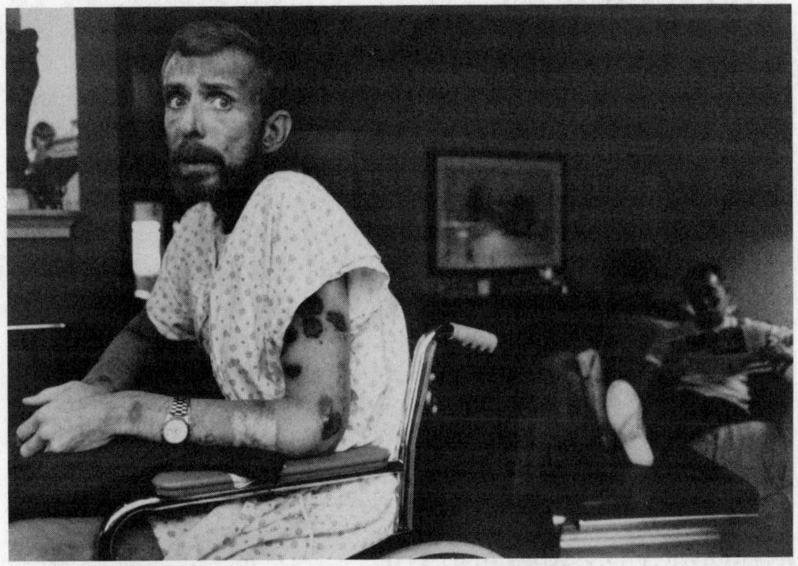

15. Patient with AIDS, Ken Meeks, being cared for by a friend. Photograph, 1986, by Alon Reininger. Contact Press Images.

This image is analyzed in the introduction to this article.

AIDS, Gender, and Biomedical Discourse: Current Contests for Meaning

Paula A. Treichler

INTRODUCTION: AIDS AND THE CHALLENGE TO SEMANTIC IMPERIALISM

Colin Douglas's 1975 novel *The Intern's Tale* (set in a teaching hospital in Edinburgh) savages virtually every aspect of modern academic medicine—including its rampant and unreflective sexism. The book betrays its satire at the end, however, when two of the interns, Campbell and his friend, Mac, hospitalized with hepatitis B, deduce that the source of their infection is that well-known villain, the sexually active, unmarried woman:

> Campbell sat silent, with a ghastly sensation of falling and accelerating and knowing that the worst feeling was still to come. When it did it was a horrible realisation.
>
> "Christ! It's bloody Maggie!"
>
> "What is?" said Mac gently.
>
> "Maggie. Spreading it. Giving us bloody hepatitis."
>
> . . ."Christ yes. It all fits." . . .
>
> "Listen," said Campbell. "This is nasty and I'm sorry but it's important. When you were stopping by with old Maggie, did you use . . . what you might call an obstructive method of contraception?"
>
> "Nope," said Mac. "Bareback."
>
> "Charming. Me too. . . . I didn't because she said something about just finishing a period."
>
> "That's not true. Not that week anyway. But she's got something far wrong with her cycle. Always dripping."[1]

It is a commonplace of feminist scholarship to claim that medical discourse represents women's bodies as pathological and contaminated.[2] But as this fictional conversation suggests, these representations bear complex historical burdens. Contamination is certainly one feature of Woman here: Maggie—an unmarried nurse generally regarded as a readily compliant sexual object—is suddenly transformed into an unruly agent of disease, actively "spreading" hepatitis to her sexual partners, including many of the hospital's medical staff. As they compare notes, the interns find she has lied to them, passing off the symptoms of serious pathology as a routine female complaint: Her lie can only succeed, of course, because both interns are ready to attribute the signs of pathology to the expected vicissitudes of the female menstrual cycle.[3] Thus, Maggie, like women elsewhere in the book and elsewhere in the history of medicine, is not what she seems.[4] From the perspective of the interns, she has tricked them into the potentially fatal risk of having intercourse "bareback," without protective contraception. Maggie's sexuality infects them with the possibility of their own mortality; at the same time, they express no concern about hers. For she who appeared to be a victim is now revealed as a deeply duplicitous perpetrator, a mimic of the symptoms and illnesses of others: Her dupes are the interns, whose only crime was to behave like "real men."[5]

The language as well as the narrative itself enacts this judgment. The carrier of "bloody hepatitis" is herself called "bloody Maggie"; the adjective *bloody,* linking the carrier, or source, of the disease with the disease itself, suggests indeed that Maggie, not a virus, causes hepatitis: she who is infect*ed* is simultaneously both infect*ious* (a state or condition) and infect*ing* (an active agent of disease). The word *bloody* also doubles as a literal description of Maggie's offcycle bleeding and as a broader cultural epithet (in American English, *fucking* doubles in a similar way). The images of diseased blood and body fluid invoke a long tradition in scientific and medical writing (see Ludvik Fleck's account of the history of syphilis, for example, where "bad blood" was a central concept).[6] With respect to the medical construction of women's bodies, a final point here is that men are the constructors, women the constructed. Despite the attribution of active agency to Maggie as a source of pathology, it is only the two male interns, the physician-scientists, who actively bring mind and knowledge to bear upon the situation. They alone have the right to analyze the situation with an appropriately trained "clinical eye" and to engage in those key activities of privileged theorizing, diagnosis of the disease, and authoritative identification of its cause.[7] Heirs of an ancient medical legacy of semantic and gendered imperialism, they define Maggie without hesitation as "bloody" and "always dripping." No longer containable through cultural pressure or moral prescription, freely infecting man after man, the sexually active container must therefore be contained. Their words contain, but also silence her.[8]

This chapter is about the ways that words, or more precisely, discourse, enact and reinforce deeply entrenched, pervasive, and often conservative cultural "narratives" about gender; it is also about how words seek, ultimately, to contain and control women's unruly and "uncontainable" properties. I will focus my discussion, first, on constructions of gender in the biomedical discourse on AIDS and, second, on the reverberations of this discourse in other writing about gender and AIDS.[9] Why AIDS? Because the discourse on AIDS—recent but already voluminous—reenacts many of the semantic battles that have characterized relations between women and biomedical science for at least the last century. AIDS takes us to the heart of feminist inquiry (indeed, of all the "human sciences"), including the question of how sex and sexuality are constructed; it also demonstrates how language can give the illusion of control. In the case of AIDS, however, the epidemic disease is so deeply complex at this point that control is out of the question.

In 1981 the official history of AIDS as a clinically defined entity began. Involving at first a small number of sexually active gay men, AIDS rapidly shifted to involve a larger and more heterogeneous male population, homosexual and nonhomosexual; by mid-1982, people with AIDS included intravenous users of heroin (and other drugs) who shared needles; Haitians; hemophiliacs; and others who had received injected blood or blood products. By early 1983 a small number of women were also diagnosed with AIDS, evidently infected via intravenous drug use or transfusions with contaminated blood, and by mid-1983 via male sexual partners with AIDS. Shortly thereafter heterosexual men with AIDS were identified whose sexual partner(s) had been infected females, demonstrating that women could both infect and be infected with HIV, human immunodeficiency virus. By 1984 there were reports from some central African countries (later fully documented) that almost as many women there had AIDS as men. A relationship between women and AIDS has thus existed for most of the known lifespan of the disease.[10]

This relationship, however, presents us with a series of mysteries. First, given the scientifically documented diagnoses of women with [illegible] why was AIDS simply assumed by the medical and scientific community to be transmitted only by gay men? Second, given the skepticism toward established science and medicine fostered for two decades by feminist activism and scholarship, why have relatively few feminists challenged biomedical accounts of AIDS or, with the exception of some lesbian writers and activists, called for solidarity with the gay male community? Finally, above all, given the intense concern with the human body that any conceptualization of AIDS entails, how can we account for the striking silence, until very recently, on the topic of women in AIDS discourse (including biomedical journals, mainstream news publications, public health literature, women's magazines, and the gay and feminist press)? As noted above, the real and imagined links between women's bodies and disease—especially infectious and sexually transmitted disease—are many and complex, and have a history reaching back many centuries. This is a subject, then, with heavy baggage—and the bags are already packed. Yet women have repeatedly been told that *this* time they would not be traveling, that they would not need the bags. If they were in the airport at all, it was for someone else's flight.

In the fall of 1986 all this changed: The Centers for Disease Control (CDC) in Atlanta reclassified a significant number of "unexplained" AIDS cases as having been heterosexually transmitted to and from women.[11] The National Academy of Sciences / National Institute of Medicine issued a blue-ribbon report warning the nation that AIDS was heterosexually transmissible both to and from women and men, making an urgent call for nationwide health education.[12] United States Surgeon General C. Everett Koop held a press conference to announce that he, too, now viewed AIDS as a potential threat to every sexually active person and to advocate the immediate institution of explicit sex education for everyone more than eight years of age.[13] The World Health Organization (WHO) confirmed what many had suspected: AIDS was devastating the populations of at least four African countries, where half of those with AIDS are women. AIDS has now been reported in more than 100 countries around the world and is now considered a pandemic health problem of catastrophic proportions.[14] In the United States, infection with HIV is estimated by some to be increasing among heterosexually active women and men (while rates of infection among sexually active gay men appear to have leveled off, though new AIDS cases and deaths remain high). "Suddenly," proclaimed the cover story of *U.S. News and World Report* in January 1987, "the disease of *them* is the disease of *us*"; and "us" is represented graphically in the magazine by a young, white, urban professional man and woman, a problematic representation to which I shall return.[15] The main point here is that the population of people with AIDS now unquestionably includes women who appear to have become infected exclusively by way of sexual contact with infected men.

So, what a surprise to find ourselves in midair over the Atlantic without even a toothbrush packed—let alone a barrier contraceptive. The mystery is: Why were women so unprepared? And why do they continue to take it so quietly?

The construction in the United States of AIDS as essentially a male-only, sexually transmitted disease depends upon the production and reproduction of gendered readings whose reasonings are so outlandish and speculative as to be dizzying. In turn, this "knowledge" of AIDS infection and who can catch it filters out counterevidence in a variety of ways, creating a cycle of invisibility in which women do not believe themselves vulnerable and therefore do not seek medical care or even confidential testing. Despite this clinical history, moreover, women with AIDS have not been readily identifiable in the scientific literature. The pie-shaped charts typically depict the classic 4-H "risk groups"—homosexuals, heroin addicts, hemophiliacs, and Haitians—plus their sex partners, gender often unspecified—plus "Other."[16] To those familiar with feminist theory of the last two decades, the placing of women with AIDS under the literal rubric of "Other" possesses considerable irony and resonates with the ongoing construction of *otherness* in the history of venereal disease.[17] But, beyond irony, such otherness is dangerous because it creates a category of invisibility and it muddles information, both for those who have been or are at risk and for those who are responsible for identifying AIDS and its multiple manifestations. Thus, even after information about AIDS was widespread, many women did not believe they were at risk. Even today, women who finally seek care from health professionals may not be properly diagnosed, either because they are simply not seen to be at risk (whatever their symptoms) or because they do not display the symptoms (defined by the natural history of the disease in gay men) that officially denote the presence of AIDS and ARC (AIDS-related complex). Women's invisibility is created in other unexpected ways: One New York City writer, having heard in 1987 that "heterosexuals" were now considered at risk for AIDS, quizzed his white, middle-class female acquaintances and reported in the *New York Times Magazine* not a case of AIDS (or HIV infection) among them; as a nurse at Brookdale Hospital in Brooklyn acerbically pointed out in a subsequent letter to the editor, the writer would have compiled quite different statistics had he explored the populations of poor people—primarily black and Hispanic, but also white—in the area surrounding her hospital.[18] Such examples of women's invisibility in the AIDS discourse reinforce the widespread perception of AIDS as an illness of sexually active gay men and of illegal-drug users; it is based, then, on scientific constructions that have glossed over the "Other" despite growing evidence that the category includes women (and men) who have been infected with AIDS by way of heterosexual intercourse of the boy-meets-girl / missionary position / no-frills variety.[19]

AIDS is debilitating, lethal, and in many respects still mysterious; some authorities regard it as the greatest health crisis of our era. The scientific label *AIDS* is normally construed to refer to a real clinical syndrome, an infectious condition caused by a virus and increasingly understood by the scientists and physicians who study it. But the relationship between language and reality is highly problematic, for scientists and physicians as well as for "the rest of us." Although we have come to accept the findings of biomedical science as accurate characterizations of material reality, scientific and medical discourses are always provisional, and only "true" or "real" in certain specific ways—in confirming prior research findings, for example, or in promoting effective clinical treatments. "AIDS" does not merely label an illness caused by a virus. In part, the name *constructs* the illness and helps us make sense of it. We cannot, therefore, look through discourse to determine what AIDS "really" is. Rather, we must explore the place where such determinations occur: in discourse itself, which is inevitably marked by our struggles to represent what we *think* AIDS really is and to conceptualize what it *really* means.

To talk of AIDS as a linguistic construction is not, of course, to claim that it exists only in the mind. Like other phenomena, AIDS is real, and utterly indifferent to what we say about it. Documented by news reports, medical records, photographs and journals, scientific research, conferences, and individual and collective experience, something is happening that real people are dying of. Whatever we call it, however we think about or represent it, we cannot wish AIDS away. Our names and representations can nevertheless influence our cultural relationship to the disease and, indeed, its present and future course. Accordingly, we struggle in many fragmentary and often contradictory ways to grasp the true nature of AIDS; yet, finally, this is neither directly nor fully knowable. It may be tempting, even irresistible, to understand the epidemic as a temporary problem involving incomplete scientific and medical knowledge—certainly many familiar cultural narratives encourage this view—and to presume that we will eventually be provided a scientific account of AIDS closer to its reality. Moreover, to speak of AIDS as a linguistic construction that acquires meaning only in relation to networks of given signifying practices may seem to be both politically and pragmatically dubious, like philosophizing in the middle of a war zone. But as I have argued elsewhere, making sense of AIDS compels us to address questions of signification and representation.[20] When we deduce from the facts that AIDS is an infectious, sexually transmitted disease syndrome caused by a virus, what is it we are making sense of? "Infection," "sexually transmitted," "disease," and "virus" are also linguistic constructs that generate meaning and simultaneously facilitate and constrain our ability to think and talk about material phenomena. Language is not a substitute for reality; it is how we know it. And if we do not know *that,* all the facts in the world will not help us.

AIDS and its related conditions present us with an unprecedentedly complex set of social and scientific problems. If we are to address these problems with foresight, intelligence, and decency, it is crucial that we take into account the nature of language and acknowledge AIDS's enormous power to generate meanings we can never fully control. This chapter seeks to illuminate the relationship of AIDS to gender through an analysis of language, meaning, and discourse; I use analytic strategies from the sociology of science, cultural studies, and feminist theory to review the evolving constructions of gender in AIDS discourse and examine how women are situated within that discourse. The chapter is organized, roughly, around the chronology of the AIDS crisis: (1) evolving biomedical understandings of AIDS (1981–1985); (2) Rock Hudson's illness and death as a turning point in national consciousness (July 1985–December 1986); (3) AIDS perceived as a pandemic disease to which sexually active heterosexuals are vulnerable (fall 1986–spring 1987); (4) diversification of discourse about women and AIDS (spring 1987–present); and (5) implications for the future.

Broadly, I seek to explain the paradox sketched above: When history, culture, and language link women to disease in many ways, why, until very recently, were these links to AIDS erased or denied? And now, finally included in the AIDS discourse, will women contest the meanings and implications offered by the past, refuse the scripts from the theater of history? I suggest that an uncompromising feminist analysis can contest the fixed notions of scientific certainty and disrupt the familiar cultural narratives. Where AIDS is concerned, for example, the entrenched division between "them" and "us"—men and women, guilty and innocent, gay men and "the rest of us"—is deeply problematic. Based on simplified, unitary identities and essentialist biological or social categories that serve only to reinscribe conceptual and ideological divisions, the "us"–"them" division represents a form of semantic imperialism we cannot afford in the present crisis.

Purporting to describe the natural world, this division at first gave women the false belief they were invulnerable. But as evidence of women's potential risk became clear, so did the theoretical schisms in accounts of AIDS. This revelation should have demonstrated how tenuous the current conceptualizations are; it should have fundamentally challenged the validity of *any* division of "the disease of them" from "the disease of us." Yet most discourse by and about women embraces this division, simply rearranging the contents of the categories to match the latest bulletins from Washington, Atlanta, or Paris, and advising "us" (women) to protect ourselves from "them" (men). It does nothing to unseat the notion that "them" (whoever they are) is an expendable category of people, while "us" is a category of people worth saving. Despite all we have learned about the social construction of sexual difference and how it has been used against women in the past, the categorization process is given little scrutiny in the case of AIDS. By questioning, therefore, what is often taken for granted in discussions of AIDS, I hope to illuminate its multiple dimensions, intricacies, and contradictions, and, in doing so, to contribute toward the development of policies that fully acknowledge the intractable complexity of this crisis.

THE EVOLVING BODY OF THE GENDERED "AIDS PATIENT" IN BIOMEDICAL DISCOURSE

The existence of AIDS as an official clinical syndrome is generally dated from the report of the deaths of five gay men in Los Angeles from *Pneumocystis* pneumonia in the June 5, 1981, issue of the *Morbidity and Mortality Weekly Report* (*MMWR*), published by the Centers for Disease Control in Atlanta. The paper, by Drs. Michael Gottlieb and Wayne Shandera of the University of California at Los Angeles (UCLA), had been routed in May by Dr. Mary Guinan to Dr. James W. Curran, head of the CDC's venereal disease division; he returned it to her with a note: "Hot stuff. Hot stuff."[21] Although Gottlieb had initially thought nothing of the fact that his first *Pneumocystis* patient was gay (he considered it equivalent to "the fact that the guy might drive a Ford"[22]), he had decided by the time the paper was written that this was an outbreak of a new illness specific to gay men. The *MMWR* bulletin put it this way: "The occurrence of pneumocystosis in these 5 previously healthy individuals without a clinically apparent underlying immunodeficiency is unusual. The fact that these patients were all homosexuals suggests an association between some aspect of homosexual lifestyle or disease acquired through sexual contact and *Pneumocystis* pneumonia in this population."[23] The men who died from these first reported cases were not only gay, they had histories of multiple sexual contacts and of multiple sexually transmitted diseases (STDs). The published report confirmed the suspicions of physicians in other cities: Some of their gay patients were contracting and even dying from very strange diseases, including rare forms of pneumonia and cancer. What had been unofficially called "gay pneumonia" and "gay cancer" and WOGS (the Wrath of God Syndrome) now provisionally came to be called GRID: Gay-related immunodeficiency.

But in the months following the report in the *MMWR* and subsequently in other journals, these same rare diseases began to be diagnosed in people who were not gay—for example, in intravenous drug users, in hemophiliacs, and in people who had recently had blood transfusions. Despite widespread reluctance to acknowledge possible connections, there were enough nonhomosexual cases to render GRID an unsuitable diagnosis, and in 1982 the name "AIDS" was selected at a conference in Washington, D.C.[24] As it evolved during 1981 and 1982, the official CDC list of populations at risk for AIDS came to consist of the "4-H" group: homosexuals, hemophiliacs, heroin addicts, and Haitians; by 1983 the sexual partners of people within these groups had been added.[25] This list structured the collection of evidence for the next several years and contributed to the view that the major risk factor in acquiring AIDS was being a particular kind of person rather than doing particular things.

Outside the narrow, controlled, official account were disturbing exceptions: reports that in Africa women and men were afflicted with AIDS in equal numbers, observations of babies with AIDS-like symptoms, rumors of AIDS in men who had never used drugs nor had sexual contact with other men, reports of lesbians with AIDS.[26] In retrospect, it makes a tidy story to identify the tensions, ambivalences, and contradictions of this period as something simple: scientific conservatism, homophobia, denial, politicians' fears. Certainly there were instances of predictable reflex behavior: the *Wall Street Journal,* like many other publications, published nothing about AIDS until "innocent victims" could be identified.[27] Some representatives of the far right were quick to seize on AIDS as new proof of the evils of a world gone soft on pleasure, communism, or both.[28] The discourse of this period and comprehensive accounts published since then demonstrate the complexity of social responses to a conglomeration of mysterious symptoms and fatal illnesses not yet well conceptualized. This is by no means to deny the profound discrimination that existed then and continues today (to which I shall return) but is rather to emphasize that at this stage many important questions were going unanswered. The conflict and contradictions among gay men, among members of the medical and scientific communities, among government officials, among reporters—all of whom by turns perceived AIDS as a gay disease and then denied that it could be, predicted a spread of AIDS to other groups and then rejected such a possibility—might also be understood as part of the process of making sense of problematic and frightening evidence.[29] It is important for the future that the past not be oversimplified. Although Randy Shilts's comprehensive book on the AIDS crisis, *And the Band Played On,* for example, demonstrates many points at which bias against and fear of homosexuals hampered public attention and fundraising, Dennis Altman notes that had AIDS first struck intravenous drug users and Haitians rather than the politically sophisticated and well-organized gay community, funding and publicity would undoubtedly have been even more meager and delayed.[30] Policy analyst Sandra Panem, reviewing charges that homophobia delayed federal research efforts, concluded that prejudice against homosexuality per se would not have deterred ambitious scientists from initiating interesting and rewarding research projects. But ignorance, she suggests, does appear to have played a role, citing as evidence a 1984 observation by James W. Curran, by then head of the CDC's AIDS task force, that among scientists there is little widespread research interest in sexuality of any kind and "not much understanding of homosexuality." Indeed, Curran went on to say that many eminent scientists during these early years rejected the possibility that AIDS was an infectious disease because they had no idea how one man could transmit an infectious virus to another; through what orifice could such a virus possibly enter a male body, lacking as it did the vaginal portal approved for the receipt of sperm?[31]

The subsequent scientific and medical obsession with the details of male homosexual practices was in part a compensatory by-product, I believe, of this dramatic ignorance among many scientists at the outset. But only in part: For a number of scientists and physicians first involved in AIDS were either gay or familiar with the gay community. Many CDC staff members had worked closely with the gay community in the course of research on hepatitis B and had few illusions about sexual practices and sexual diversity, and were aware that not all gay men were active with multiple partners. Further, as the infected population grew, it became clear that gay men were everywhere—in politics, in Congress, on Wall Street, in Hollywood, in far-right organizations. In many cases, they were silent and invisible—unlike women and racial minorities. Part of the shock of AIDS was thus the shock of identity.[32]

Whatever else it may be, however, AIDS in the United States came to be a story of gay men and a construction of a hypothetical male homosexual body. Obsession, a repeated feature of the AIDS story, is also a feature of the fact that, in some ways, the gay man is what Mary Poovey calls a "border case." A "border case" threatens a heavily invested binary division in society (such as the nineteenth-century dichotomy of women by class and how it was threatened by prostitutes) that generates the need for discourse to restore stability. (The voluminous discourse on prostitution during this period, Poovey argues, was thus fundamentally about class.)[33] The ongoing fixation with HIV testing is in part designed to put a stop to gay men's successful passing as straight; refusal to take the HIV-antibody test is therefore similar to pleading the Fifth.[34]

A number of hypotheses and speculations were put forward during this period about the nature of the AIDS epidemic: its dimensions, causes, newness, its theoretical, scientific, and political implications, and its consequences.[35] Despite lack of understanding, scientific and journalistic gatekeeping was evident from virtually the beginning—with one effect being the disinclination of editors and journals to suggest that AIDS was caused by an infectious agent.[36] When the first cases appeared in New York, Los Angeles, and Paris, the early hypotheses tended to be sociological, relating the disease directly to some feature of a supposed "gay male life-style." For example, in February 1982 it was hypothesized that a particular supply of amyl nitrate (or "poppers") might be contaminated. But "the poppers fable," writes French scientist Jacques Leibowitch, became "a Grimm fairy tale when the first cases of AIDS-without-poppers [were] discovered among homosexuals absolutely repelled by the smell of the product and among heterosexuals unfamiliar with even the words *amyl nitrate* or *poppers*."[37] Another view was that sperm itself could destroy the immune system. "God's plan for

IF...
Steve Bell
ACCURSED ARE THE MASTURBATORS; ACCURSED ARE THE FAGGOTS;
ACCURSED ARE THE BULLDYKES; ACCURSED ARE THE AC/DC WEIRDOS;
ACCURSED ARE THE GUYS IN SKIRTS AND GALS IN PANTS;
...FOR I BELIEVE IN THE ONE TRUE SUPPLY SIDE SEXUALITY THAT WHICH IS ORDAINED BETWEEN MAN AND APP- -ROVED RECEPTACLE.
© Steve Bell 1984
1863

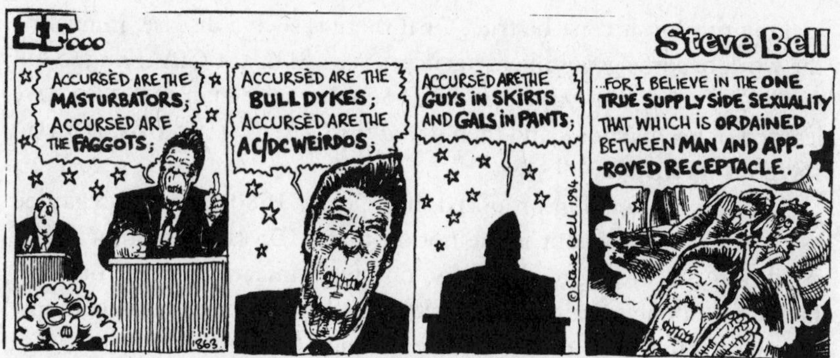

1. Steve Bell's satiric cartoon in the *Guardian* (16 October 1984, p. 29) links "supply side" Reaganomics with its sexual analogue—a position embodied nonsatirically in the deliberations of the Meese Commission for the Study of Pornography (1984–1985). Courtesy of Steve Bell.

man," after all, said conservative Congressman William E. Dannemeyer (R. Calif.), "was for Adam and Eve and not Adam and Steve."[38] A cartoon in 1984 by Steve Bell in the London and Manchester *Guardian* satirized this position by showing Ronald Reagan declaiming from a podium in similar terms (fig. 1).[39] Women, this story goes, are the "natural" receptacles for male sperm. Their immune systems have evolved over the millennia to deal with these foreign invaders; men, not thus blessed by nature, become vulnerable to the "killer sperm" of other men. AIDS in the lay press became known as the "toxic-cock syndrome."[40] Note the contrast this latter view poses to the earlier one among some scientists that infection could be transmitted only from a penis to an "approved receptacle" (i.e., a vagina); now the "natural" receptacle is somehow seen as magically resistant to infection, while the orifices of the "guys with skirts" and the "AC / DC weirdos" become the preferred targets of killer sperm. (I discuss lesbians, the "gals in pants," below.)

Although scientists and physicians tended initially to define AIDS as a problem tied to gay culture, gay men on the whole also rejected the possibility that AIDS was a new, contagious disease. Not only could this make them sexual lepers, it didn't make sense: "How can a disease pick out gays?" they asked; it had to be "medical homophobia."[41] In the gay community, the first reaction to AIDS was disbelief. A gay physician in San Francisco told Frances FitzGerald: "A disease which killed only gay white men? It seemed unbelievable. . . . I used to teach epidemiology, and I had never heard of a disease that selective. I thought, they are making this up. It can't be true. Or if there is such a disease, it must be the work of some government agency—the FBI or the CIA trying to kill us all."[42] In the *San Francisco A.I.D.S. Show,* one man is said to have learned of his diagnosis and then wired the CIA: "I HAVE AIDS. DO YOU HAVE AN ANTIDOTE?"[43]

Another explanation proposed in the early 1980s and still regarded as potentially significant is the notion that AIDS is a "multifactorial" condition. According to this view, no *single* infectious agent or other factor acts alone to cause the problem. Rather, a factor acts in conjunction with others. So-called cofactors range from the biological (e.g., various pathogens, including viruses) and biomedical (clinical history) to the social (poverty, diet), environmental (mosquitoes), psychological (guilt, stress), and spiritual (sin).[44] One hypothesis was that a person who is sexually active with multiple partners is exposed to a kind of bacterial/viral tidal wave that eventually crushes the immune system. Gay men on the sexual "fast track" would thus be particularly susceptible because of specific practices that maximize exposure to multiple pathogens.[45] Finally, a range of other possibilities has been proposed, from biological experimentation run amok to global conspiracy theories.[46] Yet the choice should not be seen as one between a single-agent theory and all other possibilities. With the growing complexity of the clinical and epidemiological picture (including the unpredictable relationship between exposure and infection, between infection and the development of clinical symptoms, and between the appearance of clinical symptoms and "AIDS") it seems, rather, that we should abandon the hope for finding a simple "cause of AIDS" and instead concentrate on making sense of what is already before us.[47]

Many were reluctant to move away from the view of AIDS as a "gay disease." For some, the name GRID would always shape their perceptions.[48] Yet what marked off the first years of AIDS from those that followed was the growing intensity of the search for an infectious agent—probably a virus—that could plausibly be implicated in the development of AIDS. Laboratories at the Pasteur Institut in Paris and at the National Cancer Institutes in the United States isolated a strain of virus that appeared to be associated with AIDS and AIDS-like conditions. I will not detail here the virus's story[49] but will say only that by the end of 1984 there was general consensus among many U.S. scientists that a virus was the major "cause" of AIDS.[50] "A virus," according to a story in *National Geographic,* "is a protein-covered bundle of genes containing instructions for making identical copies of itself. Pure information.

Because it lacks the basic machinery for reproduction, a virus is not, strictly speaking, even alive."[51] The virus is thus another "border case" that becomes the site—discursive and literal—for ongoing dispute.

Virologists and immunologists clearly considered the AIDS virus as extraordinarily interesting—a *retrovirus,* actually, that replicates "backwards," transferring genetic information from viral RNA (which becomes a template for transcription) into DNA. In turn, the DNA enters the cell's own chromosomes and, thus positioned within its infected host, may begin producing new viruses immediately or remain latent for years.[52] In the case of "the AIDS virus," now named "HIV" for human immunodeficiency virus, this dormancy can last up to (at present count) fourteen years, followed by a sudden explosion of replication that may kill the host cells (normally the helper T-cell—the conductor, it has been said, of the orchestra that is the immune system), leaving the host vulnerable to outside infections that a normal immune system would repel.[53]

The discovery of the virus by Dr. Robert C. Gallo and his research team was announced with great fanfare, and the promise of quick therapeutic measures was quickly issued by Margaret Heckler, then secretary of health and human services, who also said AIDS must and would be stopped before it spread to the "general population." For this she earned the title in the gay community of secretary of health and heterosexual services; the Reagan administration, for whatever reason, used the public outcry following the press conference as a rationale for reassigning Heckler to the post of ambassador to Ireland.[54] The incidence of AIDS in the gay community also increased, though more was becoming known about transmission, protection, and treatment. But the identification of the virus validated the authority of the Western biomedical research establishment and, as Donna Haraway suggests, enabled AIDS to be transformed from a low-status STD to the realm of High Science and High Theory. At the same time, the body was transformed from a mere combat zone to a communication, control & command center.[55] A virus, after all, is "pure information," and the body is simply the terrain on which it is transcribed.

The identification of the virus also, to some extent, put to rest so-called "spread of AIDS" stories.[56] Although the term *virus* did suggest possibilities of infection and contagion, the discovery nevertheless quickly acquired the status of a "fact" in scientific understandings of the illness and therefore fulfilled the functions of a "fact" as defined by Ludvik Fleck: "In the field of cognition, *the signal of resistance* opposing free, arbitrary thinking is called a *fact*."[57] So despite the appropriation of the virus as evidence to support many existing theories (e.g., the view that the CIA or KGB had caused AIDS), together with extant knowledge about viruses (e.g., that they cause colds, herpes, and polio), the overall effect was to concentrate speculation on modes of transmission and mechanisms of infection and destruction. Although sources of media coverage have increased and diversified since this period, particularly since late 1986, modes of representation (as suggested, for example, in a recent study of AIDS metaphors by Hughey, Norton, and Sullivan) have shifted as widespread uncertainty gave way to a better understood, if still greatly feared, illness.[58] In some cases, attempts to achieve certainty and to reduce public panic appeared to oversimplify the problem and to extend false reassurances. Other voices remained cautionary and careful, however, in assessing the data.[59]

As Jean L. Marx summarized the evidence in *Science,* "sexual intercourse both of the heterosexual and homosexual varieties is a major pathway of transmission."[60] Other articulate voices joined in warning about the public health consequences of treating AIDS as a "gay disease," and separating "those at risk" from the so-called general population.[61] Gary MacDonald, executive director of an AIDS organization in Washington, D.C., put it this way in 1985: "The moment may have arrived to desexualize this disease. AIDS is *not* a 'gay disease,' despite its epidemiology. Yet we homosexualize it, and by doing so end up posing the wrong questions. . . . AIDS is not transmitted because of who you *are,* but because of what you *do*." MacDonald went on to note that almost a fifth of AIDS patients in the United States are intravenous drug users and another 6 percent never fit any of the high-risk groups. "By concentrating on gay and bisexual men, people are able to ignore the fact that this disease has been present in what has charmingly come to be called 'the general population' *from the beginning*. It was not spread from one of the other groups. It was *there*."[62] As Ruth Bleier reminds us, questions shape answers. Thus, the question, "Why are all AIDS victims sexually active homosexual males?"—which has so dominated research—might more appropriately have been: "*Are* all AIDS victims sexually active homosexual males?"[63] But in quashing speculation and "hysteria" in the name of reason, expressions of scientific certainty also closed off considerations that women, nongay men, faithfully married couples, and so on *could* get AIDS. Statistical probabilities about what *would* happen were allowed to be read as theoretical constraints on what *could* happen.

ROCK HUDSON AND THE CRISIS IN GENDER

Ironically, a major turning point in America's consciousness came in the summer of 1985 when Rock Hudson acknowledged he was being treated for AIDS.[64] Through an extraordinary conflation of texts, Rock Hudson's illness dramatized the possibility that the disease could spread to the "general population." "I thought AIDS was a gay disease," said a man interviewed by *USA Today,* "but if Rock Hudson can get it, anyone can." Hudson was, I would argue, another "border case" (in Poovey's sense) in which such textual conflations became common: When an event contradicts the perceived natural order of things, it becomes a cultural dispute that generates vast quantities of discourse designed to shore up existing distinctions and resolve contradictions.[65]

Another site of continuous dispute is the mechanism through which the virus is transmitted, as well as the different explanations for the epidemiological finding that AIDS and HIV infection in the United States were appearing predominantly in gay men. One view holds that the prevalence among the latter is essentially an artifact ("simple mathematics") because the virus, for whatever reason, infected gay men first and gay men tend to have sex with each other. The second is that biomedical/physiological factors make sexually active gay men and/or the "passive receiver" more infectable. A third view is that the virus can be transmitted to anyone, but that certain cofactors predispose the development of infection and / or clinical symptoms in particular individuals.[66] There are also speculations about the quantity of virus that is needed to cause infection (*virus* is both a count and a mass noun). Dr. Mathilde Krim, then of the AIDS Medical Foundation, for example, suggested that because the virus "must be virtually injected into the bloodstream" male-to-female transmission is more likely.[67] Jonathan Lieberson, likewise, concluded in 1986 that infection requires "direct transfusion into the bloodstream."[68] Dr. Jacques Leibowitch, however, relates transmission patterns, on the one hand, to the fact that homosexual men have sex with other homosexual men and, on the other hand, to the male homosexual "duality." A man, that is, can be a "receiver" of the virus from one man and then be a "donor" of the virus to another, in contrast to the "relative intransitivity of heterosexual propagation." By virtue of their "natural anatomy," women receive but do not give.[69] Indeed, many scientists have come to hold the view that, as Nathan Fain put it, "infection requires a jolt injected into the bloodstream, likely several jolts over time, such as would occur with infected needles or semen. In both cases, needle and penis are the instruments of contagion."[70]

All this generated considerable confusion as to who was likely, even capable, of becoming infected and just what it was that increased or decreased that likelihood. Much of the uncertainty in the science and medical journals obviously turned (as, indeed, it still does) on the precise mechanisms of transmission. Nevertheless, even in the journal literature, and certainly as presented to the general public, questions about transmission were interpreted in part as questions—anxious questions—about sexual difference (male/female; heterosexual/homosexual; active/passive).

To the rescue came John Langone in the December 1985 issue of *Discover* magazine. In this lengthy review of research to date, Langone suggests that the virus enters the bloodstream by way of the "vulnerable anus" and the "fragile urethra." The "rugged vagina" (built to be abused by such blunt instruments as penises and small babies), in contrast, provides too tough a barrier for the AIDS virus to penetrate.[71] "Contrary to what you've heard," Langone concludes—echoing a fair amount of medical and scientific writing at the time—"AIDS isn't a threat to the vast majority of heterosexuals. . . . It is now—and is likely to remain—largely the fatal price one can pay for anal intercourse."[72] (This excerpt from the article also ran as the cover blurb.) Detailed cross-sectional drawings of anus, urethra, and vagina illustrated the article's conclusion.

The *Discover* article reassured many people about the continuing validity of the CDC's original 4-H list of high-risk categories. But categories of risk, of behavioral practice, and of identity may be quite distinct, or may overlap with each other—an ongoing problem in AIDS epidemiology and research. Sociologist Jeffrey Weeks, for example, analyzes the evolution of homosexuality as a coherent identity. "The gay identity," he writes, "is no more a product of nature than any other sexual identity. It has developed through a complex history of definition and self-definition," and "there is no necessary connection between sexual practices and sexual identity."[73] The problems with the CDC list were known to some science reporters, at least to the few who were knowledgeable and tenacious enough to take their analysis beyond the official party line. Ann Giudici Fettner, for example, pointed out in 1985 that "the CDC admits that at least 10 percent of AIDS sufferers are gay *and* use IV drugs. Yet they are automatically counted in the homosexual and bisexual men category, regardless of what might be known—or not known—about how they became infected."[74] So the "gay" nature of

AIDS was in part an artifact of the way data were collected and reported, though it was generally hypothesized until 1986 that the cases assigned to the category OTHER (or UNKNOWN, or UNCLASSIFIED) would ultimately turn out to be one of the four Hs. As Shaw and Paleo point out, however, the number of women in this category remains much larger than men; they point out, among other things, that the category "homosexual" was not broken down by sex despite potential risk for lesbians via sexual activity and artificial insemination.[75] Data from Africa were showing that women and men were infected in equal numbers; yet the practice of medicine and resources for data collection in Africa, especially outside urban areas, made the data questionable on a variety of grounds.[76] And even as evidence accumulated that transmission *could* be heterosexual (which begins with the letter H, after all), scientific and popular discourse continued to construct women as "inefficient" and "incompetent" transmitters of HIV, stolid barriers that impede the passage of the virus from brother to brother.[77]

In the discourse of this period (from approximately mid-1985 to December 1986), there were exceptions, which will probably not surprise us. As evidence of AIDS in women mounted, speculation linked the disease to prostitutes, intravenous drug users, and women in the Third World (primarily Haiti and countries in central Africa). It was not that these three groups were synonymous but, rather, that their differentness of race, class, or national origin made speculation about transmission possible—unlike middle-class American feminists, for example. American feminists also by this point had considerable access to public forums from which to protest ways in which they were represented, while these other groups of women were, for all practical purposes, silenced categories so far as public or biomedical discourse was concerned (fig. 2).[78]

Prostitutes—despite their long-standing professional knowledge of STDs and continued activism about AIDS—have long been portrayed as so contaminated that their bodies are, like "bloody Maggie's" in the passage at the beginning of this chapter, "always dripping," virtual laboratory cultures for viral replication.[79] Early failures to find AIDS cases among prostitutes, however, supported the "gay disease" hypothesis.[80] "Women in general," concluded a Johns Hopkins professor of medicine, "seem to be less efficient transmitters of the disease."[81] Immunologist Paula Strickland concurred: "I think AIDS would be containable and would pose no threat to heterosexuals if there weren't any bisexuals in our society."[82]

Commitment to this view of AIDS as a male disease was so strong

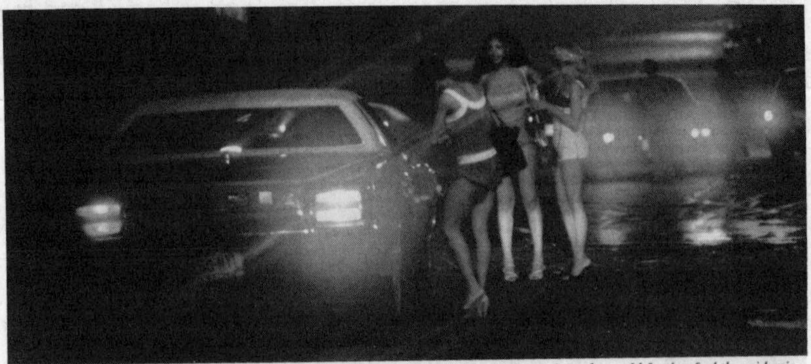

Working the streets in New York: Some experts fear that prostitutes might turn out to be carriers who could further fuel the epidemic

2. Against a dark, ominous background, prostitutes are shown "working the streets in New York." Despite many qualifiers in the caption and lack of scientific evidence, *Newsweek*'s use of this photograph (12 August 1985, p. 28) lent credibility to the familiar belief that prostitutes would inevitably figure largely in the spread of AIDS. Courtesy of Ethan Hoffmann Archive.

that when R. R. Redfield and his colleagues reported a study in the *Journal of the American Medical Association* demonstrating infection in U.S. servicemen who claimed heterosexual contact only—with female prostitutes in Germany—various attempts were made to discredit or dismiss this new evidence:[83] Servicemen, for instance, would be punished for revealing homosexual behavior or intravenous drug use; they really had gone to male prostitutes, and so on.[84] If women were merely passive vessels without the efficient capacities of a projectile penis or syringe for "efficiently" shooting large quantities of the virus into another organism, the transmission to U.S. servicemen from German prostitutes must be only apparent. Indeed, one reader suggested, transmission was not really from women to men but was rather "quasihomosexual": Man A, infected with HIV, had sexual intercourse with a prostitute; she, "[performing] no more than perfunctory external cleansing between customers," then has intercourse with Man B; he is infected with the virus by way of Man A's semen still in the vagina of the prostitute.[85] It was taken for granted that the prostitute took no preventive or cleansing measures, and, one must suppose, that the projectile penis could also function as a kind of proboscis, sucking up quantities of virus from a contaminated pool. A similar metaphor, and one we shall meet again, occurs in a study of urban prostitutes in central Africa; the prostitutes are called "major reservoir of AIDS virus," African heterosexual males are "vectors of infection."[86]

Evidence suggests, however, that prostitutes are not at greater risk because they have multiple sex partners, but because they are likely to use intravenous drugs.[87] Shaw and Paleo, for example, write:

> There is no evidence that prostitutes constitute a special risk category. . . . Some prostitutes do get AIDS. To the extent that researchers have been able to isolate prostitution and/or multiple sexual contacts from such issues as IV drug use, however, neither the number of sexual contacts nor the receipt of money . . . seems to put women at a higher risk for getting AIDS. Many women who are in paid sexual activity were concerned about sexually transmitted diseases even before the AIDS epidemic. They protected themselves and continue to protect themselves by being somewhat alert to new medical developments in sexually transmitted diseases and how to avoid them.[88]

COYOTE and other organizations of prostitutes have addressed the issue of AIDS rather aggressively for several years.[89] Some scientists have also attempted to counter the prevailing view that AIDS is predominantly and inherently a gay disease. Virologist William Haseltine, for example, dismisses exotic explanations of the African data: "To think that we're so different from people in the Congo is a more comfortable position, but it probably isn't so."[90] Haseltine successfully used this argument to obtain increased AIDS funding, citing Redfield's data on the U.S. servicemen in Germany at a congressional hearing: "These aren't homosexuals. These aren't drug abusers. These are normal, young guys who visited prostitutes. Half the prostitutes are infected, and these guys got infected."[91] Interestingly, he explicitly separates "normal, young guys" from gays and drug users, shifting in the last clause to the passive voice, a construction that reinforces their lack of culpability, representing them as innocent "receivers" of the infection, not problematic "donors." The "young guys" are the infectees, the prostitutes the infectors (compare this with the syntax of Shaw and Paleo, above, where prostitutes protect themselves and remain alert to medical news).[92]

A second exception were infected female intravenous drug users, or, as they are commonly called, "drug abusers" or "drug addicts" (though it is during *use,* not necessarily *abuse,* that transmission occurs).[93] Scientific and popular accounts have tended to show little interest in or sympathy for this group: It should be noted, however, that statistics are problematic in part because these individuals are hard to reach, and in part because drug use is compounded by other conditions. For example, HIV infection in prostitutes is often attributed to sexual contact with multiple partners (and especially to *paying* multiple partners), although, as I have noted, the sharing of needles in the course of intravenous drug

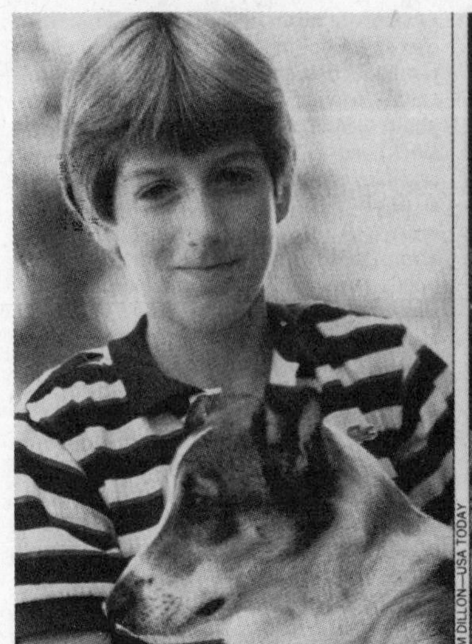

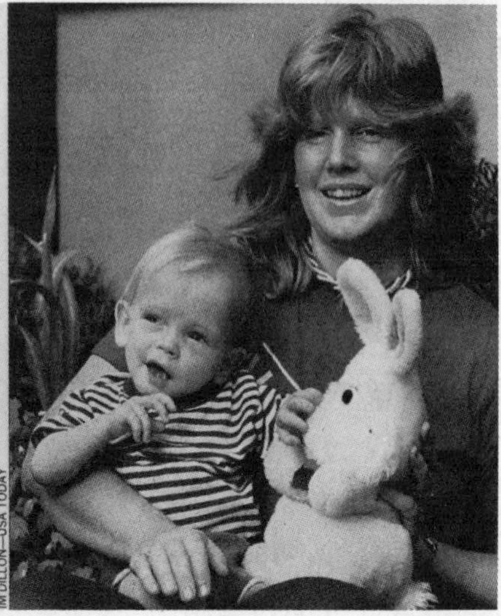

3. Live or stuffed animals in photos of persons with AIDS distinguish the "innocent" from the "guilty," or at least normalize their "otherness." After Rock Hudson's death, many publications ran sympathetic stories accompanied by photos of him playing with his dogs: He had AIDS, ran the subtext, but he was still a good person. In early stories on AIDS, researchers like the CDC's Jim Curran were often photographed with their spouses and children: He may study AIDS, but he's as heterosexual as the next guy. Photograph of Ryan White by Max Winter for Picture Group; photograph of Matthew Kozup and his mother by Tim Dillon for *USA Today*. Both ran in *Newsweek*, 12 August 1985, p. 29.

use is the more likely source of exposure. Of the women with AIDS in New York City, for example, 62 percent are intravenous drug users and most of the others are sex partners of drug users; of the 183 cases of heterosexually transmitted AIDS, 88 percent were identified as sex partners of intravenous users, and fewer than 9 percent as the sex partners of bisexual males. Of the female HIV-positive prostitutes, almost all were intravenous drug users. Of the 156 children with AIDS as of December 1986, 80 percent had one or both parents who were intravenous drug users; the number of infected babies born at risk will rise each year.[94] In San Francisco, where a different epidemiological picture exists, transfusion-related AIDS is the most common source of infection for women; drug use and heterosexual contact come second.[95] Sex partners of "drug addicts," who, like transfusion cases, are often infected without their knowledge (even knowledge that their partner may be at risk for AIDS), are sympathetic "victims"—up to the point that they become pregnant, when they become baby killers. Mothers with transfusion-caused AIDS remain sympathetic figures (fig. 3). But the CDC's James W. Curran in June 1986 pointed the finger directly at the "invidious transmission" made possible when female drug users and drug users' sex partners allow themselves to get pregnant.[96] With this act the passive receiver again becomes a culpable agent who transmits her infected blood "vertically" to her unborn child or (perhaps) after birth through breast milk. But as Shaw notes, little information is available about this phenomenon or about the effects of pregnancy on the woman herself; pregnant women may be both more likely to get infected if they are sexually active or, if already infected, pregnancy might activate the dormant virus.[97]

A third exception were women from central Africa and other areas of the world (primarily Haiti), where heterosexual transmission is more common. Again, no conceptually coherent explanation was offered for why a sexually transmitted illness should be homosexual in one country and heterosexual in another, although ad hoc speculations supported by virtually no documentation attribute the African statistics to "quasi-homosexual" transmission of the kind noted above, refusal by African men to admit to homosexuality or drug use, the practice of anal intercourse as a method of birth control, or the widespread use of unsterilized needles in clinics and hospitals.[98] A debate in the letters column of the *New York Times* over the role of genital mutilation regarding AIDS in Africa illuminates the phantasmic projections of exotica that AIDS has stimulated. Fran P. Hosken suggested in December 1986 that widespread female "circumcision" (clitoridectomy and infibulation) is the main reason why the disease pattern is different in Africa (a 1 : 1 ratio of women to men).[99] Douglas A. Feldman, acting executive director of the Queens AIDS Center, responded as follows: "Certainly, female genital mutilation is a brutal, sexist practice that should be strongly discouraged" *but,* he argued, the epidemiological pattern does not conform to the hypothesis of a relationship. In the countries where AIDS is widespread—Burundi, the Congo, Rwanda, Tanzania, Uganda, Zaire, and Zambia—clitoridectomies are rare. Where the procedure is common—from Senegal in the west to Somalia in the east—AIDS is generally not found. "However, as AIDS spreads into Kenya and eastern Tanzania, where the removal of the clitoris and labia majora is common, often resulting in genitourinary infections, it is likely that the practice may facilitate the spread of the disease." But after this potentially sensible comment—sensible because a history of infection is known to be relevant to immune-system deficiencies—Feldman embarks on his *own* speculations, suggesting that the following factors may cause higher AIDS rates in African women: (1) higher rates of prior immunosuppression (but in relation to what? the infections he has just mentioned? poverty, malnutrition?); (2) intestinal parasite infestation; (3) greater likelihood of urban African women to engage in sex during menstruation (greater than rural women, or than American women? and is it yet established that this is relevant?); (4) "possibly the common practice by prepubescent girls in parts of central Africa of elongating the labia majora through continual stretching" (does this make it thin and "fragile" like the anal tract?); and (5) possible existence of an "immunosuppressive viral co-factor" (deuces wild). "But I fear," writes the doctor, "it is just a matter of time before the pattern of heterosexually transmitted AIDS in the singles bars along First Avenue, as well as the sidewalks of Queens Boulevard, will begin to look a lot like the pandemic in Africa today."[100]

This was December 1986, and suddenly the big news—cover stories for the major U.S. news magazines—was the grave danger of AIDS to heterosexuals. Major stories on AIDS as a threat to "all of us" appeared, for example, in *Newsweek, U.S. News and World Report, Time, Scientific American, The Atlantic,* and the *Village Voice.*[101] In a four-part series beginning March 19, 1987, the *New York Times* gave front-page coverage to several dimensions of AIDS; significantly, the boilerplate explanatory paragraph in each story made no mention of gay men or intravenous drug users. Although these groups were mentioned in the stories themselves, they were no longer considered intrinsic to the definition of AIDS.[102] No dramatic discoveries in the intervening year had changed the fundamental scientific conception of AIDS. What had changed was not "the facts" but the way they were now used to construct the AIDS text and the meanings we were now allowed—indeed, at last encouraged—to read from that text.

By the fall of 1986 virtually all theories of AIDS, no matter how remarkable their semantic underpinnings, had to confront the same bottom line: AIDS *can* be transmitted through heterosexual intercourse and other sexual activities to and from both women and men. It is important to emphasize that the gay community and (especially in New York City) the black and Hispanic communities continue to be most devastated by AIDS and most urgently in need of help. This does not mitigate the need to stress the possibility of widespread heterosexual transmission, and the current obsession with precise statistics—with whether or not HIV infection is about to "explode" in the "general population," or with whether the entire epidemic itself is over—is, in my view, a dangerous diversion from questions of far greater importance.[103] My own concern continues to be with the evolution of "the facts," how these facts are constructed and represented, and, finally, how it has happened that the politically sophisticated feminist community has remained oblivious so long not simply to the potential risk to women but to AIDS as a massive social crisis.

AIDS GOES HETEROSEXUAL

Scientists commonly point out that AIDS arrived at the "right time"—that is, a time when basic science research in virology and immunology could provide a foundation for an intensive research effort on AIDS. They point out that no other epidemic disease has been analyzed so quickly nor its cause so efficiently determined.[104] Despite quarrels with this view (Randy Shilts, for example, calculates that the entire workforce assigned to AIDS was a tiny fraction of the one deployed to deal with the 1982 Tylenol scare in Illinois[105]), let us concede that a number of biomedical researchers, epidemiologists, and clinicians have greatly contributed to our understanding of AIDS and that they were able to do so in part because of scientific progress in specific fields over the last twenty years. As Simon Watney points out, however, investigations of the last two decades provide a crucial foundation for the analysis of AIDS in the human sciences as well. Such a foundation prepares us to analyze AIDS in relation to questions of language, representation, the mobilization of cultural narratives, ideology, social and intellectual differences and hierarchies, binary divisions, interpretation, and contests for meaning.[106]

Models for such analyses in relation to AIDS have primarily been carried out by members of the gay community, whose interventions have helped shape the discourse on AIDS. As gay activists contested the terminology, meanings, and interpretations produced by scientific inquiry, loaded phrases like "promiscuous" soon gave way to more neutral behavioral descriptions like "sexually active with multiple partners" (many examples of such shifts are demonstrated in the collections of AIDS papers from *Science* and the *Journal of the American Medical Association*). It is interesting that by 1986, when women were more central to the AIDS story, scientists and physicians were speaking of "sexually active" males and "promiscuous females."[107] Other linguistic practices relevant to the construction of gender and sexuality in AIDS discourse are enumerated by J. Z. Grover.[108] Although such linguistic activism is dismissed by Shilts as misguided public relations efforts on the part of the gay community, it is more accurately seen, as Watney and others have argued, as part of a broad and crucially important resistance to the semantic imperialism of experts and professionals.[109] Challenging the authority of science and medicine—whose meanings are part of powerful and deeply entrenched social and historical codes—remains a significant and courageous action. It also provides an important model for women as evidence accumulates that neither gender nor sexual preference provides magical protection from the virus.

In 1985 and again in 1986 the CDC reviewed the patients who "could not be classified by recognized risk factors for AIDS." Eve K. Nichols, analyzing the CDC review of "unexplained cases" and related research, concludes that "these facts suggest a possible association between a small number of AIDS cases and heterosexual promiscuity in this country."[110] Despite the hedging and the use of the loaded term *promiscuity,* the conclusion represents a new biomedical construction of AIDS within the official scientific establishment. In December 1986 the CDC officially reclassified 571 cases formerly classified as "none of the above."[111]

What are biomedical scientists now saying about women? In April 1987 another article on women and AIDS appeared, this in the *Journal of the American Medical Association.*[112] Coauthors Mary Guinan, M.D., and Ann Hardy, Ph.D., M.P.H., review the 1,819 cases of AIDS in women officially reported in the United States between 1981 and 1986. Within the risk group of heterosexual contacts of persons at risk, the percentage of women increased from 12 percent to 26 percent between 1982 and 1986 (heterosexual contact is the only transmission category in which women at present outnumber men). More than 70 percent of women with AIDS are black or Hispanic; more than 80 percent are of childbearing age. As to the "portal of entry" for the virus, it is unclear what is going on and will probably continue to be unclear until we know the precise mechanism(s) of transmission. The distinction between anal versus vaginal "portals," according to Guinan and Hardy, is relevant only if HIV *cannot* pass through mucous membranes and thus requires broken skin or membranes. But this is still unknown, and "if the virus can pass through intact mucous membranes, the risk of transmission through the vagina or rectum may not be different."[113]

Though its cautionary and provisional stance is welcome, this article is problematic in several ways: First, the women in risk groups are given their "status" only by virtue of their sexual partners—the men they're connected to—not by virtue of their own sexual activities. This kind of assignment appears to constitute a return to an earlier system of sociological categorization, one perhaps not fully theorized in the current situation. Second, the source of infection is determined according to a hierarchy of factors, with sexual contact taking precedence over intravenous drug use and with no dual assignments occurring; in CDC studies, therefore, infection in prostitutes has typically been assigned to contact with multiple sex partners, even though other studies, as well as prostitutes themselves, assign the source of infection to intravenous drug use.[114] And finally, above all, the *purpose* of studying women, we are told, is twofold: first, to use incidence in women as a general index to heterosexual spread of the virus, and second, to identify women at risk and prevent "primary" infection in them *in order to* prevent the majority of cases of AIDS in children that would result from these maternal risk groups without intervention.[115] There is thus no intrinsic concern for women *as women*. Yet, because pregnancy suppresses the immune system, any woman who gets pregnant increases her risk of infection with HIV or, if already infected, possibly increases her risk of developing active AIDS.

It is true that we need to be concerned about "future generations." During the Venetian plague of 1630–1631, ten thousand pregnant women were killed in a period of months, decimating the city's childbearing population.[116] As Shaw and Paleo point out, because the widespread practice of safer sex would drastically reduce the birth rate, childbearing might come under intense scrutiny by the state, and women of childbearing age might be among the *first* groups to undergo mandatory testing.[117] But surely we are also concerned about women themselves and need to give thought, in policies and practice, to *them* rather than simply treating them as transparent carriers who house either the future of humanity or small Damiens who will assist in furthering viral replication.

In other biomedical discourse, as I have noted, some scientists and physicians (including William Haseltine, Mathilde Krim, Jean L. Marx, and Constance Wofsy) have for some time noted that HIV may be heterosexually transmitted to and from women; and suggest that despite the small number of cases, woman-to-woman transmission may also be possible.[118] Because of the still-unanswered questions, these professionals emphasize caution until more is known. What about lesbians, who still figure only fitfully in the biomedical story? Lesbians appear in the abstract to be at relatively low risk for HIV infection—lesbians as a group have a very low incidence of sexually transmitted disease, although the medical literature does include isolated reports, often in letters to the editor, of HIV transmission by way of female-to-female sexual contact.[119] Despite these virtually nonexistent statistics, lesbians were lumped by the public with gay men and considered just as dangerous; although lesbians in many cities are now organizing blood drives, for example, earlier attempts to do so had been defeated by the public perception that lesbians were as likely to be infected as gay men because "AIDS is a gay disease."[120] Ironically, despite many lesbians' long-standing support for and solidarity with gay men on the AIDS question, and despite the time lesbians contribute to AIDS hotlines and task forces, very little "safer sex" literature, whether directed toward homosexuals or heterosexuals is designed specifically for women whose sexual contacts are with other women.

Concerns about women in the general press have also come relatively late in the AIDS crisis. An important exception is Cindy Patton's 1985 *Sex and Germs,* a social and political analysis of AIDS that addresses the growing connections among contamination phobia, erotophobia, and homophobia, and proposes an agenda for progressive action.[121] Also useful is the work of Ann Guidici Fettner, Katie Leishman, Marcia Pally, Nancy Stoller Shaw, and J. Z. Grover.[122] Important and informed questions about the politics of AIDS and the "risk group" mode of describing vulnerability to HIV have consistently been asked by, among others, Randy Shilts, Peg Byron, Wayne Barrett, Simon Watney, C. Carr, Larry Kramer, and Nancy Krieger.[123] These writers have been notable. Politically oriented prostitutes' organizations have also been vocal in addressing issues of AIDS as they relate to women—advocating not only individual prevention strategies but also government responsibility for assuring safe conditions in a service industry.[124] Though the subject of women and AIDS was regularly covered only by a few women writers—primarily in radical journals in New York, San Francisco, and London—by 1986 most women's magazines had run at least one "What Women Should Do" or "What Women Need to Know" article (e.g., *Vogue, New Woman*), and by 1987 mainstream feminist journals and magazines including *Ms.* in the United States and *Spare Rib* in Great Britain were providing fairly regular coverage.[125] Still, as Marea Murray had argued in a 1985 letter to *Sojourner,* some women, including lesbians, continued to perceive AIDS as a problem "the boys" had brought on themselves,[126] while heterosexual women were still tending to see AIDS as nothing to do with them or as something that "self-help" procedures would guard them against. Of course, in the absence of challenge or resistance, female roles in the AIDS story remained the traditional ones: loving mother, loyal spouse, wronged lover, philanthropic celebrity; one man with AIDS even attributed his apparent remission to "the Blessed Virgin" (figs. 4 and 5).[127] But even here a confusion was evident as to who was guilty, who innocent, who was an active agent of disease, who a victim.[128]

Why was there such resistance to acknowledging women's potential to acquire and transmit AIDS and to deal clinically with AIDS as a woman's illness? One reason is certainly denial: the sheer unthinkability of AIDS unleashed upon the entire world population because, then, as someone put it at the Paris International AIDS Conference in July 1986, "the sky's the limit." Semantic imperialism breaks down in the face of the virus's ability to replicate infinitely. Instead, there is hope that the virus will be able to be "contained" within the populations already infected—i.e., "saturating" the established high-risk groups but not spreading beyond them. Though millions would die, this is still a containable subtotal of the "general population."[129]

A second reason for resistance to the role women play in the transmission of AIDS involves the potential difficulty of feminizing AIDS at this stage, after so long an identification with gay men. Shilts notes resistance to initial reports of infants and children with AIDS because the name GRID "by definition" signified a "gay disease." Yet Shilts himself, whose own account of AIDS begins with the mysterious illness in central Africa of a Danish lesbian physician, nevertheless focuses more intensely on a sexually appetitive Canadian airline attendant, a gay man who came to be identified by the CDC as "Patient Zero." Of course, as soon as the advance publicity on Shilts's book went out, the *New York Post*'s headline blared: "THE MAN WHO GAVE US AIDS!"[130] Others have pointed out that there is no need for female representation in the AIDS saga because gay men are already substituting for them as the Contaminated Other. Conservative journals like *Commentary* preserve this place by putting forth clearly and repeatedly the thesis so boldly stated by Langone: "AIDS remains the price one pays for anal intercourse."[131] In addition, Simon Watney and Larry Kramer, among others, observe that the gay community provides most of the volunteer workforce on AIDS

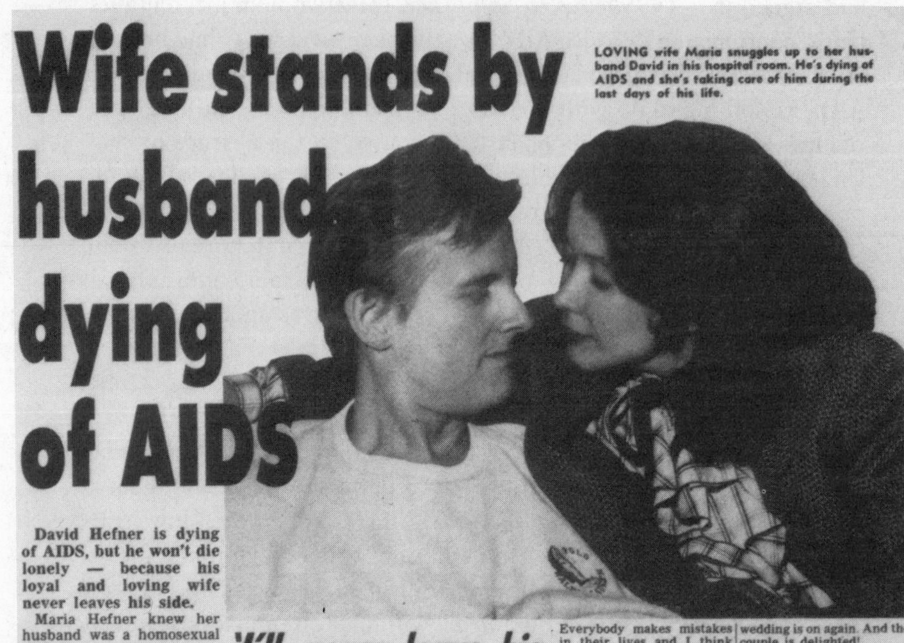

Wife stands by husband dying of AIDS

LOVING wife Maria snuggles up to her husband David in his hospital room. He's dying of AIDS and she's taking care of him during the last days of his life.

David Hefner is dying of AIDS, but he won't die lonely — because his loyal and loving wife never leaves his side.

Maria Hefner knew her husband was a homosexual before she married him in 1984. Eight months ago the New York City hairdresser found out he was sick with AIDS and broke the news to his wife with a heavy heart.

'I'll never leave his side,' vows loyal mate

"It wasn't good news," courageous Maria, 33, told *The NEWS*. "But I concentrated on the fact that I had to help him emotionally and psychologically.

"I'm not afraid for myself. I don't think about that, it doesn't help. If it happens to me, what can I do?"

Maria and her husband met and fell in love when the pretty brunette Brazilian woman became Hefner's customer in his hair salon.

Before they met, Hefner had been attracted to men — but his love for Maria changed the way he felt. The two wed in a civil ceremony and settled into a happy married life — until AIDS cast a shadow over their dreams of the future.

"We had a beautiful beginning," Maria said. "So I can't feel angry. I knew he was homosexual — he told me. But he didn't know he had AIDS. It's not his fault. Everybody makes mistakes in their lives and I think homosexuality is a mistake.

"I give him a lot of credit because he changed the way he was.

"He changed because he wanted to, not because anyone made him do it."

The Hefners made national news in January when they asked to be married in a religious ceremony in St. Patrick's Cathedral in New York City and nervous church officials turned them down.

The church reversed itself a few days later and now the wedding is on again. And the couple is delighted!

"We want to be married in the church," said Maria, who was wed in a civil ceremony three years ago.

"We've always planned to, it's not just because David is sick. After that I don't know how long it will be . . . I'm taking care of him full time. I want to make sure he's safe.

"We will do things day by day. I guess he's a lucky man to have me — but I'm a lucky woman that I met him."

— SUSAN JIMISON

4. Although cases of women with AIDS were reported early on, women rarely appeared in the official AIDS story except in secondary and traditional roles as mates and caretakers. Maria Hefner was prototypical: She knew her husband was homosexual, but love conquered all. They made national news in January 1987 after they learned he had AIDS and sought to be married in a religious ceremony in St. Patrick's Cathedral. *Weekly World News* (17 February 1987, p. 17) shows "loving wife Maria" taking care of David "during the last days of his life."

WEEKLY WORLD NEWS
May 12, 1987

Lady doc spikes mate's tomato juice with killer virus

Wife murders hubby with AIDS cocktail!

A lady physician murdered her husband by spiking his tomato juice with AIDS-tainted blood, Swedish newspapers report.

Ola Lindgren, 53, admitted that she killed Thord Lindgren, 52, with a research sample of the deadly virus and was sentenced to life in prison at the close of her trial in Goteborg, said the press.

The once-respected doctor testified that she smuggled the tiny vial of AIDS-infected blood from a Stockholm laboratory in 1982 and put it in her husband's juice "for the express purpose of killing him ever so slow and sure."

"I'd do it again," she told Judge Einar Winslof prior to her sentencing. "He was a stupid man. He was holding me back in my career.

"If anyone ever deserved to die, it was him."

The judge was stunned by the doctor's admission of guilt and lack of remorse. In sentencing her he called her husband's murder "the most bizarre of this century or any other."

"And to make matters worse, Dr. Lindgren, you took a solemn oath to preserve life — not take it."

Prosecutor Gunnar Schwartz told reporters that Dr. Lindgren would never have gone to trial had she not confessed to the murder.

"Who was to say that her husband didn't get AIDS from an illicit lover?" he said. "Who would have dreamed that he was killed by his wife?

"Prior to all this, she was a most respected physician, adored by her patients and held up as an example by her peers."

He should have had a V-8!

Lindgren, who taught history at a small college, was diagnosed as having AIDS in 1986. His health deteriorated rapidly and he died from the complications of pneumonia in July 1986.

No one suspected that he had been murdered until his wife laughingly told a friend that she had engineered his death.

That friend told police what she had heard.

"The irony of it all is that AIDS is spreading like wildfire and will eventually kill millions all on its own," said Schwartz. "But here we had a doctor who harnessed that deadly potential for her own personal use."

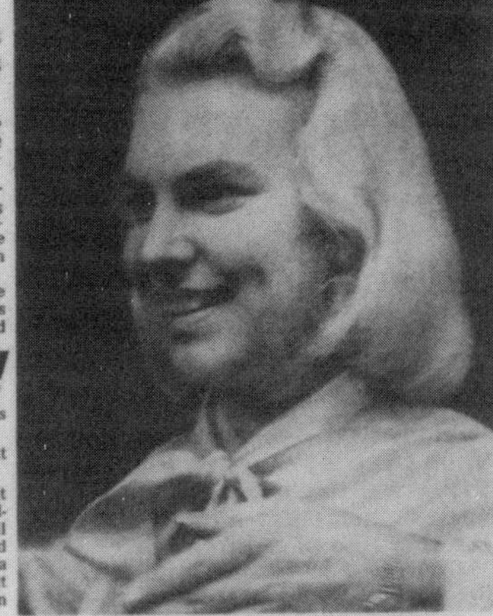

SNEAKY Ola Lindgren received a life prison term after admitting that she had murdered her husband.

5. A few months later, another wife in *Weekly World News* (12 May 1987) plays quite a different part in the AIDS story. Ola Lindgren, a Swedish physician, is reported to have murdered her husband with virus-laden tomato juice (there is little documentation that oral transmission of HIV would accomplish this). A photo shows "sneaky" Lindgren smiling, while the story tells us that this "lady doc" murdered "hubby with AIDS cocktail!" Here was evidence of a female *literally* carrying the virus home and giving it to her innocent husband, who gets the tabloid fate he deserves for having married an ambitious professional woman: an epitaph from Madison Avenue.

hotlines and other AIDS projects; when public information or television films or advertisements suggest the spread of AIDS to new groups, the "worried well" jam the phone lines beyond the capability of volunteers to answer. There are thus pragmatic reasons, until new groups of volunteers can be enlisted and trained, not to exaggerate the risk to this larger group.[132]

A third reason, I believe, essentially involves a desperate and terrorized effort to control signification. Faced with the nexus of sex and death, its fragmentation into hundreds of allied discourses, the breakdown of coherent categories of sexual identity into postmodernist "bundles of practices," and finally the virus itself with its capacities for infinite replication, who would not resist the entry of Woman, carrying the heavy baggage with which history has equipped her. As historian Allan M. Brandt notes, venereal diseases have typically been assigned a female identity; he cites a number of posters designed for U.S. servicemen, which show the equation of women with venereal disease (in one widely disseminated poster from World War II, for example, a painted prostitute walks down the street, arm in arm between Hitler and Hirohito; the caption reads: "VD: THE WORST OF THESE").[133] In this book and elsewhere, Brandt argues that AIDS has followed the historical pattern of earlier sexually transmitted diseases in generating fears of casual contact, concerns about contagion, stigmatization of victims as agents of the disease, and a search for a "magic bullet." AIDS is not yet, however, a particularly feminized disease, perhaps because, thus far, gay men have served so well as the Contaminated Other. As I have observed elsewhere, HIV is often anthropomorphized as a secret agent, but so far the gender is that of James Bond, not Mata Hari.[134] So long as the virus is characterized as "pure information," belonging to the largely male domain of perfect codes and high theory, it may resist a feminine conceptualization.

We should be aware, however, that language is already traveling from the site of the "sexually active" gay male body to the "promiscuous" female body. Numerous metaphors appearing in newspapers and scientific journals are cited by communication researchers.[135] Water metaphors appearing in 1987 ("IV drug users are the hole in the dike to the general population," "prostitutes are reservoirs of disease," and the "moist, vulnerable mucous membranes" of the female sexual organs) are reminiscent of the gendered tropes of history identified by, for example, Emily Martin and Allan M. Brandt.[136] In the *Weekly World News,* crème de la crème of supermarket tabloids, a loyal wife who stands by her husband with AIDS contrasts sharply with a new role for women: a wife—a physician—who adds an HIV-infected blood sample to her husband's tomato juice and, with apparent relish, watches him develop AIDS and die.[137] The film *Fatal Attraction,* recapitulating Alfred Hitchcock's *The Birds,* gives us a taste of the consequences of "promiscuity."[138] Meanwhile, biomedical journals record the saga of an "exotic virus" infecting "exotic" African female bodies; now we learn that like this "fragile" AIDS virus our female bodies are "fragile," too, not rugged and tough after all but penetrable, "moist and vulnerable," or riddled with cracks and potholes. Are we now to become the carriers of this epidemic, ruthlessly moving everywhere? Is the female body, in fact, meaning itself, contaminating everything with its reservoirs of possibility and death? Reservoirs breaking down and letting language flow out, uncontainable within definitions? Like the virus, wearing an innocent disguise, are we not double agents, in league with the enemy? The question is how to disrupt and renegotiate the powerful cultural narratives surrounding AIDS. Homophobia, racism, and sexism are inscribed within other discourses at a high level, and it is there that they must be disrupted and challenged.

This leads to a fourth reason for the ambiguous positioning of women in AIDS discourse: Our relative failure—as feminists and as women—to address the problem of AIDS in challenging, theoretically comprehensive, or politically meaningful ways. In a final section, I will suggest some problematic aspects of current AIDS discourse by and about women as well as some useful directions toward a more satisfactory feminist analysis.

WOMEN AND AIDS: TOWARD A FEMINIST ANALYSIS

Any analysis of AIDS based on a faith in stable boundaries between risk groups ignores everything we know about the realities of human sexual behavior and sexually transmitted infection. It further ignores the growing presence of AIDS as a dominant factor in the social life of the twentieth century in behavior, in law, in policy, in education, in health-care coverage, and in virtually all other areas of experience which, sooner or later, will touch every citizen.

Unless feminists take a broader and more active role in articulating the nature and meaning of the AIDS crisis, what is in store? One answer is that we will not understand the potential consequences of our own everyday sexual behavior, and this, I think, goes for gay as well as straight women. Sexually liberated from the hegemony of the magical projectile penis, we should not assume the absolute truth of the scientific hypothesis that an "injection" of the virus is the sine qua non of infection. Even if it turns out that a critical mass of HIV is a relevant factor, this may vary in individuals. More crucially, sexual practices vary enormously among gay women as among all other people, and some of these practices may facilitate HIV transmission.

The point, again, is that statistical probabilities should not be transformed into theoretical absolutes. A second answer, however, is that as women become aware of the potential for risk, only a collective, feminist political analysis can contest the purely self-interested, self-help perspective now beginning to emerge in many publications by and / or for women. In April 1987, for example, full-page advertisements for Mentor contraceptives appeared in several women's magazines (fig. 6). A healthy and attractive woman, in full color, looks pensively out at the camera: "I never thought I'd buy a condom." Underneath, the copy reads: "INTRODUCING MENTOR CONTRACEPTIVES. THE SMART NEW WAY TO PROTECT YOURSELF." And at the bottom of the page, under a photo in which the individually packaged condom resembles nothing so much as a container of yogurt: "SMART SEX IN THE 80'S."[139] The self-congratulatory tone of this advertisement echoes, in my view, much of what has appeared in publications for women.

Another example: "For some women," writes Erica Jong in the April 1986 issue of *New Woman,* "the AIDS crisis may be a way to come to terms with the fact that they never really liked multiple-partner sex in the first place." And, she adds playfully, "think of the time saved for working, for playing, for family, for gardening, for needlepoint!" AIDS was not even an issue two years ago, she continues, so the current flood of information on heterosexual transmission is so sudden, it is overwhelming—and hard to assimilate. Given the "plague mentality" of the media, "what's the informed woman to think—and beyond that, to do—about AIDS?" She continues:

> By far the sanest and most detailed discussion of the disease I have read was published in *Discover* magazine's December 1985 issue. Its message to women was for the most part reassuring. *Discover* concluded that AIDS is 'the largely fatal price one can pay for anal intercourse'; that the virus 'is only borne in the blood and semen'; that AIDS is a difficult disease to catch; and that vaginal intercourse is much less likely than anal intercourse to spread the disease because of the ruggedness of the vaginal lining and its relatively few exposed blood vessels.

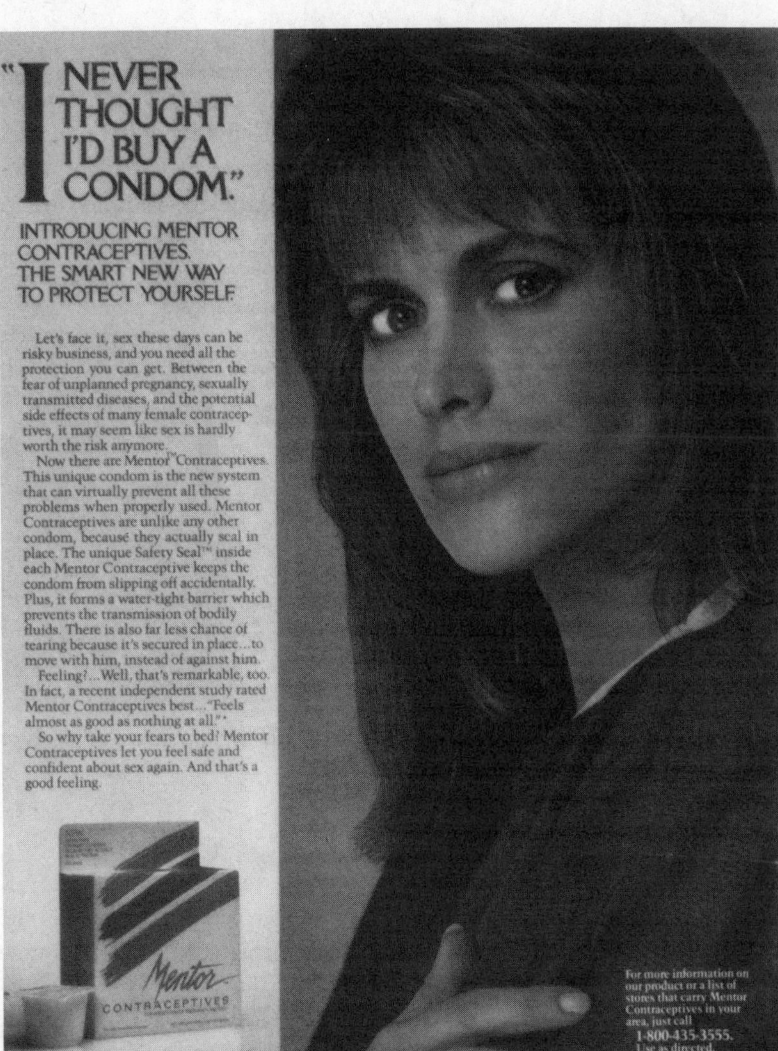

6. In ads in major U.S. women's magazines in the spring of 1987, a beautiful woman praises a condom that sounds like a Greek god and looks like a container of yogurt. It is said that AIDS has brought back the 1950s, but back then it wasn't women who bought the rubbers. DON'T GO OUT WITHOUT YOUR RUBBERS advises another ad for women, because, "if a woman doesn't look out for herself, how can she be sure anyone else will?"

So here is Langone's article, with all its problematic, false certainties reproduced intact to reassure women.[140] To make matters worse, Jong highlights a set of boxed "facts" entitled "Good News (for Women) about AIDS." She begins by contrasting our old friends, the vulnerable rectum and the rugged vagina: "moreover, the tissue in the vagina has fewer blood vessels than the rectum, and natural lubrication during intercourse lessens the chances of tears." Then come the alibis (*it's them, officer, not me; there, not here*):

1. Women with AIDS in Africa actually got it from needles, or anal intercourse (*denied by them*), or by contact with bisexuals (*also denied by them*).

But heterosexual cases in Africa are now confirmed and appear to be wiping out whole villages.

2. The AIDS virus is fragile and cannot be easily transmitted especially if "simple sexual precautions like not exchanging bodily fluids" are followed.

Considering that organizations like New York City's Gay Men's Health Crisis and the San Francisco AIDS Foundation devote entire pamphlets and videos to explicating euphemisms like "exchanging bodily fluids," it does seem that we might have expected more from the author who once brought us the "zipless fuck."

3. Most women in the United States whose cases of AIDS are attributed to heterosexual transmission are long-term partners of intravenous drug users. The small number of these cases suggests that AIDS cannot be transmitted heterosexually, but if it can be, Jong quotes a physician who argues that "women who contracted AIDS got it from steady sex partners, not from one-night stands."

The conflation of "safe sex" with monogamy is clearly problematic; and is the implication here that one-night stands are SAFER than "steady" relationships?

4. Researchers estimate that only 5 to 20 percent of those who test positive for the virus will develop the disease.

Even 5 to 20 percent is an enormous number—half a million to two million depending on who's counting—but as of January 1988 the estimate was up to 25–50 percent, and it is now considered possible that few will be entirely symptom-free forever. The fact that the virus has now been known to be dormant for as long as fourteen years means it may take some time before our understanding of the natural history of AIDS is complete. (Indeed, the large number of asymptomatic carriers is a key to the "success" of HIV: The fact that the virus does not kill quickly means there is ample time for it to be conveyed to new hosts via carriers temporarily without symptoms.)[141]

5. "Men haven't been very good to their immune systems" and therefore appear to be more susceptible to AIDS.

But this statement is apparently based on the health histories of men who already have AIDS—it is hardly fair to make it a statement about men in general (and probably not even about men with AIDS).

And here is Jong's last piece of "good news (for women)": AIDS, she writes, is like the terror of kitchen-table abortions in the 1950s. But maybe this is okay, she says, because it will make sex "a little more mysterious and precious again."

In April 1987, one year after Jong's "good news," AIDS appears in a *Ms.* magazine special issue on "The Beauty of Health." On the cover, an attractive woman in an orange shirt is eating an orange and smiling (fig. 7). "Wake up and be healthy!" the cover blurb commands, and lists what we should wake up *to:*

Skin Problems
RU-486 the Unpregnancy Pill
Exercises You Can Do In Bed
Guarding Against AIDS
Why Doncha Smile, Honey?

The two-page story by Lindsy Van Gelder (who earlier wrote a reasonably intelligent piece for *Ms.* and coauthored a competent article on "AIDS on Campus" for *Rolling Stone*) begins with an anecdote in which she asks a sexually active woman friend whether she has asked her male friend to begin using condoms: "*Rubbers??*" says the friend, "Yuck!!"[142] But, the author graphically points out, "You sleep not just with him but with all his sex partners." Should you trust him? she asks, and slips into the voice of *Seventeen* magazine in the old days: "This is a toughie." She offers some straight talk: "Brace yourself for a shocker: men *lie* to get laid." Van Gelder emphasizes some important points: The term "heterosexuals" is misleading, because "most people who contract

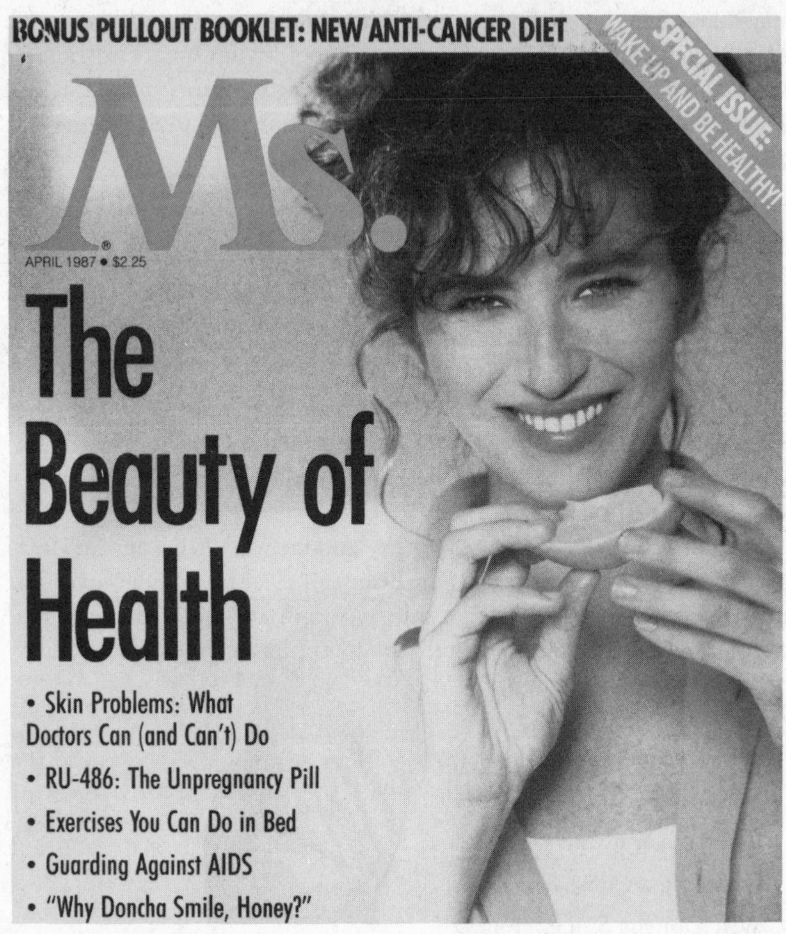

7. An attractive woman in an orange shirt eats an orange on *Ms.* magazine's April 1987 cover, which urges us to WAKE UP AND BE HEALTHY! Skin, exercise, AIDS: The special issue offers tips for all kinds of pesky health problems. "Why Doncha Smile, Honey?" the cover asks. But where AIDS is concerned, there's a better question: Why *is* this woman smiling?

AIDS heterosexually are women"; she also argues that "safe sex with many different men is less risky than unprotected sex with one [infected] man," a logical deduction, but one that many writers fail to make. But the article ends with a breezy reinscription of conventional sexual division—that outdated staple of *Ms.* magazine's version of feminism—us against them (women against men): "How much do you want to bet that if female-to-male transmission begins to be documented in great numbers, *men* will be demanding safe sex—with no wimpy worries about turning women off?"

Van Gelder's article is an example of condom journalism, a new genre that ranges from the *Village Voice*'s "Better Latex Than Never" to the safe-sex kits distributed to all Dartmouth students to the "how to" lessons of *New Woman* and *Spare Rib* to the critiques of condoms and condom advertising that have appeared in, among other places, the *New York Times*.[143] All of which prompts mention of another recent genre, the Heterosexual White Male's commentary on AIDS. Although the *New York Times,* as the "newspaper of record," has improved its coverage of AIDS (there is now a virtual AIDS page in almost every issue), even recent features in the *New York Times Magazine* leave a great deal to be desired. Peter Davis, for example, offers familiar insights about AIDS as though he had thought of them all by himself (AIDS connects "sex and death" is a sample) along with a significant amount of misleading information. In his search for heterosexuals reputed to be at risk for AIDS, for instance, he interviews what appear to be an elite assortment of investment bankers, executives, and elegant divorcées (his phrase). Already-infected heterosexual people, in the real kingdom of AIDS, remain invisible as we listen to the voices of Davis's upscale informants: "God," one woman tells him, "I wish I could have just one lunch in the Russian Tea Room where we talk about something besides AIDS." Davis quotes Dr. Mervyn Silverman's prudent advice ("just because there's no reason to panic doesn't mean there's no reason to be careful") but ultimately trivializes the gravity of the problem.[144] *Newsweek,* which has provided fairly steady coverage of AIDS and rarely downplayed its seriousness, ran a long and moving photo-story on those who died during 1987. Under the photographs ran captions that displayed what journalist Rex Wockner has called "back-door homophobia." The captions of the heterosexuals, for example, tell how they got infected (transfusion, etc.) while those of the gay people state their occupation without any transmission information. It is as though, says Wockner, even the dead must be kept clean from the suspicion of homosexuality.[145] As a final example of publications I consider problematic for women, I will mention sex therapist Helen Singer Kaplan's 1987 book *The Real Truth About Women and AIDS*. The book is both depressing and interesting. Geared toward heterosexual middle-class women and their "unborn babies," the book is depressing because it retrogressively asserts, in the name of saving women from a fate synonymous with death, that AIDS is caused by who you are, not by what you do. The advice to "avoid unsafe practices," says Kaplan, is "nonsense!" Rather: "avoid infected partners." The only way to "avoid sexual exposure to high-risk males" is to (1) make any candidate take the ELISA test; (2) wait; (3) make him get tested again; and if he's clean and you still want to (4) go ahead and have a sexual contact.[146] And then, presumably, (5) handcuff him to you for the rest of your life.

An interesting feature of Kaplan's book, however, is her inclusion, in an appendix, of the transcript of a telephone conversation between a woman caller and a New York AIDS hotline. This transcript not only graphically dramatizes the complex and, as Kaplan points out, often problematic understandings of AIDS-related concepts, but it also lets us see AIDS as it is constructed in everyday talk.[147] Likewise, a BBC special on AIDS, broadcast around the world in September 1987, wove together commentary from professionals and from women on the front lines of the AIDS crisis: A Kenyan health care worker describes her workshops on AIDS and safer sex for prostitutes in Nairobi; a British woman, who, like her roommates, formerly used drugs and now tests HIV positive, talks about living with the knowledge of infection; a woman from a prostitute's organization describes her group's concerns about AIDS and preventive techniques, pointing out that prostitutes have extensive knowledge about alternative sexual practices that they could usefully be sharing with other women.[148]

In recent months (at any rate, in the September 1987 issue), *Ms.* finally got serious and published a photo-essay called "Facing AIDS" made up of photographs and words of women with or facing AIDS (fig. 8). This is not to say that such a representation is unmediated or closer to the "true experience" of AIDS, but it is a welcome departure from the chipper good news/bad news tone of other articles. The *Spare Rib* series initiated in 1987 also expressed a determination to begin—as women and feminists in alliance with others and in a larger social and economic context—confronting and working through the numerous questions and problems that AIDS creates (fig. 9).[149] Likewise, the 1987 Gay and Lesbian March on Washington moved dramatically toward the integration of the AIDS issue with broader cultural issues: the refusal to be extinguished, the refusal to die.[150] At the same time, as AIDS moves out of scientific journals, news stories, and print journalism and becomes increasingly a focus in the arts and mass culture, we can expect the continued diversification of discourse and resources.[151]

To sum up, then. A body of evidence suggests that AIDS is like other sexually transmitted diseases, capable of infecting women and men in equal numbers and now spreading as rapidly by way of heterosexual contact as it once did by way of homosexual contact. Current data suggest, in other words, that the consequences of ignoring earlier evidence of heterosexual transmission may be devastating. Large numbers of people are already infected; many will die. Just as male homosexuals and intravenous drug users in the 1970s and early 1980s engaged in behavior that gave them pleasure without thinking it could kill them, many people today are engaging in activities that a few years from now may kill them.

My general argument is not that biomedical scientists have been "irresponsible" or that "the media" have created a sense of false security (or false terror), or that we can never truly know the biological "facts" about AIDS. What is important is that even scientific characterizations of the reality of AIDS are always partly founded upon prior and deeply entrenched cultural narratives. One step is to ask, as new narratives and new meanings are produced, such questions as the following:

How and why is knowledge about AIDS being produced in the way that it is?

Who is contributing to the process of knowledge production? To whom and by whom is this knowledge disseminated?

What are the practical and material consequences of any new interpretation? Who benefits? Who loses?

On what grounds are facts and truth being claimed?[152]

Any characterization of AIDS has a history, it has a vocabulary, origins, and consequences. Even a seemingly innocent and straightforward term like "the AIDS virus"—a term that now permeates technical and general AIDS discourse—is in fact profoundly misleading. Simon Watney, for example, scrupulously insists on calling the virus *HIV* and, speaking of a person known to be infected, *HIV-positive*. His point is not that what we call "HIV" is "real," but that this term is a much more preferable *representation*. What we call "AIDS," he argues, consists of some thirty diverse clinical entities and conditions. Although a virus may initiate the breakdown of the body's immune system, which in turn makes possible the development of one or more of the thirty diseases and conditions, it does not cause "AIDS."[153] Suppose a thief enters your house, ties you up, cuts your phone cord and burglar alarm, steals your silver, and uses your credit cards to catch the next plane to Copenhagen.

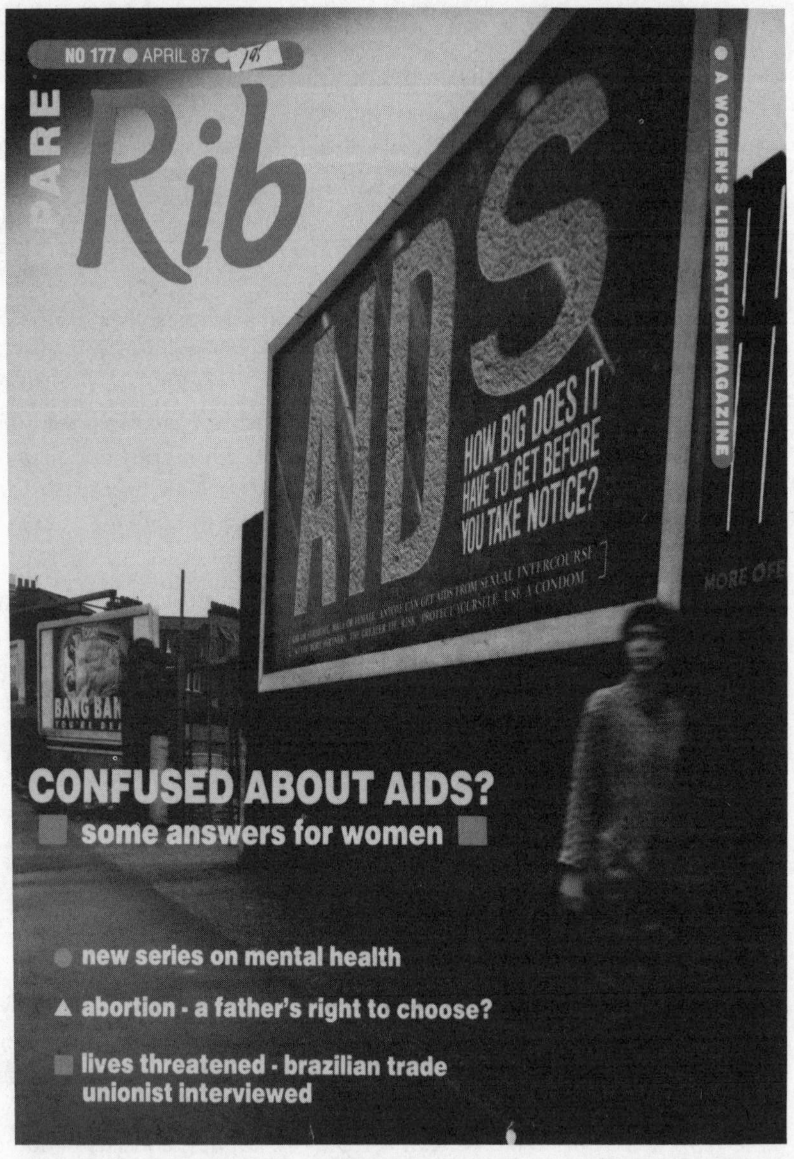

8. In April 1987 the British feminist magazine *Spare Rib* initiates a series on women and AIDS that calls for a broad analysis of the AIDS crisis and coalitions with others. Authors Susan Ardill and Sue O'Sullivan "attempt to focus on the impact AIDS is primarily having, or will have, on us as women—through our sexuality, sexual practices and sexual identities." Rather than pretending to have total knowledge and control, the authors urge readers to ask questions, and "from there to go on and ask more questions, loudly and clearly" (*Spare Rib* 177 [April 1987]: 14–19). Courtesy of *Spare Rib*, London.

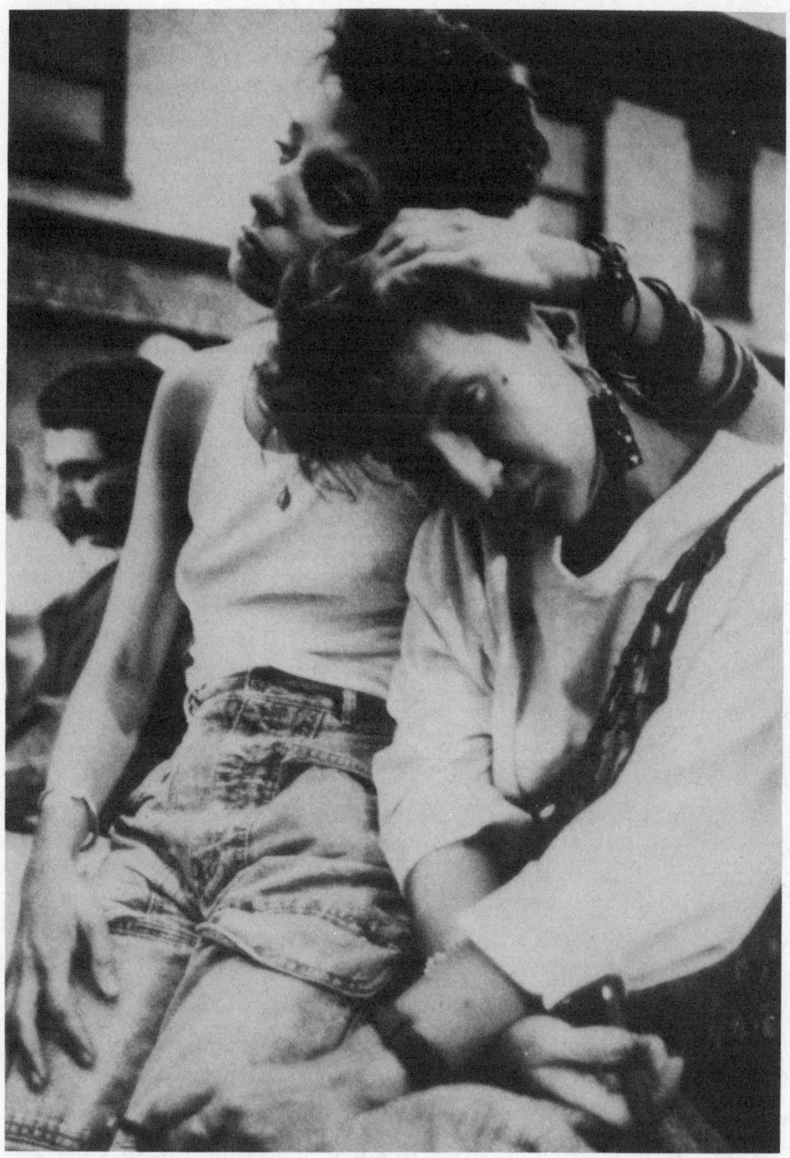

9. Ann and Juliette at New York City annual AIDS vigil, 1985. In September 1987, *Ms.* runs a different kind of story on AIDS, a photo-essay by Jane Rosett and Gypsy Ray, two women who work with AIDS; in photos and text, the darker, exhausting dimensions of AIDS emerge. Courtesy of Jane Rosett, Brooklyn.

Because you're still tied up, you can't do anything when the microwave explodes and starts a fire. Is the thief an arsonist?[154] In the end, we cannot look "through" language to obtain knowledge about AIDS. Rather, we must examine how language itself produces what we think we know; and if we are to intervene, language is one place where that intervention must take place. Thus we can also ask:

What are the origins and implications of the language used to talk about such concepts as behavior, risk, persons at risk, modes of transmission—interpersonally and "epidemically" (Greek for *among the people*)—agents of transmission, health and illness?

What is the nature of the bodies said to be most "at risk" for AIDS? How are these bodies gendered? What is their discursive history?

What are the differences between "dominant" and "oppositional" accounts of this complex phenomenon?[155]

My argument in this essay is a simple one. Contests over meaning come into stark relief in the case of AIDS, which in multiple, fragmentary, and often contradictory ways we (as feminists perhaps, certainly as global citizens) struggle to understand. The name AIDS—and indeed the entire biomedical discourse that surrounds it—in part *constructs* the disease and helps make it intelligible. The construction of AIDS as a "gay disease," for example, is not based on "material reality"—which challenges any stable division between male and female, gay and straight, "promiscuous" and monogamous, guilty and innocent. Yet the construction inscribed again and again throughout our cultural discourses radically contains and controls this diverse and contradictory data, producing and reproducing monolithic identities of those "at risk" or not at risk, depending on their official classification.

The feminist community, or the communities of feminisms, have only recently begun to address the AIDS crisis. Feminists, who have learned to analyze and theorize about complex and contradictory data, can usefully contribute to an analysis of AIDS that brings together the collective insights of feminist scholarship and feminist theory to date. These would include historical description and analysis of women's experience during past epidemics and panics over sexually transmitted disease; critiques of conventional sociological categories in which women are inexorably linked to their male partners and to the diseases they contract; the intersections of gender, race, and class in relation to an illness profiled in terms of nonintersecting categories; and theoretical work on the nature and history of gendered representation and on the evolution of Woman as a constructed identity. Finally, we might wish to ask whether the call for a "feminist analysis" is theoretically paradoxical: AIDS is complex, after all, in part because it exposes the artificiality of the categories and divisions that govern our views of social life and sexual difference. It challenges the existence of "women" as a monolithic sisterhood and as a meaningful linguistic entity. But feminist theory also suggests why a feminist analysis remains imperative: for women are both linguistic and material subjects who exist within language and history. Even as we work to deconstruct and perhaps finally to dissolve the linguistic subject, we must nonetheless keep our attention fixed relentlessly on the inequities still embodied in the material one.[156]

At the very end of *The Intern's Tale,* after the scene I quoted when I began this chapter, one of the interns—Mac—dies, and Campbell, the protagonist, suggests that Maggie should be told. He learns she has read about Mac's death in the newspaper and called the hospital to inform them that she is a carrier of the virus but never developed the full-blown disease. The following morning she is found dead from an overdose of sleeping pills. Like many of the deaths of diseased women in history and literature, Maggie's suicide destroys, in a single gesture, the treacherous host—that is, the conscious subject, the material body required for replication—of the virus, of sexuality, of children, of life, of mind, of desire. Such self-extinction is part of women's discursive and historical legacy. We must therefore be alive to its potential incarnations in this latest social crisis. Nancy Shaw and Lyn Paleo point out, for example, that as more childbearing women become infected and more babies develop AIDS, childbearing may come under even more intense scrutiny by the state: Because if everyone practices safer sex, no babies will be born at all. Women, not gay men, may thus be among the first groups tested for HIV antibodies (with, presumably, a subsequent separation of the "clean" from the "dirty"). They also note that women, as caretakers in this epidemic, have thus far not felt they could protest sexism as they would under less life-threatening conditions.[157] And what of Kaplan's message that women must refuse to be the "bridges" between one infected pool and another; is there something of an extinction process working here? Meanwhile, a film like *Fatal Attraction* recapitulates for women the message gay men received when AIDS first occurred: What you have done for twenty years is wrong, what you desire is evil, sexuality is wrong, you are sick, you are dangerous, you must be punished.[158]

Maggie's death is the symbolic conclusion we must find ways to challenge and disrupt. This means, it seems to me, that we need to refuse the appeal of "binary division," of them versus us, of distinguishing ourselves from gay men and members of other "high-risk" groups. If we, as women, are to cope with AIDS in any reasonable and intelligent way, we must unequivocally see ourselves connected to it and refuse the lie that our own identities and gender offer magical protection against the invasions of that alien Other.

NOTES

Research for this chapter was made possible in part by grants from the National Council of Teachers of English and the University of Illinois at Urbana-Champaign Graduate College Research Board and by a residency at the Ragdale Foundation in fall 1987. An earlier version was presented at the Colloquium on Women, Science, and the Body: Discourses and Representations, Society for the Humanities, Cornell University, May 1987. My thanks for comments or other assistance to Douglas Crimp, Elizabeth Fee, Daniel M. Fox, Mary Jacobus, Stephen J. Kaufman, Teresa Mangum, Emily Martin, John Mirowsky, Meaghan Morris, Cary Nelson, M. Kerry O'Banion, Eve Sedgwick, Daniel Tiffany, Simon Watney, Michael Witkovsky, and Leslie Kirk Wright. This chapter is part of an ongoing project entitled "Authority, Feminism, and Medical Discourse: Current Contests for Meaning."

1. Colin Douglas, *The Intern's Tale* (1975, New York: Grove, 1982), 180–181.

2. Two useful recent collections are Catherine Gallagher and Thomas Laqueur, eds., *The Making of the Modern Body: Sexuality and Society in the Nineteenth Century* (Berkeley and Los Angeles: University of California Press, 1987); and Susan Rubin Suleiman, ed., *The Female Body in Western Culture* (Cambridge: Harvard University Press, 1986). Mary Poovey, for example, "'Scenes of an Indelicate Character': The Medical 'Treatment' of Women," in *Making of the Modern Body,* ed. Gallagher and Laqueur, 137–168, documents the "longevity of [the] male aversion to female bodies" in quoting a nineteenth-century Boston physician who takes Hippocrates as his authority on women's illnesses ("What is woman?" asked Hippocrates: "Disease.") and adds approvingly that "the wise old physician was not far wrong in his judgment" (166). See also Alain Corbin, "Commercial Sexuality in Nineteenth-Century France: A System of Images and Regulations," in *Making of the Modern Body,* ed. Gallagher and Laqueur, 209–219. Other useful sources on the historical specificity of representations of women include G. J. Barker-Benfield, *The Horrors of the Half-Known Life: Male Attitudes Toward Women and Sexuality in Nineteenth-Century America* (New York: Harper & Row, 1976); Caroll Smith-Rosenberg, *Disorderly Conduct: Visions of Gender in Victorian America* (New York: Knopf, 1985), 197–216; Mary Jacobus, "In Parentheses: Immaculate

Conceptions and Feminine Desire" (Paper presented at the Colloquium on Women, Science, and the Body: Discourses and Representations, Cornell University, May 1987); Ludmilla Jordanova, "Nature Unveiling before Science: Images of Women and Knowledge" (Paper presented at the Colloquium on Women, Science, and the Body: Discourses and Representations, Cornell University, May 1987); Jordanova, "Natural Facts: A Historical Perspective on Science and Sexuality," in *Nature, Culture and Gender,* ed. Carol P. MacCormack and Marilyn Strathern (Cambridge: Cambridge University Press, 1980), 42–69; Judith Walzer Leavitt, ed., *Women and Health in America* (Madison: University of Wisconsin Press, 1984).

Additional discursive links between women's bodies and disease are documented by Allan M. Brandt in *No Magic Bullet: A Social History of Venereal Disease in the United States since 1880,* rev. ed. (New York: Oxford University Press, 1987). Venereal disease, in particular, has historically been given feminine personifications. One World War II army poster that Brandt reprints (following p. 164) shows the face of an attractive young woman. "SHE MAY LOOK CLEAN," the poster warns, "BUT PICK-UPS, 'GOOD TIME' GIRLS, PROSTITUTES SPREAD SYPHILIS AND GONORRHEA. You can't beat the Axis if you get VD." See also Cindy Patton, *Sex and Germs: The Politics of AIDS* (Boston: South End Press, 1985).

The characterization of women and women's bodies as diseased or pathological is not necessarily explicit. Sander L. Gilman, *Difference and Pathology: Stereotypes of Sexuality, Race, and Madness* (Ithaca, N.Y.: Cornell University Press, 1985) shows that even scientific and medical texts are pervaded by implicit cultural narratives about women's bodies (and black bodies). Emily Martin, *The Woman in the Body: A Cultural Analysis of Reproduction* (Boston: Beacon, 1987), identifies linguistic devices (metaphors, for example) in nineteenth- and twentieth-century medical texts used to describe human sexuality and reproduction; Martin's meticulous comparison of passages about women with comparable passages about men demonstrates the ways in which female functions are conceptualized negatively (for example, menopause is viewed as a breakdown in "production" or, in some recent texts, as a breakdown of "authority" and efficient communication) while male functions remain heroic and full of energy; her manipulation of the texts demonstrates how the same passages could be rewritten (but rarely are) to reverse the traditional conceptualizations.

Ruth Herschberger's *Adam's Rib* (1948; New York: Harper & Row, 1970), demonstrated earlier that a traditional—supposedly "objective"—account of male and female biological development is revealed as "patriarchal" only when a "matriarchal account" is created and placed beside it (75–82). Hilary Allen, "At the Mercy of Her Hormones: Premenstrual Tension and the Law," *m/f* 9 (1984): 19–43, draws on the language and logic of recent British court decisions to show that they are founded on an implicit assumption that women are always already pathological (thus "premenstrual tension" is essentially a permanent—and potentially disqualifying—condition). Bryan Turner, *The Body and Society* (London: Basil Blackwell, 1984), 2–3, writes that disorders of the body, especially women's bodies, are often treated as disorders of society; order is preserved by the control of women's bodies under a system of patriarchy (see also 115–176, 204–226). See also Barbara Ehrenreich and Deirdre English, *Complaints and Disorders: The Sexual Politics of Sickness* (Old Westbury, N.Y.: Feminist Press, 1973).

The long-standing deployment of the human body as an image of society takes on special apocalyptic force in some recent "postmodern" accounts: like contemporary society, the body too is increasingly commodified and diseased, and frequently this diseased society / body is conceptualized as female: see, for example, Christine Buci-Glucksmann, "Catastrophic Utopia: The Feminine as Allegory of the Modern," in *Making of the Modern Body,* ed. Gallagher and Laqueur, 220–229; Arthur Kroker and David Cook, *The Postmodern Scene: Excremental Culture and Hyper-Aesthetics* (New York: St. Martin's, 1986); and Edward Shorter, *A History of Women's Bodies,* chap. 10 (New York: Basic Books, 1982).

3. Thomas Laqueur, "Orgasm, Generation, and the Politics of Reproductive Biology," in *Making of the Modern Body,* ed. Gallagher and Laqueur, 31–32; and Martin, *Woman in the Body,* 35, cite the vivid language of Walter Heape, a nineteenth-century antifeminist, antisuffrage zoologist at Cambridge, to suggest how extreme male views of menstruation could become. In menstruation, writes Heape in the late nineteenth century, the entire epithelium is torn away, "leaving behind a ragged wreck of tissue, torn glands, ruptured vessels, jagged edges of stroma, and masses of blood corpuscles, which it would seem hardly possible to heal satisfactorily without the aid of surgical treatment" (Heape was the first to use the term *estrus,* a neologism from Latin for *gadfly* to mean "frenzy, rut, heat"). As Laqueur notes, Heape did represent an extreme, but Martin observes that the 1977 edition of a widely used textbook of medical physiology disrupts its characteristically "emotionally subdued prose" to inform the reader that "to quote an old saying, 'menstruation is the uterus crying for lack of a baby.'"

4. The duplicitous female body is also signaled in *The Intern's Tale* when another woman successfully deceives Campbell into thinking she is a virgin and still another woman's apparent indigestion turns out to be appendicitis. This long-standing equation of women with acting is echoed in filmmaker Lizzie Borden's comment on *Working Girls,* her 1987 release about prostitutes: "Men's bodies are exposed and therefore vulnerable, whereas women have this ability to conceal. On some level, women have always dealt with theater" (Katherine Dieckmann, "Lizzie Borden: Adventures in the Skin Trade," *Village Voice,* 10 March 1987, 33).

5. Poovey, "'Scenes of an Indelicate Character,'" cites a variety of ways in which women and their bodies are judged to be duplicitous, including the view of hysteria as mimicry, the "periodicity" of the menstrual cycle as creating inherent "instability," and the invisibility and mysteriousness of the origins of many "women's illnesses"; the female body, wrote one physician, "mocks the reality of truth," and another wrote of hysterics that "these patients are veritable actresses" whose lives are "one perpetual falsehood." Duplicity and changeability are also typically attributed to venereal diseases, most classically to syphilis, the "Great Imitator," with its diverse array of symptoms; "if you know syphilis," it used to be said, "you know medicine." Writes Ludvik Fleck, *Gene-*

sis and Development of a Scientific Fact, ed. Thaddeus J. Trenn and Robert K. Merton, tr. Fred Bradley and Thaddeus J. Trenn (1935; Chicago: University of Chicago Press, 1979), 12, "Syphilis is an extremely pleomorphic disease of many aspects. We read in many treatises that it is a 'proteoform' disease, since with its many forms, it reminds one of 'Proteus or Chameleon.' . . . There was hardly any disease or symptom that was not attributed to syphilis." Mark Thomas Connelly, "Prostitution, Venereal Disease, and American Medicine," in *Women and Health in America,* ed. Leavitt, 196–221, 284, argues that early twentieth-century education, conceptualization, and views on regulation of venereal disease were curiously inconsistent: On the one hand, the antiprostitution crusade and call for premarital testing for both women and men clearly assumed that both women and men could transmit disease; this assumption was contradicted by the widespread view that men are always the authors of these social crimes, women always their victims. Connelly argues that "to insist that women could not spread venereal disease simply because they were women embodied an attitude that, even by 1915, was becoming increasingly absurd."

6. Blood and other liquids figure prominently in the history of sexually transmitted diseases. Fleck, *Genesis and Development,* discusses "bad blood" as a central concept in the history of syphilis. Brandt, *No Magic Bullet,* 23, quotes early twentieth-century physician Homer Kelly's description of the city as a massive civic circulatory system, its "countless currents flowing daily in our cities" distributing morality and disease equally throughout the body politic. The "rising tide" of venereal disease was thus linked to urbanization and to immigration—the "incessant inpouring of a large foreign population." Brandt notes that a "rare blood disease" was the euphemism of choice for venereal disease in the press. Connelly, "Prostitution, Venereal Disease, and American Medicine," 214, cites early twentieth-century rhetoric that linked syphilitic blood to insanity: "The red mills grind out men's brains." Patton, *Sex and Germs,* 23, observes that as old myths about blood resurface, AIDS triggers not only homophobia but also hemophobia—fear of hemophilia. As members of a still feared and stigmatized group, many people with hemophilia have chosen to keep it a secret; getting AIDS, one man with hemophilia told Patton, had forced him out of the "clot closet." In turn, when the National Hemophilia Foundation established a "gay blood ban" in 1983, the executive director of the National Gay Task Force objected: "I don't have to tell you what 'gay blood–bad blood' could mean to a community that has been historically discriminated against" ("National Gay Task Force, Others, Decry Gay Blood Ban by National Hemophilia Foundation," *The Advocate,* 20 January 1983, 8).

7. Mary Ann Doane, "The Clinical Eye: Medical Discourses in the 'woman's film' of the 1940s," in *The Female Body,* ed. Suleiman, 152–174.

8. Poovey, "'Scenes of an Indelicate Character,'" discusses at length the role of silence in the nineteenth-century medical debates about the use of chloroform during childbirth, specifically, the value of the "quiet and unresisting body" for the physician. Above all, Poovey argues, "the silenced female body can be made the vehicle for any medical man's assumptions and practices because its very silence opens a space in which meanings can proliferate" (152); she describes this as the "metaphorical promiscuity of the female body" (153).

9. Sources for this analysis of gender in AIDS discourse are deliberately diverse, though primarily Anglo-American, and may be categorized as follows: (1) leading scientific and medical journals, (2) scientific and medical journals for general readers, (3) general circulation magazines and newspapers, (4) books and reports on AIDS and AIDS-related topics, (5) conservative journals, (6) leftist journals, (7) gay and lesbian journals and newspapers, (8) general circulation women's magazines, (9) feminist journals, (10) supermarket tabloids, (11) national radio and network television programs on AIDS; and (12) other specialized print media. By the term "biomedical discourse about AIDS" I mean, unless otherwise specified, writings and statements about AIDS found in leading U.S. medical and scientific journals as well as public statements made by AIDS researchers, clinicians, and public health officers (i.e., examples are drawn primarily from categories (1) to (4) above). It is within this discourse that what is now the Received View on AIDS (its viral etiology) has evolved. For definition and discussion of the evolution, politics, and coverage of AIDS, see Dennis Altman, *AIDS in the Mind of America* (Garden City, N.Y.: Anchor / Doubleday, 1986). David Black, *The Plague Years: A Chronicle of AIDS, the Epidemic of Our Times* (New York: Simon and Schuster, 1986) and Randy Shilts, *And the Band Played On: People, Politics, and the AIDS Epidemic* (New York: St. Martin's, 1987). (Conservative commentators typically consider "the AIDS Establishment" to include scientists and physicians, public health officials, government officials, gay activists, and the American Civil Liberties Union—all in league to sacrifice the health of "innocent citizens" for the civil rights of "AIDS victims." Nat Hentoff's list, for example, in "The New Priesthood of Death," *Village Voice,* 30 June 1987, 35, includes "public health officials and researchers, supervisory hospital personnel, bioethicists, liberal members of Congress, and a representative of the National Gay and Lesbian Task Force.")

10. A San Francisco female prostitute who died in 1978 appears to have been one of the earliest AIDS cases in the United States. Shilts, *Band Played On,* begins his chronicle of AIDS with the 1976 case of the Danish lesbian surgeon Grethe Rask, who became ill working in Zaire, describes AIDS's subsequent appearance and evolution in the United States—though in the United States only—as a "gay disease," and documents widespread resistance to evidence that women and babies could also develop AIDS. Ironically, however, the only entry for women in Shilts's detailed index is to the film *Women in Love*. Black, *Plague Years,* 74, reports one researcher who jokingly called the CDC's risk list the "4-H Club": "homos, heroin addicts, Haitians, and hookers." Several early studies explored whether prostitutes were at risk: Joyce Wallace, for example, "Acquired Immune Deficiency Syndrome (AIDS) in Prostitutes," in *The Acquired Immune Deficiency Syndrome and Infections of Homosexual Men,* ed. Pearl Ma and Donald Armstrong (New York: Yorke Medical Books, 1984), 253–258, concludes that despite normal T-cell ratios, working prostitutes in New York City could be at risk to develop AIDS; more precise studies (based on tests for HIV antibodies), however, remain inconclusive as to prostitutes' *sexual* risk because of high incidence of intravenous drug use in the same population (more on this below). When hemophiliacs and transfusion recipients started be-

coming ill, they bounced "hookers" off the 4-H list and simultaneously brought conventional "respectability" to the list. On the development of risk groups and conceptualization of AIDS, see Altman, *Mind of America,* esp. 30–37. Lawrence K. Altman, "Heterosexuals and AIDS: New Data Examined," *New York Times,* 22 January 1985, 1, 19, reports researchers' puzzlement over the heterosexual nature of AIDS in Africa as well as the small but confirmed number of heterosexually transmitted cases in the United States, and their disagreement over whether the public should be informed. There is still no real consensus among researchers or the public as to precisely *why* women may be "at risk," but evidence is now clear that women can become infected and can infect others. See Margaret A. Fischl et al., "Evaluation of Heterosexual Partners, Children, and Household Contacts of Adults with AIDS," *Journal of the American Medical Association* 257 (1987): 640–644; Mary Guinan and Ann Hardy, "Epidemiology of AIDS in Women in the United States: 1981 through 1986," *Journal of the American Medical Association* 257 (1987): 2039–2042; Constance B. Wofsy, "Human Immunodeficiency Virus Infection in Women," *Journal of the American Medical Association* 257 (1987): 2074–2076; and Marsha F. Goldsmith, "Sex Experts and Medical Scientists Join Forces against a Common Foe: AIDS," *Journal of the American Medical Association* 259 (1988): 641–643. See also Marilyn Chase's summary, "Spread of AIDS among Women Poses Widening Challenge to Medical Field," *Wall Street Journal,* 26 June 1986, and Matt Clark (with Mariana Gosnell) and Mary Hager, "Women and AIDS," *Newsweek,* 14 July 1986, 60–61. This information and more was amplified in Katie Leishman, "Heterosexuals and AIDS: The Second Stage of the Epidemic," *The Atlantic* (February 1987), 39–58. But Scott S. Smith's letter to the editor, *The Atlantic* (January 1988), 9–10, argues that the small number of women with AIDS to date hardly warrants the common "bubonic plague" comparison; Leishman replies that even with Smith's qualifiers (i.e., the "women" he counts are white, do not use intravenous drugs, never received transfusions, and are not sexual partners of high-risk men), the number represents only women with AIDS now, not the number who may be infected. A politically astute analysis is offered in Diane Richardson, *Women and AIDS* (New York: Methuen, 1987).

11. The question of how AIDS is defined by the CDC, the agency responsible for surveillance, exemplifies the nontransparent nature of language in relation to reality: as knowledge of the "reality" of AIDS increases, redefinition is regularly called for; but a new definition reorganizes the reality now under surveillance. The 1986 reclassification of AIDS cases is reported in Centers for Disease Control, "Update: Acquired Immunodeficiency Syndrome—United States," *Morbidity and Mortality Weekly Report* 35 (12 December 1986): 757–760, 765–766, and discussed in Eve K. Nichols, *Mobilizing Against AIDS: The Unfinished Story of a Virus* (Cambridge: Harvard University Press, 1986); reports in the general media include Kathleen McAuliffe et al., "AIDS: At the Dawn of Fear," *U.S. News and World Report,* 12 January 1987, 60–69; and Associated Press, "571 AIDS Cases Tied to Heterosexual Cases," *Champaign-Urbana News-Gazette,* 12 December 1986, A-7.

12. David Baltimore and Sheldon M. Wolff, *Confronting AIDS: Directions for Public Health, Health Care, and Research* (Washington, D.C.: National Academy Press, 1986).

13. U.S. Surgeon General, *U.S. Surgeon General's Report on Acquired Immune Deficiency Syndrome* (Washington, D.C.: Public Health Service, 1986).

14. See Thomas W. Netter, "Cases of AIDS Rise around the World," *New York Times,* 5 October 1986, 7. By May 1987 WHO reported at a press conference that 112 countries had reported cases of AIDS (see "Official Warns of 'Racist, Fascist' Approaches to AIDS," *American Medical News,* 12 June 1987, 19).

15. See the cover of *U.S. News and World Report,* 12 January 1987, and the story in that issue by McAuliffe et al., "AIDS: At the Dawn of Fear." Accompanying the story, a graph showing rising numbers of AIDS cases cuts across a two-page photograph of the roofs of Manhattan apartment buildings, while a boxed insert lists U.S. "Hot Spots"—cities with high numbers of cases. These dual allusions to real estate and vacation spots function to domesticate AIDS for an upscale New York City readership.

16. Pie-shaped charts (see, for example, the overview in *Issues in Science and Technology* 2 (1986): 2) "hid" cases of AIDS among women within the category "Other"—meaning unknown, no known risk factor, risk factor could not be established. Leslie Kirk Wright suggests that "Other" has moved from a benign euphemism for presumed heterosexuals in earlier publications to newly undesirable "others" (personal communication). Stephanie Poggi, "*In These Times:* With Friends Like Us, Who Nee [*sic*]," *Gay Community News,* 12–18 July 1987, 3, satirizes the ubiquitous AIDS pie-shaped charts in her attack on the leftist publication *In These Times*'s endorsement of mandatory HIV testing.

17. The extensive feminist literature on Woman as Other includes Simone de Beauvoir, *The Second Sex,* trans. and ed. H. M. Parshley (New York: Knopf, 1953); Shari Benstock, ed., *Feminist Issues in Literary Scholarship* (Bloomington: Indiana University Press, 1987); Luce Irigaray, *Speculum of the Other Woman,* trans. Gillian C. Gill (Ithaca, N.Y.: Cornell University Press, 1985); Virginia Woolf, *A Room of One's Own* (New York: Harcourt, Brace, 1929); Cary Nelson, "Envoys of Otherness: Differences and Continuity in Feminist Criticism," in *For Alma Mater: Theory and Practice in Feminist Scholarship,* ed. Paula A. Treichler, Cheris Kramarae, and Beth Stafford (Urbana: University of Illinois Press, 1985); Jonathan Culler, *On Deconstruction: Theory and Criticism after Structuralism* (Ithaca, N.Y.: Cornell University Press, 1982), 43–64; Toril Moi, *Sexual / Textual Politics: Feminist Literary Theory* (New York: Methuen, 1985); and Catherine Belsey, *Textual Practice* (New York: Methuen, 1980).

Brandt, in *No Magic Bullet,* cites "otherness" in the history of venereal diseases, which are always said to originate in other races, other places, other classes; among the poor, among immigrants; among aliens. See also Judith Walkowitz, *Prostitution and Victorian Society: Women, Class, and the State* (New York: Cambridge University Press, 1983). During the Black plague of the fourteenth century, Jews were accused of "poisoning the wells" and were massacred. In the fifteenth and sixteenth centuries, the Spanish called syphilis "the

Portuguese disease," the Portuguese called it "the Moroccan disease" (Ladislav Zgusta, personal communication). According to Leslie Kirk Wright, "A Disease of the Other: AIDS Discourse and Homophobia" (Paper presented at the International Scientific Conference on Gay and Lesbian Issues, Amsterdam, December 1987), and Jamie Feldman, "Social Dialogue, Public Dilemma: French Research Perspectives on AIDS" (Paper presented at the Medical Humanities and Social Sciences Seminar, University of Illinois College of Medicine, Urbana, January 1988), in France, where AIDS was at first called "the Moroccan plague," French researchers and clinicians have little difficulty incorporating Africans with AIDS into the French / European population of people with AIDS; American gay men, however, seem to remain the Other. In central Africa, meanwhile, AIDS is always said to have originated in one of the other countries. In Japan, "the other" is not homosexuals but foreigners; because Japan has never allowed "foreign" blood of any kind to be given to Japanese people, transfusion-related AIDS cases are nonexistent; see "AIDS Carrier's Baby Free from Virus, Gov't Confirms," *Japan Times,* 19 April 1987. On AIDS, plague, and Judaism, see Robert Kirschner, "Keeping AIDS in Perspective," *Reform Judaism* (Fall 1986): 12–14, and Angela Graboys, "The Courage of Sunnye Sherman," *Reform Judaism* (Fall 1986): 14–15, 36. Edward Albert, "Acquired Immune Deficiency Syndrome: The Victim and the Press," *Studies in Communication* 3 (1986): 135–158, reviews accounts of the general process through which communities create distinctions between the normal and the deviant; he uses this division to discuss media accounts of AIDS. For a theoretical account, see Gilman, *Difference and Pathology.*

18. Peter Davis, "Exploring the Kingdom of AIDS," *New York Times Magazine,* 31 May 1987, 32–40; Patricia M. O'Kane, R.N., letter to the editor, 28 June 1987, 78.

19. See Leishman, "Heterosexuals and AIDS"; Associated Press, "Doctors: Case Shows AIDS Can Spread Heterosexually," *Champaign-Urbana News-Gazette,* 10 April 1986, A-7; Thomas C. Quinn et al., "AIDS in Africa: An Epidemiologic Paradigm," *Science* 234 (November 1986): 955–963; Thomas A. Peterman et al., "Risk of Human Immunodeficiency Virus Transmission from Heterosexual Adults with Transfusion-Associated Infections," *Journal of the American Medical Association* 259 (1 January 1988): 55–58; L. H. Calabrese and K. V. Gopalakrishna, "Transmission of HTLV-III Infection from Man to Woman to Man," letter to the editor, *New England Journal of Medicine* 314 (1986): 987. Numerous papers on heterosexual transmission were presented at the Second International AIDS Conference, Paris, June 1986 (e.g., see the report by Lawrence K. Altman, "Study Says AIDS in Haiti Spreads Mainly by Heterosexual Activity," *New York Times,* 29 June 1986. Questions about routes of transmission continue; Daniel J. Lehmann and Suzy Schultz, "4 Women among New Cases Here in August," *Chicago Sun-Times,* 3 September 1987, 3, report that one woman was infected through heterosexual intercourse with a man who used intravenous drugs, two women were infected through blood transfusions, "and the fourth did not acknowledge risk factors for [AIDS]." To stress the potential danger of heterosexual relationships, graphic artist Milton Glaser designed a symbol for use in a World Health Organization AIDS prevention cam-

paign; the symbol shows two overlapping red hearts, and a blue skull within the intersecting space; Glaser said the image suggests that "the consequence of uncontrolled coupling is fearful" ("Official Warns of 'Racist, Fascist' Approaches to AIDS," 19).

20. Paula A. Treichler, "AIDS, Homophobia, and Biomedical Discourse: An Epidemic of Signification," *Cultural Studies* 1 (1987): 263–305. (Reprinted, *October* 43 [1987]: 31–70.) Connections between viral and linguistic contamination were paradigmatically, indeed clairvoyantly, represented by William S. Burroughs in *Electronic Revolution* (Cambridge, England: Blackmoor Head Press, 1971). In the AIDS crisis a 1987 MacNelly cartoon for the Chicago *Tribune* shows Ronald Reagan pulling on plastic gloves as he peers into a room marked "Speechwriters" and asks "The AIDS speech ready?" A 1987 AIDS public service announcement sponsored by Esprit clothing likewise links the two epidemics through its slogan "Spread the word, not the virus" (as Julian Halliday has suggested to me, this AIDS message seems to be framed by Esprit's larger interest in promoting the notion that health, like Esprit clothing, makes you look good). On the general question of the linguistic construction of scientific reality, see Susan Sontag, *Illness as Metaphor* (New York: Farrar, Straus & Giroux, 1978); Bruno Latour and Steve Woolgar, *Laboratory Life: The Construction of Scientific Fact* (Cambridge: Cambridge University Press, 1985); David Bloor, *Knowledge and Social Imagery* (London: Routledge & Kegan Paul, 1976); Barry Barnes and David Bloor, "Relativism, Rationalism and the Sociology of Knowledge," in *Rationality and Relativism,* ed. Martin Hollis and Steven Lukes (Cambridge: MIT Press, 1982), 21–47; Roger Cooter, "Anticontagionism and History's Medical Record," in *The Problem of Medical Knowledge: Examining the Social Construction of Medicine,* ed. Peter Wright and Andrew Treacher (Edinburgh: Edinburgh University Press, 1982), 87–108. With respect to the media, see Tony Bennett, "Media, 'Reality,' Signification," in *Media, Culture, Society,* ed. Michael Gurevitch, et al. (London: Methuen, 1982), 287–308; and Todd Gitlin, *The Whole World Is Watching: Mass Media in the Making and Unmaking of the New Left* (Berkeley and Los Angeles: University of California Press, 1980). Gitlin, 251, writes that news is, among other things, "the exercise of power over the interpretation of reality."

21. Shilts, *Band Played On,* 67.

22. Ibid., 43.

23. Centers for Disease Control, "*Pneumocystis* Pneumonia—Los Angeles," *Morbidity and Mortality Weekly Report* 30 (5 June 1981): 250–252.

24. Shilts, *Band Played On,* 171, describes the coining of the acronym AIDS. In Africa, posters warn against "'Slim' Disease / AIDS." Right-wing Lyndon LaRouche supporters in the Montreal airport post signs that play on the French acronym for AIDS: "Give our children SDI [Strategic Defense Initiative, or Star Wars], not SIDA." Joanne Edgar, "Iceland's Feminists: Power at the Top of the World," *Ms.* (December 1987), 30, notes that to preserve the purity of the Nordic languages, official policy in Iceland prohibits borrowed words; instead of the word AIDS, a public opinion poll chose the Icelandic word *eydni* "wasting" or "destruction." Black, *Plague Years,* 60, comments that CDC task force director James Curran called the new name "reasonably descriptive without

being pejorative"; but, Black adds, "names have power." According to Jim D. Hughey, Robert N. Norton, and Catherine Sullivan, "Confronting Danger: AIDS in the News" (Paper presented at the Annual Meeting of the Speech Communication Association, Chicago, November 1986), several companies have removed the word *aid* from their titles; Jennifer Dunning, "Suit Filed over Benefit for AIDS," *New York Times,* 27 August 1987, 20, reports that an organization that raises funds for young adults with cancer through an annual benefit called Dance for Life is suing an organization planning an AIDS benefit called Dancing for Life. A spokesperson for the Dance for Life group said, "If we lose our primary funding source and our identity because we are identified with Dancing for Life, then it is the equivalent of our death." George Whitmore, "Bearing Witness," *New York Times Magazine,* 31 January 1988, reports that some black and Hispanic people prefer the specific diagnosis of Kaposi's sarcoma or *Pneumocystic carinii* pneumonia to AIDS. Whatever term is used acquires its own power. Patton, *Sex and Germs,* 24, writes that one man put a pink triangle on his hospital door with the sign "AIDS Camp."

25. On the evolution and some of the problematic issues in characterizing "risk groups" for AIDS, see Keewhan Choi, "Assembling the AIDS Puzzle: Epidemiology," in *AIDS: Facts and Issues,* ed. Victor Gong and Norman Rudnick (New Brunswick, N.J.: Rutgers University Press, 1986), 15–24; and Ann Guidici Fettner and William Check, *The Truth about AIDS: Evolution of an Epidemic* (New York: Holt, Rinehart and Winston, 1985). Harry Schwartz, "AIDS in the Media," in *Science in the Streets: Report of the Twentieth Century Task Force on the Communication of Scientific Risk* (New York: Priority Press, 1984), 92, describes the complexity of "the Haitian connection." Catherine Ross and John Mirowsky, "Theory and Research in Social Epidemiology" (Paper presented at the Second Conference on Clinical Applications of the Social Sciences to Health, University of Illinois at Urbana-Champaign, October 1980), note that using discrete categories to measure variables that actually exist along a continuum "represents a loss of information that may make results ambiguous." Gender yields discrete categories; but sexual practice, such as heterosexual or homosexual behavior, in many cases does not.

26. See Choi, "Assembling the AIDS Puzzle"; "Update: Acquired Immunodeficiency Syndrome" *MMWR* 35 (12 December 1986); "AIDS: What Is to Be Done?" Forum section, *Harper's* (October 1985), 39–52; and Altman, "Heterosexuals and AIDS."

27. A reporter for the *Wall Street Journal* wrote a piece on the epidemic in 1981 that the editors refused to print; in February 1982 the paper did accept a story centered around twenty-three heterosexual cases, primarily intravenous drug users. According to Shilts, *Band Played On,* 126, publication thus occurred only after "bona fide heterosexuals" had been infected; the story was headlined "New, Often-Fatal Illness in Homosexuals Turns Up in Women, Heterosexual Males." Geoffrey Stokes, "Press Clips," *Village Voice,* 15 October 1985, argues that a similarly misleading focus was evident on "60 Minutes" that same month when Diane Sawyer interviewed Pat Burke, a heterosexual with hemophilia who became infected through contaminated blood products and subsequently infected his pregnant wife; their son also became infected.

Stokes suggests that Sawyer's focus undermined the fact that hemophiliacs represent a tiny percentage of the population.

Edward Albert, "AIDS: The Victim and the Press," and Brian Becher, "AIDS and the Media: A Case Study of How the Press Influences Public Opinion" (Research paper, University of Illinois College of Medicine—Urbana, 1983) discuss media treatment across a range of publications. Julie Dobrow, "The Symbolism of AIDS: Perspectives on the Use of Language in the Popular Press" (Paper presented at the International Communication Association annual meeting, Chicago, May 1986) notes the dramatic and commercial appeal of the common "cultural images" in popular press scenarios of AIDS. A theoretical analysis of media accounts in relation to questions of identity and desire is offered by Simon Watney, *Policing Desire: Pornography, AIDS, and the Media* (Minneapolis: University of Minnesota Press, 1987). Continued monitoring of AIDS coverage is provided by Geoffrey Stokes in his *Village Voice* column "Press Clips" (e.g., 11 October 1985, 3, 10).

28. In "An Epidemic of Signification," I note far-right beliefs that AIDS is God's punishment for homosexuals and that communists or the KGB introduced the virus into the United States to weaken the blood supply. See William F. Buckley, Jr., "Crucial Steps in Combating the AIDS Epidemic: Identify All the Carriers," *New York Times,* 18 March 1986, and Lyndon LaRouche, Jr. "My Program against AIDS," pamphlet (Washington, D.C.: LaRouche Democratic Campaign, 7 February 1987). As a number of commentators have pointed out, if AIDS is God's punishment to gay men, then lesbians, who are virtually AIDS-free, must be God's favorites. Hughey, Norton, and Sullivan, "Confronting AIDS." Compare Governor Lester Maddox's remark that drought was God's way of punishing everyone in Georgia.

29. For a reminder of how much was unknown in the early stages of the AIDS story, see Ruth Kulstad, ed., *AIDS: Papers from Science, 1982–1985* (Washington, D.C.: American Association for the Advancement of Science, 1986); American Medical Association, *AIDS: From the Beginning* (Chicago: American Medical Association, 1987); and Fettner and Check, *The Truth About AIDS.*

30. Altman, *Mind of America;* Black, *Plague Years.* Other comprehensive accounts include Fettner and Check, *The Truth About AIDS;* Jacques Leibowitch, *A Strange Virus of Unknown Origin,* trans. Richard Howard, introd. Robert C. Gallo (New York: Ballantine, 1984); John Green and David Miller, *AIDS: The Story of a Disease* (London: Grafton, 1986); Patton, *Sex and Germs;* Richardson, *Women and AIDS;* and Shilts, *Band Played On.* Brandt, *No Magic Bullet,* 199, summarizes the ways that AIDS thus far recapitulates the social history of other sexually transmitted diseases: the pervasive fear of contagion, concerns about casual transmission, stigmatization of victims, conflict between the protection of public health and the protection of civil liberties; increasing professional control over definition and management; and the search for a "magic bullet." Despite the supposed sexual revolution, Brandt writes, we continue through these social constructions "to define the sexually transmitted diseases as uniquely sinful" (202). This definition is inaccurate but pervasive: and as long as disease is equated with sin, "there can be no magic bullet."

31. Sandra Panem, "AIDS: Public Policy and Biomedical Research," *Hastings Center Report,* special suppl., 15 (August 1985): 23–26. Public health policy is also addressed in Office of Technology Assessment, *Review of the Public Health Service's Response to AIDS: A Technical Memorandum* [Congress of the U.S.] (Washington, D.C.: Government Printing Office, 1985).

32. See Larry Kramer, "1, 112 and Counting," *New York Native,* March 1983, 14–27; Michael Lynch, "Living with Kaposi's," *Body Politic* (November 1982), 88; and Richard Goldstein, "Heartsick: Fear and Loving in the Gay Community," *Village Voice,* 28 June 1983, 13–16. The questioning of established authority had occurred earlier in the struggle over whether homosexuality was to be officially classified as an illness by the American Psychiatric Association. See Ronald Bayer, *Homosexuality and American Psychiatry: The Politics of Diagnosis* (New York: Basic Books, 1981), as well as Jeffrey Weeks, *Sexuality and Its Discontents: Meanings, Myths and Modern Sexualities* (London: Routledge & Kegan Paul, 1985). (Albert, "AIDS," 140, notes, however, that of 2,500 psychiatrists polled almost ten years after the official change, 69 percent still defined homosexuality as "pathological.") In any case, AIDS first struck members of a relatively seasoned and politically sophisticated community (many of whom were also professionals in science, medicine, and government) at a time when American culture at large was contesting medical and scientific authority—points addressed by Altman, *AIDS in the Mind of America,* and Daniel M. Fox, "AIDS and the American Health Polity: The History and Prospects of a Crisis in Authority," *The Milbank Quarterly,* suppl., 64 (1986): 7–33. As Shilts notes, 16, 356, AIDS is a real threat to closeted gay men, serving in a sense as a "double diagnosis" that jeopardizes their anonymity and their lives. This dilemma took the form of an early AIDS sick joke, reported by Black, *Plague Years:*

> Q: What's the hardest thing about getting AIDS?
> A: Convincing your mother you're Haitian.

Elizabeth Kastor explores this problem in the case of conservative fundraiser Terry Dolan (head of the National Political Action Committee, NCPAC) and others, "The Conflict of a Gay Conservative," *Washington Post National Weekly Edition,* 8 June 1987, 11–12.

33. Mary Poovey, "Speaking of the Body: A Discursive Division of Labor in Mid-Victorian Britain" (Paper presented at the Colloquium on Women, Science, and the Body: Discourses and Representations, Cornell University, May 1987). Poovey argues that in nineteenth-century Britain, womanhood was legally categorized with regard to both property and sex. Single women could own property but could not engage in sexual activity with men; married women could have sexual relations but could not own property. Prostitutes, Poovey argues, who could both own property and have sexual relations, can be seen as a "border case"—a case that contradicts or disrupts existing conceptions and stable dichotomies and generates discourse that is designed to restore a stable dichotomy.

34. Leslie Kirk Wright suggests that some linguistic features of "the AIDS scare" seem to be modeled on the "red scare" of the McCarthy era, including

the notion of the virus as fellow traveler, secretly using cells to build power (cf. Peter Jaret, "Our Immune System: The Wars Within," *National Geographic* (June 1986), 702–735, 723, 724: "This strategy makes it even easier for the virus to pass from cell to cell undetected"; "the normal cell turns traitor"). Actor Dack Rambo drew an explicit parallel: "I am convinced we are seeing the return of witch-hunting and McCarthyism because of the fear AIDS has generated" (quoted by Scott Haller, "Fighting for Life," *People,* 23 September 1985, 28–33).

35. Hypotheses about AIDS are reviewed by Altman, *AIDS in the Mind of America;* Baltimore and Wolff, *Confronting AIDS;* Kevin M. Cahill, ed., *The AIDS Epidemic* (New York: St. Martin's Press, 1983); and Gong and Rudnick, eds., *AIDS: Facts and Issues*.

36. Journalistic gatekeeping in AIDS research is discussed by Shilts, *Band Played On;* he notes, for example, 157, that by May 1982 one paper, "hypothesizing an infectious agent as the cause of GRID, had now been rejected by every major scientific journal in the country" because it contradicted the then-dominant view that AIDS was a "life-style" problem. Dorothy Nelkin, "Managing Biomedical News," *Social Research* 52 (1985): 3, discusses the so-called Ingelfinger rule of the *New England Journal of Medicine,* which prohibits release of findings prior to publication; Arnold Relman, however, the journal's current editor, discusses suspension of the Ingelfinger rule and other changes in editorial policy designed to speed up publication of AIDS-related research ("Introduction," *Hastings Center Report,* special suppl. (August 1985): 1–2—but see also Lawrence K. Altman, "Medical Guardians: Does *New England Journal* Exercise Undue Power on Information Flow?" *New York Times,* 28 January 1988, 1, 13).

On another front, Simon Watney, in "AIDS: The Outsiders," *Marxism Today* (January 1988), discusses censorship in the United Kingdom, where the government's aggressive prevention campaign is undermined by its other activities, including the recent banning of all "safer sex" instruction materials as pornography (because they "promote homosexuality"). On the role of institutionalized scientific authority and existing scientific networks during the AIDS crisis, see David Black's discussion of "the AIDS Mafia" and AIDS "gestapo" in *Plague Years,* 113, and Shilts, *Band Played On.* Shilts obtained thousands of government documents through the Freedom of Information Act and shows that despite bitter behind-the-scenes disagreements, most of the scientists connected with federal agencies have tended to display unanimity in public. Outside the federal health-care network, evidence of gatekeeping fuels charges of an AIDS "party line" and conspiracy theories from left, right, and center. Joseph Sonnabend, M.D., for example, a discoverer of interferon and former scientific director of the AIDS Medical Foundation, founded the *Journal of AIDS Research* to print scientific articles he believed were being suppressed because they argued for a multifactorial cause rather than a single virus (see Black, *Plague Years,* 112–118, for discussion). Raymond Keith Brown, author of *AIDS, Cancer, and the Medical Establishment* (New York: Robert Speller, 1986), has chaired two symposia on controversial aspects of AIDS.

37. Leibowitch, *Strange Virus,* 5.

38. Congressman William E. Dannemeyer (R.-Calif.), October 1985, during a legislative debate on a homosexual rights bill (quoted by Langone, "Latest Scientific Facts," 29).

39. Anthropologist Carole S. Vance, who observed the Meese Commission on Pornography throughout its hearings and deliberations, analyzes the recurrent obsession with "natural receptacles" in her forthcoming book, *A Vagina Surrounded by a Woman: The Meese Commission on Pornography, 1984–1985.* Compare the position on orifices held by Lyndon LaRouche, Jr., in "My Program against AIDS": "I hold it to be true, that Creation has endowed our bodies with certain functions, including the body's orifices, each to be used in one way, and not contrary ways; . . . AIDS demonstrates afresh . . . that if society promotes the violation of the principles of our bodies' design, that society shall suffer in some way or another for this obscenity" (6). Whether blood transfusions violate "the principles of our bodies' design" is not addressed.

40. Black, *Plague Years,* 29. Jaret, "The Wars Within," 731, posits that sperm, ejaculated into a woman, are "foreigners in a hostile body" who must deploy several strategies to "accomplish their mission."

41. Black, *Plague Years,* 40.

42. Frances FitzGerald, *Cities on a Hill: A Journey Through Contemporary American Cultures* (New York: Simon and Schuster / Touchstone, 1987), 98.

43. "The A.I.D.S. Show—Artists Involved with Death and Survival," documentary produced by Peter Adair and Rob Epstein, directed by Leland Moss, based on production at Theatre Rhinoceros, San Francisco; aired on PBS, November 1986.

44. A "cofactor" is something that causes, contributes to, or makes possible an illness. Resistance and susceptibility are typically influenced by age, general health status, nutrition, exposure to environmental toxins, and presence of other infectious or parasitic agents. As Fettner observes in "Bad Science," 26, the notion really means that illness involves the interaction between unique genetic programing and a lifetime of environmental influences and cannot be analyzed in a vacuum. Reviewing the cofactors presently thought most likely to contribute to HIV infection and clinical symptoms, Fettner suggests that genetics ultimately may be most important.

45. Shilts, *Band Played On,* 131–132, reports that some gay men interviewed in the very early years were estimated to have had as many as twenty thousand sexual contacts; coupled with the likelihood of such men having a history of STDs and of going to bathhouses, the number of contacts created a network of men who were broadly exposed to numerous infectious agents. Some scientists came to use the term "amplification" to describe the role of the bathhouses in facilitating HIV infection and its geometric increase.

46. Examples of "conspiracy theories" include Gary Null with Trudy Golobic, "The Secret Battle against AIDS," *Penthouse* (June 1987), 61–68; John Lauritsen, "Saying No to HIV," *New York Native,* 6 July 1987, 17–25; and Charles L. Ortleb, "HTLV in Lake Tahoe" (subtitled: "Disease Worse than Originally Thought. Is It AIDS?"); *New York Native,* 11 May 1987, 6–8. Alternative views among scientists outside the core federal AIDS network receive little attention; several of these, including Peter H. Duesberg, "Retroviruses as

Carcinogens and Pathogens: Expectations and Reality," *Cancer Research* 47 (1 March 1987): 1199–1220, are discussed by Lauritsen, "Saying No to HIV," and Ann Guidici Fettner, "Bad Science Makes Strange Bedfellows," *Village Voice,* 2 February 1988, 25–28.

47. On the growing complexity of the clinical and epidemiological picture, see David G. Ostrow et al., "Classification of the Clinical Spectrum of HIV Infection in Adults," in *Information on AIDS for the Practicing Physician,* vol. 1 (Chicago: American Medical Association, July 1987), 7–16; Lawrence K. Altman, "AIDS Virus Always Fatal?" *New York Times,* 8 September 1987, 15–16.

48. In February 1982 Dr. Arye Rubinstein, a pediatrician at Albert Einstein College of Medicine in the Bronx, was seeing sick babies who seemed to have all the symptoms then considered characteristic of AIDS. He sent a paper on the subject to the *New England Journal,* but heard nothing; meanwhile, other scientists were calling his hypothesis "improbable if not altogether impossible. By its very name, GRID was a homosexual disease, not a disease of babies or their mothers" (Shilts, *Band Played On,* 124).

49. The titles of Nichols's *Unfinished Story of a Virus* and Leibowitch's *A Strange Virus of Unknown Origin* follow in the classic Microbe-as-Hero tradition of such biographers as Hans Zinsser, *Rats, Lice and History: The Biography of a Bacillus* (Boston: Little, Brown, 1934). In her interviews with French AIDS researchers, Jamie Feldman ("Social Dialogue, Public Dilemma") confirmed their perception of AIDS as the story of the virus (Feldman also concludes that for the French AIDS also became the story of "the underdogs outsmarting the big shots." Many famous French virologists and immunologists initially rejected the retrovirus theory of AIDS: "If it were a virus, the Americans would already have discovered it.")

50. See Treichler, "An Epidemic of Signification," for perspectives on the uncertainties, politics, and competing accounts that established the virus as the "cause" of AIDS and stabilized it as a legitimate scientific "fact"; Latour and Woolgar in *Laboratory Life* provide a fuller account of the scientific process through which facts are constructed. Self-conscious attention to the construction and interpretation of biomedical science is also provided by Black, *Plague Years;* Altman, *Mind of America;* and Marek Kohn, "Face the Virus: Essential 1980s Biology," *The Face* (April 1987), 64–71.

51. Jaret, "The Wars Within."

52. A summary of the scientific account of retroviruses is provided in my "Epidemic of Signification" as well as in many sources cited here. The HTLV-I, isolated by Gallo in 1980, was the first retrovirus to be identified with a human disease (June E. Osborn, "The AIDS Epidemic: An Overview of the Science," *Issues in Science and Technology* 2 (Winter 1986): 40–55).

53. The name HIV specifies the pathological / clinical effect of the virus (immune deficiency) rather than (as HTLV or LAV does) the type of cell it attacks. The term *HIV infection* is now sometimes used as a generic name to signify the entire spectrum of possibilities (from asymptomatic infection to full-blown AIDS). Brown, *AIDS, Cancer, and the Medical Establishment,* objects to the name *HIV* as being "conciliatory" but too nonspecific because all microbes associated with AIDS are immunosuppressive. Duesberg, "Retroviruses," also

argues that HIV is at most a precipitating agent in AIDS; Duesberg told John Lauritsen of the *New York Native* that many respected scientists agreed with him in private but were afraid to do so in public.

54. See "AIDS: What Is to Be Done?" and Shilts, *Band Played On*.

55. Donna J. Haraway, in "The Biological Enterprise: Sex, Mind, and Profit from Human Engineering to Sociobiology," *Radical History Review* 20 (Spring–Summer 1979): 206–237, suggests a transformation within the field of immunology from the military combat metaphors of World War II to postwar conceptions of the body compatible with the postmodern cold war period in which communication and information are played for the highest stakes. (Cf. Jaret, "The Wars Within," 728: "Interleukin-2 is a lymphokine, one of a dozen or so known chemical 'words' with which immune cells communicate during battle."

56. AIDS media coverage is discussed in William Check, "Public Education on AIDS: Not Only the Media's Responsibility," *Hastings Center Report,* special suppl. 15 (August 1985): 27–31; Barbara O'Dair, "Anatomy of a Media Epidemic," *Alternative Media* 14 (Fall 1983): 10–13; Jonathan Alter, "Sins of Omission," *Newsweek,* 23 September 1985, 25; Jay A. Winsten, "Science and the Media: The Boundaries of Truth," *Health Affairs* 4 (Spring 1985): 5–23; Watney, "Visual AIDS: Advertising Ignorance," *New Socialist* (March 1987), 19–21; Simon Watney and Sunil Gupta, "The Rhetoric of AIDS: A Dossier Compiled by Simon Watney, with Photographs by Sunil Gupta," *Screen* 27 (January–February 1986): 72–85; Watney, *Policing Desire*. Schwartz, "AIDS in the Media," concluded that despite problems, the press had in the end not encouraged hysteria. One deduces that Shilts, *Band Played On,* would argue that a little hysteria might have helped. Leishman, too, in the September 1987 *Atlantic,* argues forcefully that overconcern is necessary. See also Simon Watney, "People's Perceptions of the Risk of AIDS and the Role of the Mass Media," *Health Education Journal* 46 (1987): 62–65.

57. Fleck, *Genesis and Development,* 101, emphasis in original.

58. Hughey, Norton, and Sullivan, "Confronting Danger."

59. Public statements by scientists intended to reduce AIDS panic include Merle A. Sande, "Transmission of AIDS: The Case against Casual Contagion," *New England Journal of Medicine* 314 (6 February 1986): 380–382; and Erik Eckholm, "U.S. Officials Stress AIDS Is Not Spread by Casual Contact," *New York Times,* 27 June 1986, reports the strong statement issued by federal health officials asserting that "the AIDS virus cannot be spread through casual contact in the workplace."

60. "Strong New Candidate for AIDS Agent," *Science* 230 (May 1984): 147.

61. On the public health consequences of separating people "at risk" from the "general population," see Mathilde Krim, "AIDS: The Challenge to Science and Medicine," in "AIDS: The Emerging Ethical Dilemmas," *Hastings Center Report,* special suppl. 15 (August 1985): 2–7.

62. In "AIDS: What Is to Be Done?" 51.

63. *Science and Gender* (London: Pergamon, 1986), 4.

64. Rock Hudson permitted a statement to be made in Paris confirming his diagnosis on 25 July 1985; Michael Gottlieb, his physician in Los Angeles, issued an official confirmation on 30 July, and it is at this point that Shilts ends *And the*

Band Played On, for he considers it the major turning point in public perception of and response to the AIDS epidemic. Hudson died on 2 October 1985.

65. The treatment of Hudson's illness and death in the tabloids is revealing in this respect. The perceived natural division between the sexes ("women are women and men are men") is obviously challenged by the knowledge that Rock Hudson, a highly masculine screen actor, was homosexual. Discourse devoted to rendering this contradiction unproblematic takes the form of stories detailing Hudson's suffering from his gayness ("The Hunk Who Lived a Lie"), his supposed desire for a "normal" life with a wife and children, and his wish to be reunited with his mother. His underlying "normalcy" is often signaled by showing him with his dogs (e.g., George Carpozi, Jr., "Rock: His Years of Triumph and Tragedy—In His Own Words," *Star,* 15 October 1985, 27–30). Indeed, a key figure in AIDS redemption stories is a pet; the presence in a photograph of a dog or a cat, or even a stuffed animal, seems designed to infantilize and render sympathetic the person with AIDS. In reporter George Whitmore's personal account of his struggle with HIV infection ("Bearing Witness"), a teddy bear functions as a recurrent talisman of hope, while a large color photograph shows Whitmore with his cat.

66. Both sexual transmission and blood-borne transmission continue to raise questions, primarily because no consensus about the actual mechanisms of transmission has been achieved. See the report of recent public surveys in *Science* (January 1988).

67. Krim, "AIDS: The Challenge to Science and Medicine," 4.

68. Jonathan Lieberson, "The Reality of AIDS," *New York Review of Books,* 16 January 1986, 44.

69. Leibowitch, *Strange Virus,* 72–73.

70. Nathan Fain, "AIDS: An Antidote to Fear," *Village Voice,* 1 October 1985, 35.

71. John Langone, "AIDS: The Latest Scientific Facts," *Discover* (December 1985), 40–41.

72. Langone, "The Latest Scientific Facts," 52. Though more vivid and apodictic (i.e., presented as unarguable), Langone's conclusion parallels the conclusions of many scientists. (Joan K. Kreiss et al., "AIDS Virus Infection in Nairobi Prostitutes: Spread of the Epidemic to East Africa," *New England Journal of Medicine* 314 [13 February 1986]: 417, suggest that a history of STDs in homosexual men may "cause mucosal or squamous epithelial discontinuity or bleeding," thus compromising "epithelial integrity" as a barrier to viral transmission.)

73. Weeks, *Sexuality and Its Discontents;* see also Jeff Minson, "The Assertion of Homosexuality," *m/f* 5–6 (1981): 19–39; Wright, "A Disease of the Other"; and Mariana Valverde, *Sex, Power and Pleasure* (Philadelphia: New Society, 1987), ch. 4; "Bisexuality: Coping with Sexual Boundaries," 109–120. Valverde's discussion supports an argument that bisexuality, by challenging the binary normal / deviant model, furnishes another "border case."

Some health professionals and AIDS counselors avoid the word "gay" because for many people this implies a kind of identity or life-style; even "bisexual" may mean a kind of life-style. Although "homosexually active" is officially defined as having a single, same-sex sexual contact over the past five years, many who have had such contact do not identify themselves as "homosexual," and therefore as not at risk for AIDS. Nancy S. Shaw, "Women and AIDS: Theory and Politics" (Paper presented at the Annual Meeting of the National Women's Studies Association, University of Illinois, Urbana, June 1986), suggests that for women, too, the homosexual / heterosexual dichotomy confuses diagnosis and treatment in addition to the perception of risk. Many other examples of this fact have emerged in the course of the AIDS crisis.

74. Fettner, in "AIDS: What Is to Be Done?" 43.

75. Shaw and Paleo, "Women and AIDS."

76. Langone, "The Latest Scientific Facts," summarizes why many were skeptical about the African data. See also Patton, *Sex and Germs;* Lieberson, "The Reality of AIDS"; and Altman, "Heterosexuals and AIDS."

77. Leibowitch, *Strange Virus,* 72–73.

78. The question of silence pervades discussions of venereal disease. The "medical secret" of Victorian society referred to the collusion of "physicians and male patients, either husbands or prospective husbands, which resulted in unsuspecting women being infected with venereal disease" (Connelly, "Prostitution," 202). Feminist challenges to traditional medical conceptions of women and women's health—designed to make women's voices heard—have long since entered the mainstream of American society to change standard medical practice in such areas as breast-cancer treatment, childbirth, and prescription of psychoactive drugs. This is an extensive body of literature, yet one in which the voices of middle-class white women continue to predominate. As general background for the present discussion, see Elizabeth Fee, "Women and Health Care: A Comparison of Theories," in *Women and Health: The Politics of Sex in Medicine,* ed. Elizabeth Fee (Farmingdale, N.Y.: Baywood, 1982), 17–34. For Fee, and others in this collection, "women" is not taken as a white, middle-class category but one that is, rather, continually intersecting with race and class.

79. The history of prostitutes in disease discourse is reviewed by Brandt, *No Magic Bullet.* Connelly, "Prostitution," 196, quotes Lavinia Dock's 1910 nursing manual which states that prostitution "is now as certainly the abiding place and inexhaustible source of . . . venereal disease, as the marshy swamp is the abode of the malaria-carrying mosquito, or the polluted water supply of the typhoid bacillus." The idea of marriage, Connelly argues, 200, and especially the middle-class married woman, was at the focal point of early twentieth-century discussions of venereal disease: "It was the fate of the married woman that became a master symbol of the disastrous consequences of venereal disease, its transmitters—profligate men—and its source—prostitution."

80. Shaw and Paleo, "Women and AIDS"; Erik Eckholm, "Prostitutes' Impact on Spread of AIDS Debated," *New York Times,* 5 November 1985, 15, 18; Lawrence K. Altman, "Study Examines Prostitutes and AIDS Virus Infection," *New York Times,* 27 March 1987; Centers for Disease Control, "Antibody to HIV in Female Prostitutes," *MMWR* 36 (27 March 1987): 157–161.

81. Quoted in Langone, "The Latest Scientific Facts," 51–52.

82. Quoted in ibid., 50.

83. See R. R. Redfield et al., "Heterosexually Acquired HTLV-III / LAV Dis-

ease (AIDS-Related Complex and AIDS): Epidemiologic Evidence for Female-to-Male Transmission," *Journal of the American Medical Association* 254 (1985): 2094–2096; and R. R. Redfield et al., "Female-to-Male Transmission of HTLV-III," *Journal of the American Medical Association* 255 (1986): 1705–1706.

84. John J. Potterat, Lynanne Phillips, and John B. Muth, "Lying to Military Physicians about Risk Factors for HIV Infections," letter to the editor, *Journal of the American Medical Association* 257 (3 April 1987): 1727, offer plausible evidence that servicemen do lie to officials. As I have indicated above, however, independent evidence exists for female-to-male transmission; lying, in other words, can account for only a portion of cases thought to be heterosexually transmitted.

85. Harold Sanford Kant, "The Transmission of HTLV-III," letter to the editor, *Journal of the American Medical Association* 254 (1985): 1901.

86. Kreiss et al., "AIDS in Nairobi Prostitutes," warn that urban prostitutes may well "constitute a major reservoir of AIDS virus in such African capitals as Nairobi, Kigali, and Kinshasa," with "heterosexual men serving as vectors of infection" throughout the African continent (417). See also L. J. D'Costa et al., "Prostitutes Are a Major Reservoir of Sexually Transmitted Diseases in Nairobi," *Sexually Transmitted Disease* 12 (1985): 64–67; P. Van de Perre et al., "Female Prostitutes: A Risk Group for Infection with Human T-cell Lymphotropic Virus Type III," *The Lancet* 2 (1985): 24–27; P. Piot et al., "Acquired Immunodeficiency Syndrome in a Heterosexual Population in Zaire," *The Lancet* 2 (1984): 65–69.

87. Studies continue to suggest that HIV infection in U.S. prostitutes is brought about primarily by intravenous drug use and not by sexual contact with multiple partners (see Shaw and Paleo, "Women and AIDS"). Kreiss et al., "AIDS in Nairobi Prostitutes," found, similarly, that among the ninety female prostitutes they studied in Nairobi, HIV antibody was not significantly associated with the number of sexual encounters per year; other nonrelevant factors included age, duration of prostitution, nationality, history of immunizations, injections of medication within the past five years, transfusions, scarification, operations, induced abortions, or dental extractions. Sexual exposure to partners of different nationalities, however, was associated with HIV seropositivity.

88. Shaw and Paleo, "Women and AIDS," 144.

89. Stephanie Salter, "AIDS, Rights," *San Francisco Examiner,* 16 August 1987, quotes Carol Leigh, a representative of COYOTE (Call Off Your Old Tired Ethics, a prostitutes' activist organization based in San Francisco) and of Citizens for Medical Justice. Leigh argues that studies linking HIV infection in prostitutes to multiple sexual contacts are not borne out by empirical evidence. Brandt, *No Magic Bullet,* reviews the historical links of prostitutes to disease and the conceptual separation of infected prostitutes (and other voluntarily sexually active women) from "innocent victims." In her important 1975 essay on sociological discourse, "She Did It All for Love: A Feminist View of the Sociology of Deviance," Marcia Millman observes that studies of male deviance often portray their subjects (e.g., jazz musicians) as interesting and articulate people; in contrast, studies of prostitutes (for researchers, the primary category

of "deviance" in women) silence their female subjects by quoting male "authorities" as often as the women themselves—even "in a supposedly empathetic study of prostitutes, the pimps are treated as more intelligent, observant, and trustworthy than the subjects of the study themselves!", in *Another Voice: Feminist Perspectives on Social Life and Social Deviance,* ed. Marcia Millman and Rosabeth Moss Kanter (Garden City, N.Y.: Anchor / Doubleday, 1975), 261; 251–279.

90. Quoted in Langone, "The Latest Scientific Facts," 50.

91. Associated Press, "AIDS Funding Boost Requested: Increase Would Bring $200 Million to Bear on the Disease," *Daily Illini,* 27 September 1985, 7. See also *AIDS Hearing, House Committee on Energy and Commerce, Subcommittee on Health and the Environment,* 17 September 1984, serial no. 98–105 (Washington, D.C.: Government Printing Office, 1985).

92. John Green and David Miller, *AIDS: The Story of a Disease* (London: Grafton, 1986), 110, urge "extreme caution" in interpreting evidence that anal intercourse is more efficient than vaginal intercourse and that therefore male-to-male transmission is more efficient than male-to-female. Wofsy, "HIV Infection in Women," points out that we must be concerned for women both as potential "infectees" and "infectors."

93. On terminology and stereotyping connected with intravenous drug use, see Barrett, "Straight Shooters," Peg Byron, "Women with AIDS: Untold Stories," *Village Voice,* 24 September 1985, 16–19, and Steve Ault, "AIDS: The Facts of Life," *Guardian,* 26 March 1986, 1, 8. The list of drugs that can be "used" intravenously is long and by no means confined to either illegal or street drugs (e.g., prescription medications may also be injected). And as students of medical history–taking have long known, both the vocabulary and placement of questions can influence a client's answers (e.g., "Do you use medications?" and "Do you use drugs?" are not interchangeable, nor is the latter understood the same way when grouped with questions about the patient's current illnesses as opposed to questions about smoking and alcohol use).

94. Studies in New York and San Francisco show a greater increase in HIV infection among intravenous drug users than among gay men. Stephen C. Joseph, "Intravenous-Drug Abuse Is the Front Line in the War on AIDS," letter to the editor, *New York Times,* 22 December 1986, 18; Ronald Sullivan, "Addicts' Deaths from AIDS Are Termed Underreported," *New York Times,* 26 March 1987, 15; "Pro and Con: Free Needles to Addicts," *New York Times,* 20 December 1987, 20; Chris Anne Raymond, "Combatting a Deadly Combination: Intravenous Drug Abuse, Acquired Immunodeficiency Syndrome," *Journal of the American Medical Association* 259 (January 1988): 329, 332. Francis X. Clines, "Via Addicts' Needles, AIDS Spreads in Edinburgh," *New York Times,* 4 January 1987, 8, describes a situation in which the demographics of intravenous drug use and AIDS infection are very different from those of New York; with blacks and Hispanics most heavily infected in New York and white working-class youth in Edinburgh, Clines notes that, in Glasgow, heroin addiction in this population is high but AIDS infection is low, presumably as a result of the decision to provide free sterilized needles—a decision recently reversed in response to conservative pressure.

95. Shaw and Paleo, "Women and AIDS," discuss differences in AIDS epidemiology among women across the United States. Blood products and artificial insemination, for example, are the leading factors in HIV infection among women in California, whereas intravenous drug use is the leading factor in New York.

96. Quoted in Robert Pear, "Tenfold Increase in AIDS Death Toll Is Expected by '91," *New York Times,* 13 June 1986, A1, A17.

97. Shaw, "Women and AIDS: Theory and Politics."

98. Restrained discussions of the statistics and potential causes of AIDS and HIV infection in Africa include Lawrence K. Altman, "Linking AIDS to Africa Provokes Bitter Debate," *New York Times,* 21 November 1985, 1, 8; Kreiss et al., "AIDS in Nairobi Prostitutes"; Jean L. Marx, "New Relatives of AIDS Virus Found"; *Science* 232 (April 1986): 157; June E. Osborn, "The AIDS Epidemic"; Patton, *Sex and Germs;* Sam Siebert with Alma Guillermo and Ruth Marshall, "An Epidemic Like AIDS," *Newsweek,* 27 July 1987, 38; Blaine Harden, "AIDS May Replace Famine as the Continent's Worst Blight," *Washington Post Weekly Review,* 15 June 1987, 16–17. More problematic accounts include Jonathan Lieberson, "Reality of AIDS," and Robert E. Gould, "Reassuring News About AIDS: A Doctor Tells Why *You* May Not Be at Risk," *Cosmopolitan* (January 1988), 146–204; the latter is a particularly reckless example of unfettered speculation reassuring *Cosmo* readers that "ordinary sexual intercourse" would not place them at risk for infection. According to Gould, heterosexual AIDS in Africa exists because "many men in Africa take their women in a brutal way, so that some heterosexual activity regarded as normal by them would be closer to rape by our standards."

99. Fran P. Hosken, "Why AIDS Pattern Is Different in Africa," letter to the editor, *New York Times,* 15 December 1986.

100. Douglas A. Feldman, "Role of African Mutilations in AIDS Discounted," letter to the editor, *New York Times,* 7 January 1987.

101. See, for example, *Newsweek,* 3 November 1986, 66–67, and 24 November 1986, 30–47; Jennifer Dunning, "Women and AIDS," *New York Times,* 3 November 1986, 22; McAuliffe, "AIDS: At the Dawn of Fear"; and Mortimer B. Zuckerman, "AIDS: A Crisis Ignored," *U.S. News and World Report,* 12 January 1987, 76; Leishman, "Heterosexuals and AIDS," and "Science and the Citizen," *Scientific American* 256 (January 1987): 58–59.

102. James W. Carey, "Why and How? The Dark Continent of American Journalism," in *Reading the News,* ed. Robert Karl Manoff and Michael Schudson (New York: Pantheon, 1986), 146–196, discusses the reduction in continuing news stories of explanations to "boilerplate, a continuing thread of standard interpretation inserted in every story" (185). In a number of publications, including the *New York Times,* the boilerplate paragraph for AIDS began in 1984 to include mention of a viral etiology and in 1987 to talk about "sexual" rather than "homosexual" transmission.

The public's understanding of AIDS and HIV infection remains tenuous. By late 1987 an astonishing 99 percent of the cross-section of U.S. citizens surveyed had heard of AIDS, yet a substantial percentage expressed the belief that one could "catch" AIDS via giving blood, toilet seats, physical proximity to an infected person, or mosquitoes. The AIDS story is complicated and fluid enough to require regular reporters assigned to "the AIDS beat." This was clear when Jeffrey Levi, director of the National Gay and Lesbian Task Force, addressed the National Press Club on 9 October 1987 during the Gay and Lesbian March on Washington, D.C. Following Levi's address, a clear but essentially generic review of familiar AIDS facts and issues, at least two reporters in the audience were uninformed enough to ask the following questions: (1) "Isn't AIDS a media disease? A few years ago the government tried to give people shots for Barré . . . Gwillian . . . and they got paralyzed. Isn't AIDS a media invention?" and (2) "What is an 'op-por-tu-nis-tic infection'?" The first question presumably referred to the government's swine flu vaccination program in which a small number of people developed Guillan-Barré syndrome as a side effect; the second question was asked with heavy skepticism, as though to imply that Levi had concocted the term for political purposes.

103. As of January 1988 reported cases of AIDS in the United States totaled 50,265, 1,987 of which were reported to be caused by heterosexual transmission; 1,074 of this group were women. For a review of knowledge, statistics, and estimates of HIV infection in the United States as of December 1987, see *MMWR* 36, 18 December 1987, 801–804; the full report is available as *MMWR,* suppl., 36, 18 December 1987, S–6. Interviewed in January 1988, James W. Curran, director of the AIDS program at the CDC, predicted that although current "estimates of the total number of people infected remains complex and inexact, and the approaches used to compute a national HIV prevalence cannot be considered definitive. . . . The epidemic will get much worse before it gets better, both here and throughout the world." He continued: "We can expect the number of American AIDS cases to increase for the rest of this decade and that the problem will be with us for the rest of this century. Our best estimate is that between one million and 1.5 million Americans have been infected with the human immunodeficiency virus, and I am confident that this figure is neither too high nor too low." "Interview with James W. Curran," *American Medical News,* 15 January 1988, 1, 33–35. For more on current estimates and their potential consequences, see Klemens B. Meyer and Stephen G. Pauker, "Screening for HIV: Can We Afford the False Positive Rate?" *New England Journal of Medicine* 317 (July 1987): 238–241; and Gene W. Matthews and Verla S. Neslund, "The Initial Impact of AIDS on Public Health Law in the United States—1986," *Journal of the American Medical Association* 257 (January 1987): 344–352.

The CDC has never predicted that AIDS or HIV infection would "explode" in the heterosexual population; though Harold Jaffe's denial of such an explosion was widely quoted in such a way that it appeared to reflect new evidence, Jaffe himself stressed that he was making "deductions" from current known evidence that 4 percent of AIDS cases were heterosexual, primarily in IV drug users; in line with previous CDC statements, Jaffe predicted that "the virus is more likely to spread gradually over a period of years, rather than explosively, into the heterosexual population." Lawrence K. Altman, "Anxiety Allayed on Heterosexual AIDS," *New York Times,* 5 June 1987, 11. See Redfield et al., "Heterosexuals and AIDS," and Warren Winkelstein, Jr., et al., "Sexual Practices and Risk of Infection by the Human Immunodeficiency Virus: The San Francisco Men's Health Study," *Journal of the American Medical Association* 257 (January 1987): 321–325, for predictions based on current distribution of HIV antibodies.

104. See Relman, "Introduction"; June E. Osborn quoted in Erik Eckholm, "Broad Alert on AIDS: Social Battle Is Shifting," *New York Times,* 17 June 1986, 19–20; Morton Hunt, "Teaming Up Against AIDS," *New York Times Magazine,* 2 March 1986, 42–51, 78–83; "AIDS: Science, Ethics, Policy," Forum section, *Issues in Science and Technology* 2 (Winter 1986): 39–73; Robert C. Gallo, "The AIDS Virus," *Scientific American* 256 (January 1987): 47–56. Jaret, "The Wars Within," 723, writes: "Indeed, had AIDS struck 20 years ago, we would have been utterly baffled by it."

105. Shilts, *Band Played On,* 191.

106. Simon Watney, "A.I.D.S. U.S.A.," *Square Peg* (Autumn 1987), 17.

107. Kulstad, ed., *AIDS: Papers from Science;* AMA, *AIDS: From the Beginning.*

108. J. Z. Grover, "The 'Scientific' Regime of Truth," *In These Times,* 10–16 December 1986, 18–19. Grover points out a number of problematic terms and assumptions that recur in scientific writing about AIDS: (1) the term "AIDS victim" presupposes helplessness (the term "person with AIDS," or PWA, was created to avoid this), prevention and cure are linked to a conservative agenda of "individual responsibility," sex with multiple partners and / or strangers is equated with "promiscuity," and "safe" sexual practices are conflated with the cultural practice of monogamy; (2) it emphasizes the differences between "caregivers" and "victims," between scientific / medical expertise and other kinds of knowledge, between "those at risk" and "the rest of us"; and (3) it notes but fails to challenge existing inequities in the health care system.

109. On the subject of "AIDSspeak," see Richard Goldstein, "Visitation Rites: The Elusive Tradition of Plague Literature," *Voice Literary Supplement* 59 (October 1987); Leibowitch, *Strange Virus;* Walter Kendrick, "AIDSspeak," *Voice Literary Supplement* 59 (October 1987); Patton, *Sex and Germs;* Shilts, *Band Played On,* esp. 315–316; and Watney, "AIDS: The Cultural Agenda." Nor are texts the only point of debate. Some members of the San Francisco gay community complained early that public health warnings used euphemistic language ("avoid exchange of bodily fluids") and through innocuous pictures subverted the fact that AIDS was a deadly and physically ravaging disease (FitzGerald, *Cities on a Hill*).

110. Nichols, ed., *Mobilizing against AIDS.*

111. Centers for Disease Control, "Update: Acquired Immunodeficiency Syndrome," *MMWR* 35 (December 12, 1986): 757.

112. Guinan and Hardy, "Epidemiology of AIDS in Women."

113. The mucous membrane is revisited by Helen Singer Kaplan, *The Real Truth about Women and AIDS* (New York: Simon and Schuster, 1987), 78: "the moist vulnerable mucous membranes" of the female genital organs. ACT-UP (AIDS Coalition to Unleash Power) protested an article by Dr. Robert E. Gould in the January 1988 *Cosmopolitan* magazine (described in n. 98) for promoting a sense of false security in women readers by claiming that there was

virtually no danger of contracting AIDS through "ordinary heterosexual intercourse." Condoms, Gould noted parenthetically, were relevant only to "anyone not sure whether she has any open vaginal lesions or infections." ACT-UP's protest flyer, however, counters that "in fact, most women have infections and internal lacerations that are asymptomatic and often caused by childbirth, IUDs, tampons, Herpes II, sex without lubrication, and other sexually transmitted diseases." Similarly, Ann Johnson, a London AIDS specialist quoted on the August 1987 BBC radio special, emphasized that "No trauma need be seen. . . . There may be tiny areas of bleeding such as erosion on the neck of the womb which would be quite adequate for the virus to get into the bloodstream."

114. Shilts, *Band Played On,* describes the CDC's discussions of how to establish categories and classifications for AIDS, how to arrange risk factors in a hierarchy, what to do about overlapping categories, and how to keep track of phenomena with no official relationship as yet to AIDS. Guinan and Hardy, "Epidemiology of AIDS in Women," demonstrate some of the consequences of these decisions. The question of how best to define and classify AIDS and AIDS-related conditions—which involve some thirty different clinical entities and a spectrum of symptoms—also complicates the identification of health problems and assessment of the scope of the crisis. Not only has the CDC's initial surveillance definition been revised and broadened, but continuum models of symptoms (not necessarily progressive in time) have in general replaced former classifications by discrete disease (e.g., Kaposi's sarcoma).

An overview of current systems is given by David G. Ostrow, Steven L. Solomon, Kenneth H. Mayer, and Harry Haverkos, "Classification of the Clinical Spectrum of HIV Infection in Adults," in *Information on AIDS for the Practicing Physician,* vol. 1 (Chicago: American Medical Association, July 1987), 7–16. The authors remark, however, that "none [of these systems] satisfies all of the criteria required by public health officials, epidemiologists, clinicians, and researchers. . . . The desire to have an ironclad system that fully explains the progression of immunodeficiency and clinical symptomatology after HIV infection is understandable; however, it is not realistic at this time" (14–15).

115. The relatively few studies of women and AIDS are typically justified on the grounds that infected women may bear infected children and / or that measurement of infection in women provides an "index" to the spread of heterosexual AIDS. Guinan and Hardy, "Epidemiology of AIDS in Women," and the several studies by Redfield et al. use these justifications; similarly, Virginia Lehman and Noreen Russell, "Psychological and Social Issues of AIDS," in *AIDS: Facts and Issues,* ed. Gong and Rudnick, 246–263, mention women in a number of contexts but always under another heading—e.g., *Children,* or *AIDS and Minorities.* In part, this has to do with the politics of publishing and the convention of beginning scholarly articles with a clear and accepted raison d'être; thus, because research builds on other research, the invisibility of women in the AIDS narrative to date reinforces their invisibility in the future.

It is therefore important that researchers—those, at any rate, who do believe in the intrinsic importance of women—break this lineal citation pattern and insist on inserting women *as women* into biomedical discourse on AIDS. But the politics of pregnancy is also at work here. This emerges in a letter to *JAMA* regarding the evolution of the CDC guidelines for preventing transmission of perinatal AIDS in HIV-positive women; Dr. David A. Grimes describes a series of meetings in which recommendations for counseling women about abortion as an option were progressively watered down and finally omitted altogether in the published version (*MMWR* 34 [6 December 1985]: 721–726). Grimes's letter appeared in *Journal of the American Medical Association* 259 (January 1988): 217–218.

116. Stephen R. Ell, "The Venetian Plague of 1630–1631: Assessment of a Human Disaster," *Medical Heritage* 2 (March–April 1986): 151–156. "The disease spared no one," writes Ell (155); "primitive epidemiologic data" indicate that in Venice and its surrounding area there were 93,661 mortalities (or about one-third of the total population), among them 11,486 pregnant women, "a catastrophic blow to the reproductive capacity of the city. Yet, this inclination toward pregnant women is quite in keeping with the fact that pregnancy acts as a non-specific immune-suppressant." Barbara Tuchman, *A Distant Mirror: The Calamitous 14th Century* (New York: Ballantine, 1978), 92–125, provides a dramatic account of the Black Death, tracing the social and economic consequences of curtailed reproduction (consequences borne out by modern epidemiology).

117. Shaw and Paleo, "Women and AIDS," 150. We do not really know the clinical relevance of pregnancy, though one recent study of 120 pregnant women, reported in *Center to Center* 1 (1987): 5, concluded that HIV did not affect the clinical course of pregnancy, or vice versa.

118. See Patton, *Sex and Germs*. In January 1983 the CDC officially added heterosexual partners of people with AIDS to the list of high-risk groups. The *MMWR* cited two known cases of AIDS in women who were long-time partners of men with AIDS, noting also forty-three reports of previously healthy women who had developed *Pneumocystis* or other AIDS-related conditions, primarily after sexual contact with intravenous drug users—none of whom, however, had yet developed AIDS. Shilts, *Band Played On,* 225, suggests that this was one turning point in AIDS media coverage.

119. Reports of female-to-female transmission of HIV include Maria T. Sabatini, Kanu Patel, and Richard Hirschman, "Kaposi's Sarcoma and T-cell Lymphoma in an Immunodeficient Woman: A Case Report," *AIDS Research* 1 (1984): 135–137, on the case of a non-Haitian, non-drug-using thirty-seven-year-old black female who was a "lifelong homosexual" (as was her partner), and conclude that "this would suggest that females may harbor the AIDS agent as healthy carriers"; Michael Marmor et al., "Possible Female-to-Female Transmission of Human Immunodeficiency Virus," letter to the editor, *Annals of Internal Medicine* 105 (December 1986): 969. See also Vada Hart, "Lesbians and AIDS," *Gossip* 2 (1986); and Ann Bristow, Andrea Devine, and Denise McWilliams, "AIDS and Women in Prison," *Gay Community News*, lesbian prisoner suppl., 23 August–5 September 1987, 10–11, who provide safer-sex guidelines for lesbians.

120. In 1983 the women members of a San Francisco gay Jewish congregation, Sha'ar Zahev, donated blood as a way of expressing solidarity with gay men. In 1984 the Blood Sister Project of San Diego collected blood from hun-

dreds of lesbians to contribute to the diminishing supply in blood banks. As a group with virtually no cases of AIDS-related disorders, lesbians were among the very safest of donor groups. Nevertheless, the association of "gay" with "blood supply" triggered gender-blind homophobia: Not only were there objections within individual communities to this contamination of the blood supply by homosexuals but conservative groups flooded the White House with telegrams demanding that Assistant Secretary for Health Edward Brandt be fired if he attended a Fund for Human Dignity dinner to present the award to the San Diego group. See Altman, *AIDS in the Mind of America,* 95; Shilts, *Band Played On,* 455–456; and Richardson, *Women and AIDS,* 88–89. Today, Blood Sisters chapters exist in many cities.

121. Altman, *AIDS in the Mind of America,* 94, notes both the "enormous energy and generosity" with which many lesbians have responded to the AIDS crisis. At the same time he suggests that solidarity has not been the uniform response: "Many lesbians feel resentment that gay men, who never showed any interest in questions of women's health, now seem to expect total commitment to AIDS activity from them."

122. Examples include Cindy Patton, "Feminists Have Avoided the Issue of AIDS," *Sojourner* (October 1985), 19–20, Cindy Patton and Janis Kelly, *Making It: A Woman's Guide to Sex in the Age of AIDS* (Boston: Firebrand, 1987); Richardson, *Women and AIDS;* Byron, "Untold Stories"; Grover, "Scientific Regime of 'Truth',"; Katie Leishman, "Two Million Americans and Still Counting," *New York Times Book Review,* 27 July 1986, 12; Katie Leishman, "Heterosexuals and AIDS: The Second Stage of the Epidemic," *The Atlantic* (February 1987), 39–58; Marcia Pally, "AIDS and the Politics of Despair: Lighting Our Own Funeral Pyre," *The Advocate,* 24 December 1985, 8; Nancy S. Shaw, "California Models for Women's AIDS Education and Services," Report, San Francisco AIDS Foundation [333 Valencia St., 4th fl., San Francisco, CA 94103], 1986, and "Women and AIDS."

123. Examples include Altman, *Mind of America;* Wayne Barrett, "Straight Shooters: AIDS Targets Another Lifestyle," *Village Voice,* 26 October 1985, 14–18; Richard Goldstein, "The Hidden Epidemic: AIDS and Race," *Village Voice,* 10 March 1987; Cindy Patton, "Resistance and the Erotic: Reclaiming History, Setting Strategy as We Face AIDS," *Radical America,* 68–78; Kramer, "Taking Responsibility for our Lives," Nancy Krieger and Rose Appleman, *The Politics of AIDS* (Oakland: Frontline Pamphlet, 1986). Kramer remains regularly enraged in print at what he perceives is the gay community's failure to play hardball politics (see, for example, "Taking Responsibility," as well as Watney's critique of it) and, after leaving Gay Men's Health Crisis, helped found ACT-UP, an activist zap group whose motto is SILENCE = DEATH. Both Patton and Watney have critiqued the left's general failure (despite differences in the United States and Britain) to contribute meaningfully to an AIDS political agenda.

124. See Background Paper, 1985 COYOTE convention summary, San Francisco, 30 May–2 June 1985; *World Wide Whores' News,* report of the 1985 conference; Laurie Bell, ed., *Good Girls / Bad Girls: Feminists and Sex Trade Workers Face to Face* (Seattle: Seal Press Toronto: Women's Press, 1987); Frederique Delacoste and Priscilla Alexander, eds., *Sex Work: Writings by*

Women in the Sex Industry (Pittsburgh: Cleis, 1987); Lizzie Borden, *Working Girls;* Judith Miller, "Prostitutes Make Appeal for AIDS Prevention," *New York Times,* 5 October 1986, 6. See also Barrett, "Straight Shooters." In the BBC AIDS special on women and AIDS, Louise Hansen, a British prostitute, reports the growing desire by clients for alternatives to high-risk sex, including condoms, "nonpenetrative sex," fantasy scenes, lesbian scenes, and argues—as does Carol Leigh (interviewed in Salter, "AIDS, Rights")—that "people can learn a lot from the working skills that prostitutes have—like how to be assertive and alternative sexual practices." Prostitutes, they argue, should be seen as a valuable resource for information about sexual practices.

125. Erica Jong, "Women and AIDS," *New Woman* (April 1986), 42–48; Ellen Switzer, "AIDS: What Women Can Do," *Vogue* (January 1986), 222–223, 264–265; Jane Sprague Zones, "AIDS: What Women Need to Know," *The [National Women's Health] Network News* 11 (November–December 1986): 1, 3.

126. "Too Little AIDS Coverage," letter to the editors, *Sojourner* 10 (July 1985): 3.

127. Traditional roles available to women in the cultural narratives of AIDS include mother, spouse, lover, celebrity, Blessed Virgin, and, in the words of conservative Theresa Crenshaw (member of the White House AIDS commission), "mainstays in the resistance to this epidemic."

128. Confusion as to innocence and guilt in relation to infection is evident in a 12 April 1987 story in *Japan Times,* reporting that a baby born to an infected woman did not itself appear to be infected ("Baby Born to AIDS Carrier Infection Free," 2); in an odd sentence construction that appears to separate "the AIDS carrier" from "the mother," the report added that the government's "public health division said that there is little danger that Japan's first baby born to a [AIDS] carrier was infected in the mother's womb." The story indicates that after the infected woman insisted on bearing her child against medical advice, a special medical team was appointed both to reduce the chances that the virus would be transmitted to the baby during delivery and to protect the mother from AIDS; but the story describes only the procedures and rationale for protecting the baby.

129. On "saturation," see Altman, "Heterosexual Fears Allayed."

130. Shilts, *Band Played On,* 124, reports that scientific papers about pediatric AIDS were rejected in 1982 by scientific and medical journals because of the widespread conception that "by its very name, GRID was a homosexual disease, not a disease of babies or their mothers." Yet even in 1987, when Shilts's book was published and publicized, attention was given to "Patient Zero," a figure of gay sex rampant in the person of a Canadian airline flight attendant who, Shilts suggests—and the media at large appear to have concluded—was the "man who brought us AIDS."

Yet Shilts's account begins in December 1976 with the story of the Danish lesbian physician Grethe Rask, who contracted *Pneumocystis carinii* pneumonia working in Zaire and died in December 1977; though her case was reported in a letter to *The Lancet* 2 (1983): 925, by her medical colleague and friend Dr. Ib Bygbjerg, her case has received little attention. For further analysis of Shilts's book, see Douglas Crimp, "How to Have Promiscuity in an Epidemic," *October* 43 (1987). (In his letter, Bygbjerg, citing Robin M. Henig's discussion of AIDS as a tropical disease ["AIDS: A New Disease's Deadly Odyssey," *New York Times Magazine,* 6 February 1983, 28], notes the existence of endemic disease related to three "acutely deadly viruses of central African origin" as well as Rask's exposure, through her work as a surgeon, to "blood and excretions of African patients"; he suggests possible connections to AIDS and urges investigation by U.S. and European epidemiologists and virologists.)

131. A growing literature documents the placement of gay men in AIDS writing as the Contaminated Other, and there seems evidence that in some respects they do fill the role that women, especially prostitutes, have played in the past. It is not clear what effect AIDS is having on notions of masculinity and femininity in the gay community. Gay men's creation of the term "AIDS widows" to designate the men who survive their lovers is a small but positive use by men of a "feminine" linguistic form. On the other hand, sexism remains entrenched. Ned Weeks, the author's persona in Larry Kramer's play *The Normal Heart* (New York: Samuel French, 1985), denounces the members of Gay Men's Health Crisis for preferring deathbed scenes over politics: "I thought I was starting a bunch of Ralph Naders or Green Berets, and at the first instant they have to take a stand on a political issue and fight, almost in front of my eyes they turn into a bunch of nurse's aides" (62). Shilts, *Band Played On,* 556–557, discusses the play but makes no comment on the implicit sexism in lines like these.

In "Taking Responsibility," Kramer charges that gay men's failure to demand their rights "proves they are the sissies people have always accused them of being." Michael Musto, "Mandatory Macho," *Village Voice,* 30 June 1987, 30, deplores the repressive effect of this compulsory masculinity on the flamboyant drag tradition within gay life. On the general topic of relations among the sexes within the gay community, see Donald Mager, "The Discourse about Homophobia, Male and Female Contexts" (Paper presented at the Annual Meeting of the Modern Language Association, New York, December 1986), and Craig Owens, "Outlaws: Gay Men in Feminism," in *Men in Feminism,* ed. Alice Jardine and Paul Smith (New York: Methuen, 1987), 219–232.

132. Watney observes that after any media message to heterosexuals, the phone hotlines—still staffed primarily by gay volunteers—are jammed far beyond their capacity by the mainly straight "worried well"; the same thing occurred after a 20 May 1987 front-page story by Robert Pear appeared in the *New York Times:* "3 Health Care Workers Found Infected by Blood of Patients with AIDS." Wofsy, "HIV Infection in Women," argues that although media representations of AIDS striking middle-class white women provide an important message to be careful, they reinforce the invisibility of, and may thus promote denial among, members of the groups most at risk—black and Hispanic women.

133. *No Magic Bullet,* following p. 164.

134. Treichler, "Epidemic of Signification," 281–282, 297, n. 28. The tendency of male scientists to keep themselves textually clean is well-documented. Martin, for example, in *Woman and the Body,* 50, notes that menstruation is commonly described in medical and scientific texts as a form of hemorrhaging,

and menstrual flow as "blood mixed with endometrial debris"; Martin points out that seminal fluid, too, picks up shredded material as it moves through various male ducts but is never characterized by so negative a term as "debris."

135. Various metaphors in AIDS discourse are identified in Hughey, Norton, and Sullivan, "Confronting Danger"; Dobrow, "Symbolism of AIDS"; and Albert, "AIDS: The Victim and the Press."

136. June E. Osborn, quoted in Clark et al., "Women and AIDS," called intravenous drug users "the great gaping hole in the dike," and compared the spread of the virus through the drug-using community to "dropping red dye into a pond." Turner, *Body in Society,* 221, writes that "venereal disease is popularly conceptualized as an invasion of the body by alien germs, but the mechanism which, so to speak, opens the sluice-gates permitting nature to invade culture is the deviance of human populations from morality." Other common liquid metaphors about AIDS include *waves, pools, islands, oceans, streams, reservoirs, pouring, spilling,* and *icebergs.* Metaphors about liquid appear to flow easily into metaphors about women and disease: drain the red-light district, it was frequently argued in the venereal disease debates, and you drain the swamp (Brandt, *No Magic Bullet,* 72). Corbin, "Commercial Sexuality," 87, notes that the prostitute was considered to have a body that smelled bad and had rotten blood. One nineteenth-century analogy likened the body to a house and the prostitute to the house's cesspool; more broadly, her body is the sewer into which the social body excretes its excess (as a nineteenth-century physician put it, "the seminal drain"). Prostitutes therefore serve a crucial function in keeping the surrounding countryside clean.

137. These roles are played out most graphically in the supermarket tabloids.

138. The resurgence of discourse on "female promiscuity" raises pressing questions about women's health and women's pleasure. Opening a panel discussion on the erosion of civil rights and affirmative action under Reagan, Betty Friedan pointed to the film *Fatal Attraction* to suggest a widespread backlash against "liberated" women and the feminist agenda (The Sag Harbor Initiative, Maine, 10–12 October 1987). Gould, "Reassuring News," recycled data and old theories to reassure *Cosmo* readers that "ordinary sexual intercourse" would not place them at risk for AIDS; as noted above (n. 98), he explains heterosexual AIDS in Africa as the result of rough sexual practices. The inaccuracy, irresponsibility, racism, and sexism of Gould's article provoked ACT-UP to organize an international boycott of the magazine, asking women and men everywhere to "SAY NO TO COSMOPOLITAN." The need for such feminist commentary, activism, and discussion is pressing. Neither the search for safety nor the search for pleasure should be abandoned. As Carole S. Vance has eloquently argued on many occasions, "It is not safe to be a woman, and it never has been. Female attempts to claim pleasure are especially dangerous, attacked not only by men, but by women as well." "Pleasure and Danger," in *Pleasure and Danger,* ed. Carole S. Vance (New York: Routledge & Kegan Paul, 1984), 1–27.

139. Leslie Kirk Wright reports that in early 1987 a small company introduced a device that enables women to urinate standing up. Advertisements appearing extensively in the MUNI Metro System (and particularly aimed, apparently, at the Financial District crowd) urged women to "Stand UP! for hygiene,"

and showed a smartly (but sedately) dressed woman holding a smallish box suggestive of tampons. Wright suggests to me that, like the condom ads aimed at women, this may reflect an appeal to the "new freedom."

140. Other publications were quick to spread Langone's word. Speaking to audiences and friends (gay and straight, in many cities) who do not stay daily apprised of AIDS developments, I have found Langone's argument still widespread.

141. HIV is believed to be a relative newcomer on earth (the presence of antibodies in stored blood now goes back to 1959 in samples collected in Africa, to 1973 in U.S. blood—though a case in St. Louis in 1968 has recently been verified). Though, from our perspective, the AIDS virus is indeed virulent, killing quickly, in fact, the long latency between infection and the appearance of clinical damage provides plenty of time—often years—for the virus to replicate and infect a new host. For the time being we are sufficiently hospitable so that this virus can live off us relatively "successfully"; if mutation occurs, our relationship to the AIDS virus could evolve into something relatively benign or mutually disastrous.

142. "AIDS," *Ms.* (April 1987), 64–71. (See, in contrast, Lindsy Van Gelder and Pam Brandt, "AIDS on Campus," *Rolling Stone* (December 1986), 89–94.

143. For examples of this burgeoning genre, see Mary Cantwell, "Who's Responsible for 'Safe Sex'?" *New York Times,* 8 July 1987, 26, and Anna Quindlen, "For Women, the Condom Campaign Is a Bit Tardy," *New York Times,* 17 June 1987, 17, 19.

144. Heterosexual white male commentary about AIDS comes from left and right. See Peter Davis, "Exploring the Kingdom of AIDS," and Nat Hentoff, "The New Priesthood of Death" for the former; William F. Buckley, Jr.'s, "Crucial Steps" and other columns on AIDS, and Michael Fumento's articles in *Commentary.*

145. Peter Goldman, "The Face of AIDS," *Newsweek,* 10 August 1987, 22–37. Rex Wockner, "Back-door Homophobia," *Chicago Outlines* (Summer 1987). In contrast, Michael Shnayerson, "One by One," *Vanity Fair* (April 1987), 91–97, 152–153, uniformly captions each photo with occupation and age only.

146. Chris Norwood, *Advice for Life: A Woman's Guide to Aids Risks and Prevention* (New York: Pantheon, 1987) and Helen Singer Kaplan, *The Real Truth about Women and AIDS: How to Eliminate the Risks Without Giving Up Love and Sex* (New York: Simon and Schuster, 1987). The two books are similar in their orientation toward white middle-class heterosexual childbearing women, for whom they recommend safe partners over safe practices. Kaplan is less skeptical in her analysis of official sources. For Norwood, one "risk" of AIDS for women is that they will find its name, in those four big capital letters, frightening, so she forswears the acronym in favor of user-friendly *Aids.*

147. Kaplan, *The Real Truth,* app. C, 157–164. Kaplan does not provide information about the circumstances of the call.

148. "Women and AIDS," radio program produced in London by the BBC, aired 13 September 1987 in central Illinois.

149. Susan Ardill and Sue O'Sullivan, "AIDS and Women: Building a Feminist Framework," *Spare Rib* (May 1987), 40–43 (first in a projected series).

150. Increasingly, other voices are demanding a forum for discourse on AIDS. Minority and women's organizations and journals now cover AIDS conferences, and do so vocally. An August 1987 federal conference on AIDS and minorities, for example, provoked nearly 100 of the black delegates to adopt and make public a resolution critical of the level and quality of information made available; as one spokesperson said, "They gave us a lesson in AIDS 101 when all of us traveled here for a graduate course" (Jon Nordheimer, "U.S. Officials Criticized on Efforts to Curb AIDS among Minorities," *New York Times,* 10 August 1987, 1, 9).

The involvement of intravenous drug users is also beginning. Though as William Check wrote in 1985 ("Public Education on AIDS," 28), that "it sometimes appears that the only risk group that hasn't raised a ruckus is the IV drug users, who are not organized," some organization is now taking place—in New York at any rate. Gay Men's Health Crisis, aware that some drug users may avoid AIDS information centers perceived as gay, as well as medical authorities, has been working with former addicts, who in turn go to "shooting galleries" and other hangouts and teach drug users how to clean needles with bleach.

151. Only a suggestion of this diversification of AIDS discourse can be included here. Dooley Worth and Ruth Rodriguez, "Latina Women and AIDS," *Radical America* 20 (1987): 63–67, argue that AIDS education and risk reduction for U.S. Hispanics must begin using appropriate cultural forms: "Writers, newscasters, artists, actors, and producers, who successfully reach Latino households through Spanish language radio and television soap operas, 'foto-novelas' (a popular comic-book style depicting romantic stories with photographs), posters, and printed materials, must be tapped in developing an education campaign that is based on a firm understanding of the cultural possibilities for adaptive behavior," 67. Archie Comic Publications, Inc., plans a year-long AIDS education campaign in 1988.

Lisa H. Towle, "Learn to Read with 'Word Warriors,'" *New York Times,* 31 January 1988, 21. Jaret, "Wars Within," 705, describes a "Killer T-Cell Video Game" for cancer patients. *AIDS: You Can't Catch It Holding Hands,* written and illustrated by Niki de Saint Phalle (San Francisco: Lapis, 1987), is essentially an AIDS education and prevention manual, suitable for kids, with laminated jacket and drawings that are something like a combination of Matisse, subway graffitti, and the Babar books. AIDS is beginning to figure centrally in novels; several that feature women who are infected through heterosexual contact are Joseph Hansen's *Early Graves* (New York: Mysterious, 1987), Armistead Maupin's *Significant Others* (New York: Harper & Row, 1987), and Margaret Atwood, *The Handmaid's Tale* (Boston: Houghton Mifflin, 1986).

152. Knowledge about AIDS is being produced, interpreted, and put to use in vastly diverse contexts, and to assume a simple, linear model of communication is not useful. Watney, in "AIDS: The Outsiders," writes that "for those of us living and working in the communities most devastated by AIDS it seems as if the rest of the population are like tourists, wandering casually through the

height of a blitz, totally unaware of what is going on all around them," and, indeed, stumbling through a blitz may be a more useful image when we try to account for the multiplicity of understandings and unpredictable cultural realignments that the AIDS crisis continues to generate. A well-known media researcher, for example, commenting on the unexpected consequences of his own research on AIDS, said, "I never dreamed as a communications scholar I'd be teaching people how to shoot up correctly with heroin" (Annual Meeting, International Communication Association, Chicago, May 1986).

The crisis has created widespread interest, even obsession, with scientific and medical information. Many journals, for example, have provided a short course in virology (Kohn, "Face the Virus"). As a gay composer in New York said to me recently, "Whoever thought I'd be reading about the glucose coatings on viruses and how to interpret T-cell ratios." Meanwhile, however, CDC interviews with members of two heterosexual singles clubs in Minneapolis documented that as of late 1986 this already-infected population had made virtually no modifications in their sexual practices (Centers for Disease Control, "Positive HTLV-III / LAV Antibody Results for Sexually Active Female Members of Social / Sexual Clubs—Minnesota," *MMWR* 35 (14 November 1986): 697–699. Ralph J. DiClemente, Jim Zorn, and Lydia Temoshok, "Adolescents and AIDS: A Survey of Knowledge, Attitudes and Beliefs about AIDS in San Francisco," *American Journal of Public Health* 76 (1986): 1443–1445, found that many adolescents in San Francisco, a city where public health information about AIDS has been extensive, were not well informed about its seriousness, causes, or prevention.

153. See Simon Watney, "A.I.D.S. U.S.A.," for comments on the noncritical use of AIDS-related terminology among U.S. gay activists.

154. See J. Z. Grover, "A Critique of AIDS Terminology," *October* 43 (Winter 1987).

155. Models for this kind of attentive questioning, which is at once dense, critically self-conscious, and politically informed, can be found in writing about women and AIDS by Cindy Patton, Donna J. Haraway, and Diane Richardson. Far from being "idealist," it seems to me such questions set the stage for materialist interventions.

156. The following "joke" illustrates a disjunction between women as ideal and socially constructed entities and women as "real people" who are subject to particular historical conditions:

> A guy named Joe was a regular at his neighborhood bar and one night he told his drinking buddies he was going to have sex-change surgery. "I just feel there's a woman inside me," he said, "and I'm going to let her out."
>
> Joe showed up at the bar a few months later transformed into a woman who introduced herself to her old buddies as Jane. The regulars recognized her, gave their welcomes, bought her a beer, and began asking questions about the surgery.
>
> "What hurt the most?" they asked. "Was it when they cut your penis?"
>
> "No," said Jane, "that wasn't what hurt the most."
>
> "Was it when they cut your testicles, then?"
>
> "No, that wasn't what hurt the most."

> "Well, what *was* it that hurt the most?"
> "What hurt the most was when they cut my salary."

See Christine Brooke-Rose, "Woman as a Semiotic Object," in *Female Body in Western Culture*, ed. Suleiman, 305–316, and Teresa De Lauretis, *Alice Doesn't: Feminism, Semiotics, Cinema* (Bloomington: Indiana University Press, 1984).

157. Shaw and Paleo, "Women and AIDS," discuss society's view of the preciousness of childbearing women and their likelihood of being among the first groups tested. They cite women's current reluctance, as caretakers in this life-and-death crisis, to raise concerns about sexism.

158. Laurie Stone, "The New Femme Fatale," *Ms.* (December 1987), 78–79, 79, writes that *Fatal Attraction* "says good women stay at home . . . while single, working women are damaged, barely even human, and want to destroy the family they secretly covet. . . . This is a fairy tale for the age of AIDS if there ever was one," she concludes, and observes of the pathological femme fatale character that "we're meant to hate her so much we want her dead."

In the Eye of the Storm: The Epidemiological Construction of AIDS

Gerald M. Oppenheimer

At the beginning of an article on the human immunodeficiency virus, (HIV, the putative causal agent of AIDS that he and others isolated), Dr. Robert C. Gallo observes without comment that epidemiologists had named the new disease "acquired immune deficiency syndrome."[1] By attributing the power to name the disorder to them, Dr. Gallo shows us how prominent a part epidemiology has played in defining and ordering this "medical mystery."

In this chapter I examine the role of epidemiology in characterizing HIV infection.[2] Faced with a new disease of unknown origin, epidemiologists and their collaborators constructed, over time, hypothetical models to explain the disorder in order to contain it. Prior to the isolation of a putative causal agent, HIV, epidemiologists played a central role in defining the new syndrome, first developing a "life-style" model and, later, a model based on hepatitis B. Although later supplanted from their special position by virologists and other "bench" scientists working in laboratories, epidemiologists have continued to define important dimensions of the disorder and to raise disquieting questions. Specifically, they were concerned with defining the natural history of HIV infection, the extent to which it had spread within population groups, and the factors that affected the rates of disease—factors beyond the virus itself.

Epidemiology, unlike virology, has a strong social dimension in that it explicitly incorporates perceptions of a population's social relations, behavioral patterns, and experiences into its explanations of disease processes. Given their training, epidemiologists fairly consistently defined HIV infection as a biological process occurring within a determinate social matrix. That the infection was first identified among young, male homosexuals and intravenous drug users certainly reinforced that professional proclivity.[3]

The results of this exercise in epidemiological imagination were complex and equivocal. On the one hand, the epidemiologists' approach may have skewed the choice of models and hypotheses, determined which data were excluded from consideration until later in the epidemic, and offered scientific justification for popular prejudice, particularly against gay men. On the other hand, the epidemiological approach gave the new disease a human face. By defining the behaviors and the multiple social experiences of groups as risk factors for the disease, epidemiology countered attempts to reduce the etiology of HIV infection to a virus alone. In addition, epidemiology offered the possibility of primary prevention in the form of health education and follow-up, particularly important in the absence of a vaccine or a successful therapy.

The various characterizations of HIV infection examined in this essay will span the period from early 1981, when physicians first encountered anomalous medical facts, to mid-1987, when epidemiologists had begun to work out the causal associations between a new retrovirus isolated in 1983–1984 and the natural history of the new disease. This chapter draws almost entirely on the medical literature of the period.

EPIDEMIOLOGY AND PUBLIC HEALTH

Epidemiology played a key role in the AIDS epidemic for at least two reasons, one institutional, the other scientific. The institutional link was the Centers for Disease Control (CDC) in Atlanta. Part of the Public Health Service, which falls under the jurisdiction of the U.S. Department of Health and Human Services, the CDC is responsible for, among other things, monitoring morbidity and mortality trends in the United States and for responding to acute outbreaks of disease—infectious disease in particular. The CDC depends heavily on case reports, surveillance, and epidemiological investigations in order to fulfill its mission. Its investigations are conducted both by the permanent staff and by officers in the Epidemic Intelligence Service (EIS), who are young physicians or Ph.D.s who exchange two years of service for training in epidemiological techniques.

Epidemiology, in comparison with most other medical disciplines, is particularly well-suited to explore, portray, and explain new medical phenomena. It seeks to measure and analyze the occurrence and distribution of diseases and other health-related conditions, acting both as a sentinel who warns of shifts in disease patterns and as a scout who seizes on such shifts to discover their etiology.[4]

For example, by systematically collecting data on the frequency of disorders in populations or subgroups through surveillance programs, epidemiologists can discern changes in the distribution of diseases in the community. Observations of these distributions, and their variation in subgroups, lead to hypotheses concerning the relationship between the disease and variables that may affect its natural history and clinical course. Using various study designs, epidemiologists attempt to measure, reject, or refine the relative significance of such hypothetical associations. The ultimate objective of these studies is to isolate the causal variables of the disease in question. An intermediate goal is to discover a point in the natural history of the disease where intervention might alter its course, even if its etiology remains unknown.[5]

Epidemiologists tend to believe in multifactorial disease models. They assume, that is, that intervention is possible at several points, even in the absence of a known "first cause." The major premise of the multifactorial model is, as the name implies, that a given disease may have a number of causes or antecedents, a combination of which may be needed to produce the disorder. The "web of causes," therefore, may be interdicted at more than one vulnerable point.[6]

The power of the multifactorial model is that it can incorporate any measurable factor relevant to and statistically associated with the disease or disorder of interest. Unlike the reductionist paradigm of the germ theory, the multicausal model embraces a variety of environmental and social factors. The model's strength, however, is also its weakness. The multifactorial model allows the researcher to cast a very wide net. Scientists may attempt to incorporate many possible explanatory variables whose putative causal connections with a given disease may be plausible for a number of reasons—scientific, logical, historical, experiential, and so forth. Variables may be drawn in (or left out) as a function of the social values of the scientist, the working group, or the society. When included in the model, embraced by the professionals, and published in the scientific press, such value judgments appear to be objective, well-grounded scientific statements.

Epidemiology is an applied science that responds to two kinds of disorder within the community, one caused by the disease directly, and the other the product of the very fears it has aroused. Consequently, epidemiology bore the initial responsibility of outlining the direction of research, of generating hypotheses, and of synthesizing the results. In the face of a fatal disorder of unknown origin and indefinite proportions, such as HIV infection, epidemiology offered a set of procedures (e.g., case definition, verification, and count) that swiftly generated results and then authenticated them, giving the public a sense of definite progress. The content of this science, by providing and naming concepts ("risk groups," "life-style hypothesis"), made the epidemic potentially less frightening by making it appear more likely that it would eventually be known and controlled.

CASE-FINDING AND SURVEILLANCE

The initial discoveries heralding a new disorder of unknown origin were made by physicians treating patients in Los Angeles. Dr. Michael Gottlieb and his colleagues alerted the CDC that between October 1980 and May 1981 five young, previously healthy homosexual men had been treated in local hospitals for biopsy-confirmed *Pneumocystis carinii* pneumonia (PCP). Two of the patients had already died. An investigation by an EIS officer confirmed the diagnosis of PCP, a protozoan-produced condition that occurs almost exclusively in persons with severely suppressed or defective immune systems. On June 5, 1981, a short paper describing the patients was published by the CDC in its *Morbidity and Mortality Weekly Report* (*MMWR*).[7]

Gottlieb's communication to the CDC was closely followed by another from both New York City and San Francisco, which reported that in the thirty months prior to July 1981, Kaposi's sarcoma (KS) had been diagnosed in twenty-six male homosexuals between twenty-six and fifty-one years of age.[8] A rare cancer in the United States, KS had historically occurred in this country primarily in elderly males and immunosuppressed transplant recipients. Its manifestation in a relatively large number of young men was considered highly unusual, as was the appearance of PCP in individuals without a clinically apparent cause for immunodeficiency disease.

An editorial note in the *MMWR* issue that had published Gottlieb's paper hypothesized that "the fact that these patients were all homosexuals suggests an association between some aspect of a homosexual life-style or disease acquired through sexual contact and *Pneumocystis* pneumonia in this population."[9] The conjecture that some aspect of homosexuality predisposed the patients to immune dysfunction and infections was made on the basis of five cases from a single community—a broad generalization indeed to formulate from so small a sample.

The basis for that sweeping hypothesis lay in a rough mixture of analysis and opinion. The CDC had just completed a cooperative study with a number of gay community health clinics. It was a multiyear, multisite study of risk factors for hepatitis B, a disease that can be sexually transmitted and whose prevalence is very high among homosexual men.[10] In analyzing the interrelation of life-style and hepatitis B, the researchers found that blood markers for the disease were significantly associated with, among other factors, the number of male sexual partners and with sexual practices that involved anal contact. On average, the subjects tended to have a high mean number of partners. Nonetheless, because these were younger men (with a mean age of twenty-nine years), all of whom were attending clinics that specialized in sexually transmitted diseases, they were not necessarily representative of homosexual men.

The CDC-associated study took place against a background of other investigations that suggested an increase in the incidence as well as the types of sexually transmitted diseases (STDs) in homosexual men.[11] Analysts linked this epidemic of STDs among gay men to gay liberation and the attendant life-style of bars, discos, and bathhouses and of anonymous sexual partners.[12] These charges reinforced a set of assumptions, often expressed in medical texts (discussed in greater detail below) by venereologists, that gay men, because of their "pathetic promiscuity" and supposed hedonism, are more vulnerable to sexually related diseases than are heterosexual men and women.[13]

The combination of the CDC's recent work on risk factors for hepatitis B transmission, which had increased its awareness of gay sexuality, and its knowledge of the epidemicity of STDs among subgroups within the gay community, probably accounts, in part, for the hypothesis suggested in the *MMWR*. A greater awareness of homosexual life-style and disease patterns alone cannot explain the CDC's proposal of a hypothesis on the strength of so few actual cases and without seeking evidence that other segments of the U.S. population might be at risk. One might fairly infer that the CDC was prematurely ready to find the etiology of this mysterious disorder in an exotic subculture. This inference is strengthened by the ensuing scientific work undertaken by epidemiologists within and outside the CDC to find in gay culture—particularly in its perceived "extreme" and "nonnormative" aspects (that is, "promiscuity" and "recreational" drugs)—the crucial clue to the cause of the new syndrome.

Part of the reason for the CDC's speedy adoption of the "life-style" hypothesis was, most likely, that in certain previous outbreaks of diseases of uncertain origin (in particular, Legionnaires' disease in 1976), CDC officials had been criticized for having committed themselves too strongly to a microbial hypothesis without having paid sufficient attention to alternative causative theories.[14] This probably influenced their desire to throw a wide causative net in the case of HIV infection.[15]

A special task force on KS and opportunistic infections was established at the CDC in mid-1981 and charged with the surveillance of all new cases. According to Dr. James W. Curran, head of the task force, the purpose of surveillance was to confirm that the observed disorder was new, that it was occurring in the specific populations and geographic areas reported, and that all cases were verified.[16]

Prior to surveillance, the CDC had to define what constituted a case. It initially described a case as "a person who (1) has either biopsy-proven KS or biopsy-proven, life-threatening opportunistic infection, (2) is under age 60, and (3) has no history of either immunosuppressive underlying illness or immunosuppressive therapy."[17] By September 1982, when the CDC first used the term "AIDS" in the *MMWR*, it refined this description to define an AIDS case as one with "a disease at least moderately predictive of a defect in cell-mediated immunity, occurring in a person with no known cause for diminished resistance to that disease." Included among the diseases were KS, PCP, and a specific list of "other opportunistic infections," a list that the CDC has amended over the years.[18] The surveillance definition, whose prime purpose is to assist national reporting of the disorder, has, with as much precision as possible, been limited to the more severe manifestations of the disease.[19]

To establish a count of, and to verify, all cases, the task force and EIS officers conducted a letter and telephone survey of physicians in eighteen U.S. metropolitan areas. In addition, by August 1981 all state health departments had formally been asked to notify the CDC of all suspected cases.[20]

To determine if Kaposi's sarcoma had occurred before 1980 in individuals less than sixty years of age, the task force contacted epidemiologists at state or local tumor registries. Because the CDC was the sole supplier of pentamidine, a drug used in the treatment of PCP, its own files could reveal whether the infection had been seen in adults without underlying illness. Both investigations suggested that the disease was new, the first documented community-acquired epidemic of immunosuppression.[21]

What caused this disorder? With limited clinical data at hand, the CDC did a "quick and dirty" survey of 420 males attending STD clinics in San Francisco, New York, and Atlanta with the intention of finding cases with KS or PCP. The thirty-five cases culled from the sample (biased, or unrepresentative, in that such patients may be more active sexually than the general population) were interviewed on many subjects in the hope that a lead might be discovered.

The researchers found two patterns of behavior that "fell out": sex and drugs. The cases, all homosexuals, had had many sexual partners in the past year (the median number of partners was eighty-seven) and had frequently used marijuana, cocaine, and amyl or butyl nitrite—inhalant sexual stimulants.[22] Were sex and drugs independent of each other, however? The rate of nitrite use, for example, was closely associated with the number of sexual partners, suggesting that nitrite inhalation might be associated with other hypothetical causal variables, including STDs or the medications used to treat them, or types of sexual behavior, or attendance at gay bathhouses.[23] It was also possible that nitrite use was not an etiological factor, but appeared to be one because it was associated with a causal, or "confounding," variable like sexual behavior.

"There are a lot of theories . . . at the start," James W. Curran is quoted as saying:

> You get heterosexual doctors examining gays, and they jump on the first possible hypothesis, that it must be due to the sexual behavior of homosexuals. Because gays are involved, there is also the assumption that they are doing drugs. There were suggestions that it had something to do with amebiasis, a type of dysentery that poses a particular threat to gay men because the guilty protozoa can be spread through anal contact. There wasn't any evidence for this either.[24]

Despite the dearth of clinical evidence, amyl nitrite (AN) became one of the first hypothetical causal variables to be investigated. The "quick and dirty" survey had found that 86.4 percent of homosexual or bisexual men had used nitrite in the previous five years, compared to 14.9 percent of male heterosexuals.[25] As a clue, amyl nitrite seemed worth pursuing, particularly as it appeared to be a component of the "gay life-style" thesis that was posited in the *MMWR* and was riveting the epidemiological researchers. Studies in which nitrite inhalant was a variable will be evaluated below.

Published scientific papers in 1981 were mainly case and surveillance reports—attempts to define the new syndromes and the patients, that is, to formulate what constituted a "case." By describing the population at risk in terms of person, place, and time, and by learning from physicians the clinical details of the disorder, epidemiologists could grope for etiological clues they might use to design formal studies.

One of the first clinical clues the CDC pursued was the possibility that the new syndrome was caused by the cytomegalovirus (CMV), a microbe suspected of being both sexually transmitted and a cause of KS. In September 1981 the British medical journal, *The Lancet,* published a clinical study of Kaposi's sarcoma in eight homosexual men hospitalized in New York City; the investigation found that of four patients tested, all were positive for CMV.[26] Three months later Michael Gottlieb and his colleagues reported in the *New England Journal of Medicine* that four previously healthy men with PCP were both infected with cytomegalovirus and were suffering from a marked decrease in white blood cells, particularly of a kind known as "T4 helper cells."[27] Although acknowledging that CMV infection might result from T4-cell deficiency and the reactivation of a dormant infection, Gottlieb and his colleagues preferred to hold CMV highly suspect. Their position was based on previous studies that had shown that exclusively homosexual men had a higher rate of CMV infection than heterosexual men attending the same STD clinic (94 percent versus 54 percent), that the virus could shed in the semen for prolonged periods of time, and that some evidence existed that CMV produced immunosuppression. Consequently, the authors reasoned that CMV might be responsible for immune-system defects, leaving its victims susceptible to opportunistic infections such as PCP and to cancers such as Kaposi's sarcoma.

CMV was also cited by the CDC as one of three possible etiological agents in its year-end summary on the epidemic.[28] Other putative causes, perhaps more closely related to the "life-style" hypothesis, were amyl nitrite and opiate addiction (a recent investigation of eleven immunocompromised men with PCP treated in New York City had found that seven of the patients, including five heterosexuals, were drug "abusers"[29]). Did any of these agents bear a relationship to any other? How did CMV fit into the "life-style" hypothesis? An editorial in the *New England Journal of Medicine* addressed these issues in December 1981.

Ignoring the heterosexual cases of PCP and other opportunistic infections, the editorialist noted that "the question of cause is obviously central. What clue does the link with homosexuality provide?",[30] positing that the answer was a high incidence of sexually transmitted diseases, including viral infections such as CMV and hepatitis B, which might cause immunosuppression and KS. But because neither homosexuality nor CMV is new, the author suggested that a new factor may have modified the host–agent relationship: recreational drugs, particularly amyl nitrite. Based on this reasoning, he postulated a possible multifactorial disease model,[31] proposing that the joint effects of persistent, sexually transmitted viral infection (presumably from CMV) and a recreational drug like amyl nitrite precipitated immunosuppression in genetically predisposed males. From this followed a clinical course that included minor illnesses, then KS or other neoplasms, and serious opportunistic infections. In essence, the model was an elaboration of the hypothesis originally proposed in the editorial note appended to the first *MMWR* on the new disease.

THE "LIFE-STYLE" HYPOTHESIS: EXPERIMENTAL WORK

To refine hypotheses generated by case reports, "quick and dirty" surveys, and surveillance, researchers compared patients with a group of healthy men possessing comparable sociodemographic characteristics, experiences, or behaviors. Such research designs, which begin with outcome (the disease) and attempt to discover factors retrospectively that can account for the different health status of the two groups, are known as "case-control studies." The early case-control studies were meant, in part, to test whether suspected agents like CMV or amyl nitrite might be causative factors.

One of the first such studies, by James Goedert and his colleagues at the National Institutes of Health (NIH) and the Uniformed Services University of the Health Sciences in Bethesda, Maryland, explored the relationship between KS and amyl nitrite.[32] Goedert attempted to assess the new disorder (the outcome) by collecting clinical, virological, and immunological information on two male homosexuals with KS and fifteen healthy homosexual volunteers. The researchers hypothesized that CMV hyperinfection and / or the chronic use of amyl nitrite might be causal variables. In presenting their results and assessing the implications, the investigators suggested that amyl nitrite inhalation may predispose homosexual men to immune deficiency.[33]

This investigation had some serious limitations. The small number of subjects in the study, for example, deprived it of the power to find statistical significance if significance existed. Moreover, there was no internal evidence to link CMV with Kaposi's sarcoma or amyl nitrite. Though amyl nitrite was correlated with immune defects, the researchers did not report any controls for the effects of possible "confounders," that is, alternative causal variables such as the number of sexual partners, duration of homosexual experience, or any other proxy for infectious transmission of a disease. Notwithstanding its defects, the study by Goedert and his colleagues was cited by others as evidence for the plausibility of amyl nitrite as a causal variable, a tribute, in part, to the power of the "life-style" hypothesis.[34]

Almost simultaneously with the investigation by Goedert and his colleagues in Bethesda, researchers in New York City interviewed twenty gay men with biopsy-confirmed KS and forty gay male controls, matched for age and race, eliciting information on sociodemographic characteristics, medical history, sexual practices, and drug consumption. The cases were twenty of the twenty-one men, aged fifty-two or younger, with biopsy-confirmed Kaposi's sarcoma attended to by New York University Medical Center between March 1979 and August 1981. Controls were selected from the private patients of a Manhattan physician who mainly treated homosexual men. A third of those asked to be controls refused, raising the possibility that the control group was skewed in some indeterminate way. Using multivariate analysis, the investigators found that of all the study variables, only amyl nitrite and "promiscuity" (as measured by number of different sexual partners per month in the year before onset of disease) appeared to have an independent, statistically significant association with KS. The results, like those of Goedert's, were published in the *Lancet,* under the title "Risk Factors for Kaposi's Sarcoma in Homosexual Men."[35]

In October 1981, which was approximately when the New York City investigation began, the CDC undertook a multisite case-control study to identify risk factors for Kaposi's sarcoma and *Pneumocystis* pneumonia in gay men who lacked predisposing clinical factors for either. The results of the study were published in August 1983.[36] Its authors chose as controls male homosexuals without KS or PCP, matched to the cases by age, race, and metropolitan area of residence. Mindful that private-practice controls might not be drawn from precisely the same population, with equal risk of exposure to any number of factors as the cases, the researchers used, where possible, multiple controls—that is, patients from both private practice and STD clinics.

The study found that KS and PCP were associated with certain aspects of male homosexuality, in particular, numerous sexual partners per year. Other significant variables were attendance at bathhouses, a history of syphilis, the use of illicit drugs (excepting nitrites), and exposure to feces during sex. The strong implication was that a subgroup of the male homosexual population, those who were most sexually active, were at greatest risk for KS or PCP. Based on the appearance by then of similar opportunistic diseases in other segments of the U.S. population, including hemophiliacs, the authors concluded that an infectious agent might be the necessary cause.

Nonetheless, the CDC was unwilling to disengage itself from the "life-style" hypothesis or to commit itself to a microbe theory alone. In the second part of the study report, the authors summarized that position: "Although the cause of the acquired immune deficiency syndrome in homosexual men remains unknown, the study presented here and in the companion paper has identified a distinctive lifestyle as an important risk factor."[37]

In their exploration of the "life-style" model, CDC researchers asked detailed questions regarding diet, residence, drugs, and sex, then generated hypotheses based on the associations discovered. As KS and PCP were first seen in persons identified by their sexual orientation, research into sexual behavior followed logically. But the term "promiscuity" implied more than this; it implied moral judgment. Why was this term used so frequently in scientific articles? The Marmor study of 1982, for example, repeated the term "promiscuity" six times.[38]

Promiscuity denotes behavior that is casual, careless, indiscriminate, or irregular. "Irregular" means behaving without regard for established laws, customs, or moral principles, failing to accord with what is usual, proper, accepted, or right.[39] Not surprisingly, the term has been closely associated with sexuality, referring to persons who willfully violate the moral code, who lack self-control. The notion of promiscuity has been applied to groups at the "margin" of society, those who, like immigrants, the working class, the criminal, or blacks, are also seen as intemperate and prone to disease.[40]

Despite its heavy moral freight, "promiscuity" is traditionally used in medical texts to signify sexual behavior involving multiple partners. For example, in an important article in *Annals of Internal Medicine* in 1975, researchers reported the results of a retrospective study testing the validity of the hypothesis that serum hepatitis might be sexually transmitted. In the monograph, five subpopulations were compared, including one composed of male homosexuals and one of male and female heterosexuals attending STD clinics in New York City. In the body of the article and in the initial abstract, both groups are described as "high promiscuity populations," although gays are singled out by the statement that "a well-known feature of homosexual behavior, primarily in men, is an extraordinary degree of sexual promiscuity," with the Kinsey work on *Sexual Behavior in the Human Male* cited as evidence.[41]

Other examples can be adduced. An article published in the *British Journal of Venereal Disease* in 1976 states that "the high proportion of homosexuality among men with syphilis and gonorrhoea has been ascribed to such factors as the promiscuous behavior of homosexuals."[42] A 1981 study in the same journal comments that "male homosexuals appear to be more prone to these [venereal] conditions than female heterosexuals because a large minority are indiscriminately promiscuous."[43]

Although it appears often in a "clinical" context, the concept of "promiscuity" retains its moral dimensions, even in a medical dialogue or text. For example, Dr. Joyce Wallace, an internist and AIDS researcher interviewed by the *Journal of the American Medical Women's Association* in 1982 observed that "during the last year we have become aware of an unusual number of infections and cancers in formerly healthy homosexuals who admit to a promiscuous lifestyle."[44] She went on to say that "both monogamous homosexuals and those who are not sexually active have absolutely normal [T cell] ratios. It seems to be the promiscuity that's the culprit."[45] When asked "what does this epidemic mean?", she responded: "That promiscuity can kill you. These people don't have enough T-lymphocytes to ward off serious diseases such as tuberculosis, *Pneumocystis carinii* pneumonia or Kaposi's sarcoma."[46] In brief, as the title of the piece suggests ("Medical Sequelae of a Life-style"), the predisposing cause of the epidemic appeared to be unbridled behavior as much as a microbe or immunosuppression.

Sensitivity to the use of "promiscuity" in a clinical context was expressed in a letter to the *Journal of the American Medical Association* by two members of the American Association of Physicians for Human Rights, an organization consisting primarily of gay doctors. The writers noted that the use by medical personnel of a term like *profound promiscuity* to describe multiple sex partners was strongly judgmental. It did not belong in the scientific medical literature, and its continued use adversely affected homosexual patients, who hesitated to discuss sexually related issues frankly with their physicians, fearing their disapprobation.[47]

"Promiscuity" as a moral expression implied that the patients bore direct responsibility for their condition. Integrated into the life-style model, the term inadvertently muddied an already difficult inferential problem; namely, whether the risk factors isolated by researchers were indirect causes of the disease, lone direct causes, or cofactors. In effect, the use of the term "promiscuity" confused a scientific problem (*what factors are causally responsible?*) with a moral and political one (*who is accountable?*). Perhaps more important, use of the term reflected how skewed the life-style model had become; that is, the degree to which its adherents had limited the spectrum of patients to homosexual men.

The first heterosexual patients, including the first woman, were reported by the CDC in August 1981.[48] The first clinical descriptions of immunosuppression in heterosexual intravenous drug users appeared in December 1981.[49] By June 1982 the *MMWR* had reported that 22 percent of patients with KS and / or PCP were heterosexuals, the majority intravenous drug users.[50] Almost a third of the heterosexual patients were women. Despite the early appearance and growing number of heterosexual patients, epidemiologic studies of this group were significantly underrepresented in the literature prior to 1984.[51]

Would investigations of heterosexual patients, paralleling those done of gays, have offered a different cast to the life-style model? We will never know for certain. The model probably would have placed less emphasis on multiple sexual partners, on "promiscuity." Perhaps chemical toxicity or the immunosuppressive power of heroin, nitrites, and other drugs might have had more significance, at least at the start. But inasmuch as women—some of whom were *not* intravenous drug users—were among the earliest patients, investigators might possibly have hypothesized much earlier on that a microbe was *the* direct cause, explaining the appearance of the new disorder in all affected groups.

Why, we might well ask, were heterosexual intravenous drug users not studied? There is no simple answer. One reason, a structural one, is that at the federal level the National Institute of Drug Abuse (NIDA) had principal responsibility for investigating issues related to intravenous drug use and had a staff of epidemiologists just for that purpose. NIDA's traditional focus, however, was only on drug abuse, eschewing investigations of diseases such as hepatitis B and endocarditis that were endemic or epidemic in their target populations. The leadership of

NIDA decided that AIDS would be treated like any other disease, thereby leaving the research initiative to other centers at NIH or the CDC.[52] Unfortunately, the CDC, lacking previous experience and expertise, shied away from studying the drug-using population, leaving a lacuna.[53]

Another reason drug users were not studied was the relatively small number of research subjects available, particularly outside the New York metropolitan area.[54] That problem was alleviated, however, by the development during the summer of 1984 of a blood test measuring antibodies to HIV. The test created a much larger pool of potential research subjects by identifying individuals who were infected but who did not have AIDS or serious, related illnesses.[55]

A final answer to the question posed was the unwillingness of epidemiologists to study this group.[56] Partly justified by the disinclination of addicts to cooperate in interviews and with follow-up, it may also, in part, be explained by a feeling among many clinicians and researchers (in this respect reflecting the attitudes of the public at large) that addicts are of less social consequence than other patients.[57] In a striking reflection of that lack of interest, at all levels of government and in the universities few epidemiologists had expertise in drug addiction when the HIV epidemic began.

Despite its appeal, the life-style hypothesis was eventually undercut as a sufficient explanation. During 1982 epidemiological surveillance and case reports made it clear that in addition to homosexual males, others were at risk for AIDS. As an article in *JAMA* observed in September of that year: "If lifestyle is the key, the question still remains: Why has AIDS also occurred in heterosexual men (84 cases so far), women (32 cases so far), mostly heterosexual Haitians, and hemophiliacs?"[58] A new model was required.

AN UNKNOWN TRANSMISSIBLE AGENT

On March 4, 1983, after a year of suggestive data, a Public Health Service interagency report (published in the *MMWR*) marked a major shift in the conceptualization of the disorder.[59] What caused that shift was in part the kind of evidence cited by *JAMA:* Case reports to and surveillance by the CDC made it clear that the disease was more than a syndrome of homosexual men and promiscuity.

On July 9, 1982, the CDC had reported that thirty-two Haitian immigrants to the United States, seven of them women, showed immunological, morbidity, and mortality patterns similar to those in homosexual men and intravenous drug users.[60] Although the *MMWR* had previously published two general updates on the increased incidence of the new disease—updates that had included data on heterosexual patients—the article on Haitians constituted the first complete report focusing directly on persons outside the "homosexual" category.

A week later, and again in December 1982, the *MMWR* alerted its readers that patients with hemophilia but no other underlying disease had contracted PCP.[61] The CDC observed that inquiries concerning the patients' sexual activities, drug usage, travel, or residence offered no evidence that the cases were in contact with each other, with homosexuals, intravenous drug users, or Haitian immigrants. What the hemophilia patients shared was a dependence on Factor VIII, the clotting substance they lacked, usually derived from the pooled blood of two thousand to twenty thousand donors.[62]

The possibility of blood as a vector for AIDS was heightened by a CDC report of unexplained immunodeficiency and opportunistic infection in a twenty-month-old infant who had received multiple transfusions, including platelets from a donor subsequently diagnosed with AIDS.[63] The sibling of the infant was in good health and his parents were described as "heterosexual non-Haitians" without a history of intravenous drug use.

Summing up the new cases, the March 4 *MMWR* observed that current epidemiological data indicated four groups were at increased risk of contracting AIDS: homosexual men with multiple sexual partners, users of intravenous drugs, Haitians who had emigrated to the United States in the previous few years, and hemophiliacs. In addition, unexplained immunodeficiency and life-threatening opportunistic infections had occurred in the female sexual partners of bisexual or intravenous drug-using men, and the children born of their unions.

Instead of life-style, the report hypothesized that the cases shared exposure to a transmissible agent. Though the agent was unknown, the pattern of cases mimicked that of a known pathogen, one that epidemiology had studied and helped control in the years before AIDS:[64]

> The distribution of AIDS cases parallels that of hepatitis B virus infection, which is transmitted sexually and parenterally. Blood products or blood appear responsible for AIDS among hemophilia patients who require clotting factor replacement. The likelihood of blood transmission is supported by the occurrence of AIDS among IV drug users. Many drug abusers share contaminated needles, exposing themselves to blood-borne agents, such as hepatitis

> B virus. Recently an infant developed severe immune deficiency and an opportunistic infection several months after receiving a transfusion of platelets derived from the blood of a man subsequently found to have AIDS.[65]

In adopting the hepatitis B analogy, epidemiologists posited an alternative organization of known variables, one which stressed a biological agent whose vector was blood and/or its constituents. Although "life-style" factors could be incorporated, they had lost some of their cachet. In the CDC national case-control study, for example, Harold W. Jaffe and his colleagues, reporting their results in August 1983, suggested that life-style factors are indirect causes of AIDS, with a microbe, probably a virus, as the direct cause.[66]

Although epidemiologists had not yet identified an agent, the model of hepatitis B supported the introduction of public health measures. Stated somewhat differently, the model offered a putative point of intervention in the multifactorial "web of causes," even in the absence of a known pathogen. Recommendations previously developed for hepatitis B were applied, with the Public Health Service recommending no sexual contact with persons suspected or known to have AIDS. In addition, members of groups at risk were asked not to donate blood or plasma, and doctors were encouraged to recommend autologous transfusions to their patients. Finally, the Public Health Service called for the development of blood-screening procedures.

On March 4, 1983, for the first time in the *MMWR,* the CDC referred to "high-risk groups," attesting to the spread of AIDS into multiple segments of the U.S. population and to the relationship between the concept of "high-risk group" and hepatitis B. High-risk groups were those whose members were at greater risk of infection *and* of infecting others, carrying a microbe that was capable of spreading through sexual and blood-borne traffic. The *MMWR* underscored that "each group contains many persons who probably have little risk of acquiring AIDS."[67] Nonetheless, no calibration of degree-of-risk was introduced, so no distinction could be drawn. As no microbe had been isolated, risk designation was, in effect, synonymous with carrier status, even among scientists, not to speak of the news media and among the general public.

Some months later the CDC justified its use of risk groups, arguing that classification of individuals was intrinsic to any epidemiological investigation.[68] Classification should not be taken to mean, however, that groups at higher risk for AIDS could transmit the disease through nonintimate contact, because casual transmission was a view unsupported by available evidence. To use the likelihood of casual transmission as a basis for social and economic discrimination was unfair.

The apology of the CDC missed the point. Grouping individuals may be traditional in epidemiology, both as a means of intervention and as an analytic prerequisite. The political or social consequences of such grouping are rarely examined. In this instance, even if the fear of casual transmission could be eradicated, the groups identified would still be seen as bearing a strong negative relationship to the life-sustaining blood supply. They were created, qua groups, to signify their potential status as carriers of tainted blood and as contaminators. Moreover, the analogy with the highly contagious hepatitis B virus reinforced the association of casual or vertical transmission, particularly for health-care providers, because hepatitis B is transmitted through close personal contact, through all secretions, through wounds and lacerations.[69]

A further consequence of creating "high-risk groups" was to reinforce the relationship between the disease and "marginal" members of the population. This tendency to attribute blame for disease to socially marginal groups is discussed in greater detail in the chapters by Guenter B. Risse, Elizabeth Fee, and Paula A. Treichler. In the case of HIV, although each of the groups ostensibly threatened the remainder of the community through the medium of blood or sex, public health recommendations were intended to inhibit such contamination. Consequently, the disorder could be contained at the boundaries, among people who were "different" from the majority but undifferentiated within each of the "high-risk groups."[70]

One of the dangers of a scientific classification of people based on stereotypes was that it defined the questions raised and thus answered. Such categorization created a Procrustean mind-set evident from the beginning of the epidemic. In early 1982 researchers, in an act of political and scientific oversimplification, designated the new disorder with the acronym GRID (gay-related immunodeficiency), even though the CDC and the *New England Journal of Medicine* had published reports of heterosexual intravenous-drug-using patients with the new syndrome. At a major conference Michael Gottlieb and his colleagues could report, in a paper entitled "Gay-Related Immunodeficiency (GRID) Syndrome: Clinical and Autopsy Observations," that of the ten adult males in the study with the syndrome, two were exclusively heterosexual.[71]

In 1983, when researchers seriously began to consider the diagnosis of AIDS in patients outside the previously defined high-risk groups, they attempted to fit them into the current categories. How, for example, should children with immune-deficiency syndrome be categorized? One approach was to link them to established classifications through their mothers, who were characterized as either drug-addicted or, like gay men, promiscuous.[72] Although the researchers did not define promiscuity, it was assumed to exist and to be directly or indirectly explanatory. One subject, "the mother who denied sexual promiscuity or drug addiction," therefore left a lacuna in the case report.[73]

A second article, appearing in the same issue of the *Journal of the American Medical Association* (*JAMA*), offered an alternative explanation of the same phenomenon. Noting that "until recently, AIDS seemed to be limited to adults, predominantly in those with aberrant life styles or exposure to blood products," the authors observed that the children each experienced "household exposure" to one or more individuals in the high-risk groups, including homosexuals, Haitians, and intravenous drug users.[74] As no evidence existed that the children had either been drugged or sexually abused, the investigators proposed the possibility that the patients had been infected through routine close contact. When Anthony Fauci of the National Institute of Allergy and Infectious Diseases repeated the hypothesis in an editorial in *JAMA*, he raised a firestorm of public fear and confusion.[75]

Ultimately, the hepatitis B metaphor assumed the existence of a highly contagious, infectious agent, probably a virus. Though some favored a new variant of the cytomegalovirus, others, including James W. Curran of the CDC task force, supported the notion of a new infectious agent.[76] In the long run, either hypothesis rested on detecting a pathogen that had hitherto proved elusive.

AIDS: "THE STORY OF A VIRUS"

From 1981 until the isolation of a new virus, epidemiology played a central role in the characterization of HIV infection. That discipline, using specific case definitions, surveillance, and case-control studies, identified "high-risk groups" and offered suggestive models and similes. Although epidemiology formulated the social context and morphology of the new disorder, it could not discover its microbial cause. That function was filled by virologists at the Pasteur Institut in Paris and in laboratories in the United States, at the National Cancer Institute (NCI) in particular.

In May of 1984 the journal *Science* published four reports authored by Robert C. Gallo of the NCI and his colleagues and a fifth by Luc

Montagnier of the Pasteur Institut.[77] These reports established a strong case for a causal link between AIDS and a newly discovered retrovirus that the NCI called HTLV-III and the French called LAV. Later, an international agreement was made to call the retrovirus human immunodeficiency virus (or HIV).

With the isolation of this putatively causal virus, the relative importance of epidemiology in the definition of the disease lessened. Epidemiologists continued to play an important, although somewhat more peripheral role, providing supporting evidence for the viral hypothesis and developing information in areas outside the reach of microbiology and its techniques.

Increasingly, the "bench" scientists—virologists, immunologists, cancer researchers—determined the definition of HIV infection. In effect, they redefined AIDS as a set of biomedical problems open to a chemical resolution in the form of drugs and vaccines. These scientists removed the disorder to a considerable degree from the stigma of its original social matrix, placing it instead into a context resembling that of the supposedly more purely clinical crusades against cancer or polio.

The change in the type of professionals studying HIV infection and in their defined fields of observation and analysis effected a subtle shift in the characterization of the disorder. The disease was increasingly conceptualized in terms of the infectious agent, the virus. Interest in cofactors or a multifactorial model diminished.[78]

One marker of this shift was the title of a book copublished by the Institute of Medicine and the National Academy of Sciences in 1986: *Mobilizing Against AIDS: The Unfinished Story of a Virus;*[79] four years earlier an article in *JAMA* had observed that "it seems unlikely that a virus alone is inducing AIDS."[80] Another marker was the dearth of studies on cofactors—of events or states independent of the virus but necessary to cause HIV infection in general or AIDS in particular. In early 1987 an article prospectively evaluating cofactors for HIV could cite only one published report on cofactors after 1984.[81] A few months earlier another volume cosponsored by the Institute of Medicine and the National Academy of Sciences, although acknowledging the importance of cofactors, suggested "there are no data to support the concept [of cofactors], with the possible exception of genital ulcers in Africa."[82] The authors called for well-controlled laboratory and epidemiologic investigations.[83]

The increasingly biological definition of the disease was reinforced by the successful development of serological procedures for the detection of antibodies to the virus. These tests—the enzyme-linked immunosorbent assay (ELISA) and the Western blot technique—allowed epidemiologists and other scientists to outline the biological parameters of the new disorder.

A first step was to demonstrate that the newly discovered retrovirus was the cause of AIDS. To do so, studies cumulatively had to meet the current formulation of Koch's postulates.[84] The first two postulates—(1) that a specific viral pathogen, or its particles, must be found in almost all patients with AIDS-like syndromes, and (2) that antibodies to the virus must form "in constant temporal association with the development of AIDS"—were partially met by the initial studies reported in *Science* in May 1984.[85] The third postulate (that transmission and illness must be demonstrated in a previously uninfected person) was increasingly fulfilled by epidemiologic investigations, first, by studies of patients with transfusion-associated AIDS and their blood donors, and, second, by serological investigations of the spread of HTLV III/LAV from high- to low-risk areas.[86]

In July 1986 the CDC reported that epidemiologists, using the new blood tests, had confirmed that persons at higher risk of AIDS in the previously defined groups showed a greater prevalence of HTLV-III/LAV viral antibody.[87] Epidemiologists also found that AIDS and a number of less full-blown conditions, including lymphadenopathy and AIDS-related complex (ARC), had the same underlying viral cause. In addition, antibody tests demonstrated the existence of the viral infection in persons without clinical symptomatology, a not unusual pattern in infectious-disease epidemiology. These data suggested to the CDC that the spectrum of human response to the virus was wider, thus requiring careful study.[88]

Standardized blood tests thus initially provided a biological justification for the previously defined high-risk groups. At the same time, antibody testing could distinguish within the risk groups between those who were seropositive and those who were not. As a result, group membership and carrier status could theoretically be separated. Given the logic of the biological model, moreover, the concept of high-risk membership should actually have withered away, replaced by the notion of *high-risk activities* that made infection more likely. Despite logic, a shift in emphasis from "status" to "act" did not occur until "mainstream" heterosexuals were targeted as a population at risk.[89]

Since 1984 epidemiologists have also contributed to knowledge of the natural history and transmission of HIV infection. The particular strength of epidemiology in these areas has in part derived from the "bench" scientists' inability to uncover suitable nonhuman animal models, and in part from epidemiologists' technical ability to transcend the ethical limitations on human experimentation by studying disease patterns occurring in populations.

Overall, these epidemiologic studies are attempting to enlarge our knowledge of the biological/clinical dimensions of HIV infection, but to develop that knowledge, wherever possible, within the social matrix or behavioral history of the populations involved. By so doing, epidemiologists are maintaining the vitality of a multifactorial, social conception of AIDS in the face of a narrower biological definition.

To date, most epidemiologic studies of AIDS have prospectively followed a defined cohort of individuals, usually homosexual men. The purpose of these investigations has in general been to establish the risk factors for HIV infection or to describe the pathologic state of those already infected—to estimate, in particular, the proportion of individuals who, over time, develop AIDS. In addition to defining the natural history of the disorder, the researchers aim to find determinative variables that may be open to clinical or social intervention.

For example, Cladd Stevens and her colleagues at the New York Blood Center tested the blood of 212 volunteers for HIV in order to assess its spread and to determine the impact of any changes in sexual behavior.[90] Part of a cohort of 4,394 male homosexuals residing in New York City who had participated in hepatitis B studies beginning in 1978–1979, the 212 had had sera drawn every six months from the time of their entry into the investigation until early 1984. Behaviors that proved to be significant predictors of HIV infection included being the receptive partner in anal intercourse and having sexual contact with a person known to have AIDS. The researchers also reported that 48 percent of the 212 had detectable antibodies to HIV in 1984, compared to 6.6 percent in 1978–1979; this resulted in an annual incidence that varied from 5.5 to 10.6 percent, but was highest in 1983 through early 1984. Because seroconversion (a positive test result indicating probable HIV infection) increased despite a reported curtailment of sexual activity by the study subjects, the authors inferred that "the risk of exposure from a sexual encounter is now much greater than it was early in the epidemic, and indicates that precautions taken by many homosexual men thus far are not adequate to prevent transmission."[91]

Somewhat similar results were obtained in a Dutch longitudinal study composed of 741 male homosexuals with multiple sexual partners.[92] Risk factors for seropositivity (31 percent tested positive when the first serum samples were collected in 1984–1985) included the number of sexual partners with whom one was anal-receptive, and the use of recreational drugs like cannabis and nitrite.

Anal-receptive sex, after adjusting for number of sexual partners, was also identified as a risk factor for HIV infection in homosexual males in a San Francisco study;[93] implicated as well was a history of dildo or anal-douche use. This investigation, unlike the previous two, was based on a random population sample.[94]

The three studies cited and others now appearing suffer from distinct limitations: They are restricted to high-risk groups, homosexual men in particular, and they depend primarily on volunteers, some of whom are drawn from STD-clinic populations. It is consequently possible that the prevalence of HIV infection reported may be unrepresentatively high.[95]

Despite these methodological problems, consistent results have obtained, raising the possibility of behavioral-intervention strategies. Specifically, probability of HIV infection varies in homosexual / bisexual men with the number of sexual partners with whom specific acts are performed. In particular, those who engage in anal-receptive sex are at greater risk of infection than those involved in other sexual behavior, including masturbation and oral-genital or insertive-anal sex.[96] In the population studied, HIV infection is an STD in which anal mucosa, traumatized by frequent contact or douching, appears to be an inefficient barrier to infection.[97] How drugs are associated with infection, if at all, remains conjectural.

When epidemiologists have researched the natural history of HIV-associated disorders in infected persons, they have provided information on incidence and prevalence rates and, in the main, on biological markers and disease status. Their attempts to isolate cofactors for AIDS has yielded little solid data. In addition, these investigations, like those discussed above, suffer from limitations. For example, most studies cannot specify the dates of HIV infection in their study subjects. Consequently, endpoint diseases (lymphadenopathy, for example, or AIDS itself) cannot be linked to and measured from a precisely defined date of HIV infection. This lacuna often prevents researchers from determining if a statistically significant variable is actually a surrogate for duration of infection; it also inhibits comparisons of findings across studies and the prediction of time-measured outcomes.

One of the first epidemiologic studies of the course of HIV infection was that of Harold Jaffe and his colleagues, which followed a cohort of

6,875 male homosexuals and bisexuals recruited originally between 1978 and 1980 from STD patients at San Francisco City Clinic.[98] The researchers found that by 1984, 87.4 percent of a putative random sample[99] of the cohort were seropositive, compared to 4.5 percent in 1978, and that 28.9 percent of the sample either had AIDS or a related condition. For each case of AIDS, 7.5 men had generalized lymphadenopathy, 1.1 had other prodromal signs of the syndrome, and 0.8 had blood-related abnormalities.

Similarly distressing results were obtained in a 1984 study of the long-term effects of HIV seropositivity in a cohort of 134 Danish men, a segment of a larger group of male homosexuals followed since 1981.[100] Two of the twenty-two initially healthy, albeit seropositive, men developed AIDS, and 92 percent of those seropositive for more than twenty-nine months developed a T-cell count indicative of immunological defects. Although the authors did not know if those defects were predictive of AIDS, they cited unpublished data that supported the possibility.

The study of B. Frank Polk and his colleagues, unlike the previous two studies, attempted to define predictors of AIDS in seropositive men by studying a cohort of 1,835 male homosexual volunteers recruited by centers in four cities, Los Angeles, Chicago, Pittsburgh, and Washington / Baltimore.[101] When each of the fifty-nine AIDS cases (developing over a median time of fifteen months) were matched to five seropositive controls from the same study center, the researchers found that a decreased number of T helper cells, a low level of HIV antibody, increased titers (concentration of antibodies) to CMV, and a history of sex with someone who subsequently developed AIDS were each independent predictors of the syndrome. The first three predictors, however, are probably biological markers of disease progression to AIDS rather than determinants or causes of that progression.[102] Perhaps useful for diagnostic purposes, they offer little in the way of intervention or prevention. The last predictor—history of sex with someone who subsequently developed AIDS—may in fact be a marker of an infection long-standing enough for AIDS to develop in both partners.

Polk's investigation is limited in that it cannot specify the date of seroconversion in cases and controls. An exception to this study and others is one by Goedert and his colleagues, who followed a cohort of hemophiliacs with documented dates of seroconversion.[103] The results derived from this study suggest that, in adults, AIDS usually appears more than two years after the initial infection, with new cases continuing to develop more than five years later.[104]

Why does AIDS have such a variable incubation period? This fact intrigues researchers, and suggests the possibility of cofactors—exogenous or endogenous exposures that might modulate the rate of HIV-induced immunodeficiency.[105] Some have suspected that a history of microbial infections, leading to immunological alterations, may put individuals at greater risk of infection and of disease progression.[106] Others have suggested genetic factors, a hypothesis bolstered by a recent report that inheritance of one form of a protein (group-specific component) appears to protect against HIV, whereas inheritance of another form of the protein leaves individuals susceptible.[107] There are also epidemiologic indications that age-related variables may be important, because infants and older homosexual men have higher rates of disease progression than other groups;[108] pregnancy may also increase the rate of AIDS, pointing to hormones as possible cofactors.[109]

The possible role of cofactors testifies to the terrible complexity of HIV infection and justifies the reluctance of epidemiologists to reduce AIDS and related conditions to an agent–host phenomenon. Epidemiologic researchers have consistently held up the possibility of nonviral factors to the "bench" scientists. Since 1981 they have rooted biological or clinical events in the matrices of human behavior and social experience. In a 1987 study on the role of cofactors in HIV infection, the authors put the epidemiologists' position quite well.[110] Citing the viral etiology common to all patients with AIDS, they stressed the multiple determinants probably responsible for HIV infection and disease progression, including cultural differences, the presence of other endemic illnesses, and host and viral genetic factors. Their position reaffirms the multifactorial model as central to an understanding of HIV infection and to its control.

In 1988, with no vaccine available and only one drug approved for treating AIDS in the United States, the most effective intervention is that of primary prevention—that is, the elimination or reduction of behavior that increases risk of HIV infection. Epidemiology has traditionally been associated with primary prevention—for example, in the nineteenth-century campaigns for clean water and the proper disposal of waste and sewage, and more recently in the elucidation of the link between chronic diseases and "life-style" factors, such as diet or exercise. The multifactorial model itself, with its genealogic web of causes, assumes interdiction points that ideally occur prior to infection or the onset of disease.

Epidemiologists and their collaborators have already gathered the information needed in order to implement programs of primary prevention. Such programs recommend limiting the number of sexual partners taken and the types of sexual acts engaged in, an end to sharing needles or syringes, and counseling infected women about the consequences of pregnancy.[111] Epidemiologists must now evaluate the efficacy of these programs, a task they have already begun in a rather limited fashion.[112]

Can a massive campaign of public health education alter intimate habits, physical addictions, or the desire of women infected with the HIV to be mothers? Unequivocal answers are impossible: One major problem is that programs to modify high-risk behavior will inevitably run up against socially powerful attitudes toward "deviance" that may require wrenching public-policy choices. Another important issue is the paucity of scientific knowledge regarding human sexual behavior, limiting the effectiveness of educational programs. Here epidemiology can be of some assistance. Having raised the "life-style" issue originally, having maintained the importance of social experience and behavior in the scientific understanding of disease processes, epidemiology can commit itself to studying such issues that, long taboo, have now been "normalized" by the epidemiologic approach to the HIV epidemic.

CONCLUSION

In this chapter I have tried to show how epidemiologists, drawing on the unique perspectives of their profession, reacted to the outbreak of a new disease of unknown cause. These scientists constructed explanations for the syndrome with equivocal results. Almost from the beginning of the epidemic, epidemiologists conceptualized HIV infection as a complex social phenomenon, with dimensions that derived from the social relations, behavioral patterns, and experiences of the population at risk. On the one hand, the epidemiologists' approach may have skewed the choice of models and the hypotheses pursued and may have offered some justification for homophobia. On the other, by defining HIV infection as a multifactorial phenomenon, with both behavioral and microbial determinants, epidemiologists offered the possibility of primary prevention, a traditional epidemiological response to infectious and chronic diseases. Epidemiologists, in effect, laid the basis for an effective public health campaign, and, through publications and conferences, helped make AIDS a concern of policymakers and the public.

Primary prevention, including blood screening, health education, and behavior modification, is currently the only effective social response to the spread of HIV infection. Recent evidence from San Francisco indicates that the rate of HIV infection has begun to decline, possibly because of a reduction in high-risk sexual activities among homosexual males.[113] Another investigation shows major changes in the sexual behavior of gay males in New York City.[114] These results—hopeful signs—have not yet been linked to a decrease in HIV-associated mortality. They may presage, however, a parallel between HIV and infectious-disease history.

Historical epidemiology has shown that medical interventions, both chemotherapeutic and prophylactic, have had little impact on the overall decline in infectious-disease mortality in this century. For example, John and Sonja McKinlay found that since 1900 new medical measures have had almost no detectable effect on U.S. disease-specific mortality rates, as such measures usually occurred some decades after significant declines in death rates had already set in.[115] Thomas McKeown and his colleagues have obtained similar results in a study on the mortality trends of England and Wales. According to McKeown, the observed secular decline was mainly attributable to community factors, particularly better nutrition and hygiene.[116] It remains to be seen whether HIV-related mortality will also decline as a result of community-directed hygiene (condoms, clean needles, blood screening) before a vaccine or new chemotherapy can be introduced. If it does, the history of HIV infection will offer a powerful vindication of the epidemiologists' multifactorial social definition of disease and of the public health actions that followed from it.

NOTES

This chapter is a considerably revised version of a paper first presented at the annual meeting of the American Historical Association in December 1986. It has been much improved by the generous comments of Ronald Bayer, Benjamin Brody, Don C. Des Jarlais, Elizabeth Fee, Daniel M. Fox, Robert Padgug, Zena Stein, Anne Stone, and Mervyn Susser.

1. Robert C. Gallo, "The AIDS Virus," *Scientific American* 256 (1987): 47. The descriptive term "acquired immunodeficiency syndrome," or AIDS, became synonymous with the new disorder; it has recently been replaced by "human immunodeficiency virus" (HIV) infection, named after the putatively causal virus. Though, in general, this essay uses the new acronym, in discussing specific studies it will employ whatever term was used by the investigators reporting.

2. This essay was completed before the publication of Randy Shilts's *And the Band Played On: Politics, People and the AIDS Epidemic* (New York: St.

Martin's Press, 1987), a broad account of the HIV epidemic based almost entirely on interviews and written in a diary-like format. Where Shilts writes of the work of epidemiologists (the CDC in particular), his narrative complements this essay, providing political information and descriptions of personalities that could not be inferred from the scientific literature, the primary source for this chapter. Consequently, where appropriate, reference will be made to Shilts's book in the notes.

3. Neither inductive nor deductive logic can account for the origins of explanatory hypotheses in science. These hypotheses may have their sources in intuition, based on experience. See Douglas L. Weed, "On the Logic of Causal Inference," *American Journal of Epidemiology* 123 (1986): 965–979.

4. Jennifer L. Kelsey, W. Douglas Thompson, and Alfred S. Evans, *Methods in Observational Epidemiology* (New York: Oxford University Press, 1986), 3.

5. Brian MacMahon and Thomas F. Pugh, *Epidemiology* (Boston: Little, Brown, 1970), 25.

6. Ibid. Also, John M. Last, ed., *A Dictionary of Epidemiology* (New York: Oxford University Press, 1983), s.v. "multiple causation."

7. U.S. Department of Health and Human Services, Public Health Service, Centers for Disease Control, *Reports on AIDS Published in the Morbidity and Mortality Weekly Report, June 1981 through February 1986* (Springfield, Va.: National Technical Information Service, 1986), 1–2 (hereafter cited as *MMWR*). For Shilts's account of the background to the *MMWR* report, see *Band Played On,* 63, 66–69.

8. *MMWR,* 2–4.

9. Ibid., 2.

10. David G. Ostrow, "Homosexuality and Sexually Transmitted Diseases," in *Sexually Transmitted Diseases,* ed. Yehudi M. Felman (New York: Churchill Livingston, 1986), 210. See, too, M. T. Schreeder et al., "Hepatitis B in Homosexual Men: Prevalence of Infection and Factors Related to Transmission," *Journal of Infectious Diseases* 146 (1982): 7–15.

11. William W. Darrow, "Sexual Behavior in America," in *Sexually Transmitted Diseases,* ed. Felman, 269–271.

12. Terry Alan Sandholzer, "Factors Affecting the Incidence and Management of Sexually Transmitted Diseases in Homosexual Men," in *Sexually Transmitted Diseases in Homosexual Men,* ed. David G. Ostrow, Terry Alan Sandholzer, and Yehudi M. Felman (New York: Plenum Medical Book, 1983), 5.

13. For "pathetic promiscuity" see "No Need for Panic About AIDS," *Nature* 302 (1983): 749. It is worth noting that the CDC never used the words "promiscuous" or "promiscuity" to describe homosexual life-styles.

14. See House Subcommittee on Consumer Protection and Finance, Committee on Interstate and Foreign Commerce, *Hearings on Legionnaires' Disease,* 23–24 November 1976, 94th Cong. For a defense of the CDC, see Barbara J. Culliton, "Legion Fever: Postmortem on an Investigation that Failed," *Science* 194 (1976): 1025–1027.

15. Stephen Schultz, M.D., deputy commissioner, New York City Department of Health, former EIS officer, personal communication with the author, 22 July 1987.

16. House Subcommittee on Health and the Environment, Committee on Energy and Commerce, *Hearings on Kaposi's Sarcoma and Related Opportunistic Infections,* 13 April 1982, 8 (hereafter, *Hearings*).

17. *MMWR,* 9.

18. Ibid., 18.

19. Ibid., 95–97.

20. Centers for Disease Control Task Force on Kaposi's Sarcoma and Opportunistic Infections, "Epidemiologic Aspects of the Current Outbreak of Kaposi's Sarcoma and Opportunistic Infections," *New England Journal of Medicine* 302 (1982): 248 (hereafter, "Task Force Report").

21. *Hearings,* 9–10. Also, Shilts, *Band Played On,* 80–81.

22. *Hearings,* 10; "Task Force Report," 252; see, too, Gerald Astor, *The Disease Detectives* (New York: New American Library, 1983), 56.

23. "Task Force Report," 252.

24. Astor, *Disease Detectives,* 56.

25. *MMWR,* 4–5.

26. Kenneth B. Hymes et al., "Kaposi's Sarcoma in Homosexual Men—A Report on Eight Cases," *Lancet* 2 (1981): 508–600.

27. Michael S. Gottlieb et al., "*Pneumocystis Carinii* Pneumonia and Mucosal Candidiasis in Previously Healthy Homosexual Men," *New England Journal of Medicine* 305 (1981): 1430.

28. "Task Force Report." In the early, or descriptive, stages of epidemiological investigations, studies are made of the frequency of the disease in various places, among different groups of people, and, if possible, during different periods of time. Knowledge of the relative frequency of a disease in specific groups gives rise to hypotheses and analytic case-control or cohort studies. See Judith Mausner and Shira Kramer, *Epidemiology—An Introductory Text,* 2d ed. (Philadelphia: W. B. Saunders, 1974), 119–153.

29. Henry Masur et al., "An Outbreak of Community-Acquired *Pneumocystis Carinii* Pneumonia," *New England Journal of Medicine* 305 (1981): 1431–1438. The CDC published its first report of a heterosexual case, a woman, in August 1981; see *MMWR,* 4–5.

30. David T. Durack, "Opportunistic Infections and Kaposi's Sarcoma in Homosexual Men," *New England Journal of Medicine* 305 (1981): 1466.

31. A model can be defined as "a description, a collection of statistical data, or an analogy used to help visualize often in a simplified way something that cannot be directly observed"; see *Webster's Third New International Dictionary,* unabr. (1986), s.v. "model." According to Susser, a model is a system reduced to a set of related variables for the purpose of prediction or representation; see Mervyn Susser, *Causal Thinking in the Health Sciences* (New York: Oxford University Press, 1973), 32. In the present essay, the models discussed perform a representational function in that they "represent existing or postulated relationships in simplified form" (ibid., 33).

32. James J. Goedert et al., "Amyl Nitrite May Alter T Lymphocytes in Homosexual Men," *Lancet* 1 (1982): 412–416.

33. The authors found that seven of the eight volunteers who were frequent amyl nitrite users, but only one nonuser, had a reduced number of T4 cells and

an inverted ratio of T4 to T8 cells, indicating immunosuppression. CMV antibodies were at a similar (high) level in the user and nonuser groups, and were not correlated with the low T4/T8 ratios, suggesting that repeated CMV infection does not uniformly cause immunosuppression. Unwilling to jettison the CMV hypothesis, the investigators postulated instead a joint effect: "These data provide preliminary evidence that [amyl nitrite]-induced immunosuppression, together with repeated CMV exposure, predisposes homosexual men to *P. carinii* pneumonia and to KS. . . . Further study is needed to disentangle the roles of [amyl nitrite], viruses, and other factors in the development of immunodeficiency, opportunistic infections, and KS" (ibid., 415).

34. As a causal factor, nitrite continues to attract research attention. A CDC study found that nitrite inhalants were not a cause of immunosuppression in AIDS, but would not rule out nitrite as a cofactor for some AIDS-associated illnesses; see *MMWR,* 44. Other studies that could not find a significant association between nitrite and illnesses associated with HIV infection include: Michael Marmor et al., "Kaposi's Sarcoma in Homosexual Men," *Annals of Internal Medicine* 100 (1984): 809–815; Harold W. Jaffe et al., "National Case-Control Study of Kaposi's Sarcoma and *Pneumocystis Carinii* Pneumonia in Homosexual Men: Part 1, Epidemiologic Results," *Annals of Internal Medicine* 99 (1983): 145–151; James J. Goedert et al., "Effect of T4 Count and Cofactors on the Incidence of AIDS in Homosexual Men," *New England Journal of Medicine* 316 (1987): 61–66.

Those who do find an association include Michael Marmor et al., "Risk Factors for Kaposi's Sarcoma in Homosexual Men," *Lancet* 1 (1982): 1083–1087; Mads Melbeye et al., "Seroepidemiology of HTLV-III Antibody in Danish Homosexual Men: Prevalence, Transmission and Disease Outcome," *British Medical Journal* 289 (1984): 573–575; Usha Mathur-Wagh, Donna Mildvan, and Ruby T. Senie, "Follow-up at Four and a Half Years on Homosexual Men with Generalized Lymphadenopathy" [letter], *New England Journal of Medicine* 313 (1985): 1542–1543; and Harry W. Haverkos et al., "Disease Manifestation among Homosexual Men with Acquired Immunodeficiency Syndrome: A Possible Role of Nitrites in Kaposi's Sarcoma," *Sexually Transmitted Diseases* 12 (1985): 203–208.

35. Marmor et al., "Risk Factors," 1083–1087. With great care, the researchers assessed the different pathways by which nitrites might be linked to the new disorder. Amyl nitrite could itself be an immunosuppressor, leaving the body susceptible to a cancer-causing sexually transmitted disease. Alternatively, multiple and repetitive infections of sexually transmitted diseases might result in immunosuppression, thereby allowing a carcinogenic agent (possibly amyl nitrite) to act on the body. A third possibility was that amyl nitrite inhalation was not a cause so much as a marker for a true or "confounding" causal variable, perhaps an oncogenic virus, transmitted sexually.

In a follow-up study (Michael Marmor et al., "Kaposi's Sarcoma in Homosexual Men," 809–815) that integrated questionnaire and laboratory data, investigators found, using stepwise logistic regression analysis, that nitrite use was no longer statistically significant after CMV or the number of partners per month with whom one had anal-receptive intercourse or "fisting" were entered into the model. To explain immunodeficiency and KS in the cases, Marmor and his colleagues posited an unknown infectious agent transmitted through anal-genital intercourse and "fisting." In this hypothesis, CMV either jointly caused immunosuppression with the unknown agent or bore a responsibility for the development of KS in the compromised host. The authors suggest that if further studies confirmed the hypothesis of disease transmission through anal-genital intercourse, then preventive methods might follow which could decelerate the spread of the new disorder within the gay community.

36. Harold W. Jaffe et al., "National Case-Control Study," 145–151. For background to the study, see Shilts, *Band Played On,* 96–97, 106–107, 125.

37. Martha F. Rogers et al., "National Case-Control Study of Kaposi's Sarcoma and *Pneumocystis Carinii* Pneumonia in Homosexual Men: Part 2, Laboratory Results," *Annals of Internal Medicine* 99 (1983): 151.

38. Michael Marmor et al., "Risk Factors for Kaposi's Sarcoma in Homosexual Men," *Lancet* 1 (1982): 1083–1087.

39. *Webster's Third New International Dictionary,* unabr., s.v. "promiscuity," s.v. "irregular."

40. Allan M. Brandt, *No Magic Bullet* (New York: Oxford University Press, 1985), 157. Also Gerald M. Oppenheimer, "Historical Models and the Social Definition of AIDS" (Paper presented at the 101st Annual Meeting of the American Historical Association, Chicago, 27–30 December 1986); and Cindy Patton, *Sex and Germs* (Boston: South End Press, 1985), 11–12.

41. Wolf Szmuness et al., "On the Role of Sexual Behavior in the Spread of Hepatitis B Infection," *Annals of Internal Medicine* 83 (1975): 491.

42. R. N. Thin and D. M. Smith, "Some Characteristics of Homosexual Men," *British Journal of Venereal Diseases* 52 (1976): 164.

43. R. R. Willcox, "The Rectum as Viewed by a Venereologist," *British Journal of Venereal Diseases* 57 (1981): 1.

44. Phyllis Shaw, "Medical Sequelae of a Lifestyle," *Journal of the American Medical Women's Association* 37 (1982): 199–200.

45. Ibid., 200.

46. Ibid.

47. Dennis J. McShane and Neil R. Schram, letter to the editor, *JAMA* 251 (1984): 341.

48. *MMWR,* 5.

49. Masur, "An Outbreak of Community-Acquired *Pneumocystis Carinii* Pneumonia."

50. *MMWR,* 10.

51. Harold M. Ginzburg, "The Human T-Cell Lymphotropic Virus, Type III (HTLV-III) and Drug Abusers" (Paper prepared for the Committee on a National Strategy for AIDS, Institute of Medicine, National Academy of Sciences), 14. See, too, Don C. Des Jarlais and Samuel R. Friedman, "AIDS Among Intravenous Drug Users: Current Research in Epidemiology, Natural History and Prevention Strategies," also prepared for the Committee on a National Strategy for AIDS, as well as Don C. Des Jarlais et al., "Kaposi's Sarcoma among Four Different AIDS Risk Groups," [letter] *New England Journal of Medicine* 310 (1984): 119, and Don C. Des Jarlais et al., "Heterosexual Partners: A Large

Risk Group for AIDS," *Lancet* 2 (1984): 1346–1347. For articles on women and AIDS published prior to 1984 (when the virus model superseded that of the "life-style" model in importance), see Henry Masur et al., "Opportunistic Infection in Previously Healthy Women," *Annals of Internal Medicine* 97 (1982): 533–539, and Carol Harris et al., "Immunodeficiency in Female Sexual Partners of Men with Acquired Immunodeficiency Syndrome," *New England Journal of Medicine* 308 (1983): 1181–1184.

52. Don C. Des Jarlais, Ph.D., coordinator for AIDS Research, New York State Division of Substance Abuse Services, personal communication with the author, 15 January 1988. As exceptions to that decision, NIDA funded some internal biomedical work in 1983, the same year it made a single extramural award to New York State to study risk factors for AIDS in drug users. In 1985 NIDA reversed itself and began to fund AIDS research extensively.

53. Stephen Schultz, M.D., personal communication with the author, 22 July 1987.

54. Don C. Des Jarlais, personal communication with the author, 15 January 1988.

55. Ibid.

56. Schultz, personal communication with the author, 22 July 1987.

57. Ibid.

58. Catherine Macek, "Acquired Immunodeficiency Syndrome Cause(s) Still Elusive," *JAMA* 248 (1982): 1426.

59. *MMWR,* 32–34.

60. Ibid., 12–13.

61. Ibid., 14–15, 24–26.

62. Ibid., 47.

63. Ibid., 26–27. For an exploration of the events leading up to the *MMWR* report of 4 March 1983, see Shilts, *Band Played On,* 95, 116, 169–171, 177, 206–207, 226.

64. W. Thomas London and Baruch S. Blumberg, "Comments on the Role of Epidemiology in the Investigation of Hepatitis B Virus," *Epidemiologic Reviews* 7 (1985): 59–79.

65. *MMWR,* 33.

66. Jaffe et al., "National Case-Control Study," 149.

67. *MMWR,* 32.

68. Ibid., 45. Whatever the scientific basis for these "high-risk groups," their existence was also open to negotiation. For a short discussion of the successful pressure applied by the Haitian government to have Haitians dropped as a risk group, see Dennis Altman, *AIDS in the Mind of America* (Garden City, N.Y.: Anchor/Doubleday, 1986), 71–73.

69. Abram S. Benenson, ed., *Control of Communicable Diseases in Man,* 12th ed. (Washington, D.C.: APHA, 1975).

70. For the newly discovered and defined groups at greater risk, Haitians and hemophiliac patients, high-risk group designation marked them with a double shame. In addition to being associated with a fatal disease that threatened the blood supply, they were associated with a "promiscuous" population of gays and intravenous drug users. Though Haitians were eventually dropped

by the CDC as a high-risk group, they suffered the consequences of stigmatization, as do hemophiliac patients, who experience what one of them dubbed "hemophobia" (see Patton, *Sex and Germs*, 23). Ironically, the ones who may have gained something by risk-group designation were intravenous drug users who, for the first time, changed from being a parenthetical clause to becoming a segment of the explanatory model.

71. Michael S. Gottlieb et al., "Gay-Related Immunodeficiency (GRID) Syndrome: Clinical and Autopsy Observations," *Clinical Research* 30 (1982): 349A.

72. Arye Rubinstein et al., "Acquired Immunodeficiency with Reversed T4 / T8 Ratios in Infants Born to Promiscuous and Drug-Addicted Mothers," *JAMA* 249 (1983): 2345–2356.

73. Ibid., 2351.

74. James Oleske et al., "Immune Deficiency Syndrome in Children," *JAMA* 249 (1983): 2347–2348.

75. Anthony S. Fauci, "The Acquired Immune Deficiency Syndrome: The Ever-Broadening Clinical Spectrum," *JAMA* 249 (1983): 2375–2376. Also William A. Check, "Beyond the Political Model of Reporting: Non-Specific Symptoms in Media Communication About AIDS" (Paper prepared for the Committee on a National Strategy for AIDS, Institute of Medicine, National Academy of Sciences).

76. Jean L. Marx, "A New Disease Baffles Medical Community," *Science* 217 (1982): 619; Gallo, "The AIDS Virus," 48. James W. Curran was showing slides demonstrating the plausibility of a viral etiology at scientific meetings as early as February 1982 (Pauline Thomas, M.D., director of AIDS surveillance, New York City Department of Health, personal communication with the author, 28 July 1987).

77. *Science* 224 (1984): 497–508.

78. That scientists concentrated on the microbe and its pathogenesis is not surprising, given the expectations raised by the new discovery and the complex scientific work required to exploit its potential. The extent to which the traditional germ theory's agent–host diad replaced the multifactorial model is noteworthy.

79. Eve K. Nichols, *Mobilizing Against AIDS: The Unfinished Story of a Virus* (Cambridge: Harvard University Press, 1986).

80. Catherine Macek, "Acquired Immunodeficiency Syndrome Cause(s) Still Elusive," 1425.

81. James J. Goedert et al., "Effect of T4 Count and Cofactors on the Incidence of AIDS in Homosexual Men Infected with Human Immunodeficiency Virus," *JAMA* 257 (1987): 334.

82. Institute of Medicine and National Academy of Sciences, *Confronting AIDS* (Washington, D.C.: National Academy Press, 1986), 45.

83. Ibid., 193, 201.

84. P. M. Feorino et al., "Lymphadenopathy-Associated Virus Infection of a Blood Donor–Recipient Pair with Acquired Immunodeficiency Syndrome," *Science* 225 (1984): 70–71.

85. Ibid.; Robert C. Gallo et al., "Frequent Detection and Isolation of Cytopathic Retroviruses (HTLV-III) from Patients with AIDS and at Risk for AIDS," *Science* 224 (1984): 500–502; M. G. Sarngadharan et al., "Antibodies

Reactive with Human T-Lymphotropic Retroviruses (HTLV-III) in the Serum of Patients with AIDS," *Science* 224 (1984): 506–508; see, too, Bijan Safai et al., "Seroepidemiological Studies of Human T-Lymphotropic Retrovirus Type III in Acquired Immunodeficiency Syndrome," *The Lancet* 1 (1984): 1438–1440.

86. Feorino et al., "Lymphadenopathy," 69–72; Harold W. Jaffe et al., "Infection with HTLV-III/LAV and Transfusion-Associated Acquired Immunodeficiency Syndrome," *JAMA* 254 (1985): 770–773; Mads Melbye et al., "Seroepidemiology," 573–575.

87. *MMWR*, 63.

88. Ibid.

89. See, for example, Institute of Medicine and National Academy of Science, *Confronting AIDS*, viii–ix.

90. Cladd E. Stevens et al., "Human T-Cell Lymphotropic Virus Type III Infection in a Cohort of Homosexual Men in New York City," *JAMA* 255 (1986): 2167–2172.

91. Ibid., 2170.

92. Godfried J. P. van Griensven et al., "Risk Factors and Prevalence of HIV Antibodies in Homosexual Men in the Netherlands," *American Journal of Epidemiology* 125 (1987): 1048–1057.

93. Warren Winkelstein, Jr., et al., "Sexual Practices and Risk of Infection by the Human Immunodeficiency Virus," *JAMA* 257 (1987): 321–325.

94. The sample was of single men aged twenty-five to fifty-four years residing in the nineteen census tracts with the highest rates of AIDS in San Francisco. Unfortunately, 40 percent of those selected refused to participate, making those who agreed quasi volunteers. The total cohort obtained consisted of 1,034 individuals, of whom 809 were homosexual/bisexual men.

95. For example, a study by Harold W. Jaffe et al., "The Acquired Immunodeficiency Syndrome in a Cohort of Homosexual Men," *Annals of Internal Medicine* 103 (1985): 210–214, which sampled a cohort of male homosexual STD patients attending San Francisco City Clinic, found that 67.4 percent tested positive for HIV antibodies in 1984. The Winkelstein study, which attempted to generate a random sample of the San Francisco gay male population in nineteen census tracts, found that a smaller proportion, 48.5 percent, had tested positive in 1984–1985.

The reported prevalence of HIV infection varies by place, time, and person. The Multicenter AIDS Cohort Study reported seropositivity for homosexual men in Los Angeles, Chicago, Baltimore/Washington, and Pittsburgh in 1984–1985 to be 51, 43, 31, and 21 percent respectively, with recruitment processes differing from center to center. See Richard A. Kaslow et al., "The Multicenter AIDS Cohort Study: Rationale, Organization and Selected Characteristics of Participants," *American Journal of Epidemiology* 126 (1987): 310–318. Among U.S. hemophiliacs, 70–85 percent were infected with HIV by the end of 1984. See Gene A. McGrady, Janine M. Mason, and Bruce L. Evatt, "The Course of the Epidemic of Acquired Immunodeficiency Syndrome in the United States Hemophilia Population," *American Journal of Epidemiology* 126 (1987): 25–30.

96. Van Griensven et al., "Risk Factors," 1052–1056; Winkelstein et al., "Sexual Practices," 324–325.

97. Ibid., 325.

98. Jaffe et al., "Cohort," 210–211.

99. Approximately a third of the sample refused to participate.

100. Mads Melbye et al., "Long-Term Seropositivity for Human T-Lymphotropic Virus Type III in Homosexual Men without the Acquired Immunodeficiency Syndrome: Development of Immunologic and Clinical Abnormalities," *Annals of Internal Medicine* 104 (1986): 496–500.

101. B. Frank Polk et al., "Predictors of the Acquired Immunodeficiency Syndrome Developing in a Cohort of Seropositive Homosexual Men," *New England Journal of Medicine* 316 (1987): 61–66.

102. Ibid., 65.

103. James J. Goedert et al., "Three-Year Incidence of AIDS in Five Cohorts of HTLV-III–Infected Risk Group Members," *Science* 231 (1986): 992–995.

104. Ibid., 994.

105. *Confronting AIDS,* 193.

106. Thomas C. Quinn et al., "Serologic and Immunologic Studies in Patients with AIDS in North America and Africa," *JAMA* 257 (1987): 2617–2621.

107. L.-J. Eales et al., "Association of Different Allelic Forms of Group Specific Component with Susceptibility to and Clinical Manifestation of Human Immunodeficiency Virus Infection," *Lancet* 1 (1987): 999–1002.

108. Donald P. Francis and James Chin, "The Prevention of Acquired Immunodeficiency Syndrome in the United States," *JAMA* 257 (1987): 1359.

109. Ibid.

110. Quinn et al., "Serologic," 2617, 2620.

111. Francis and Chin, "Prevention," 1359–1361.

112. See, for example, John L. Martin, "AIDS Risk-Reduction Recommendations and Sexual Behavior Patterns among Gay Men: A Multifactorial Categorical Approach to Assessing Change," *Health Education Quarterly* 13 (1986): 347–358.

113. Warren Winkelstein, Jr., et al., "The San Francisco Men's Health Study: III, Reduction in Human Immunodeficiency Virus Transmission among Homosexual/Bisexual Men, 1982–1986," *American Journal of Public Health* 77 (1987): 686–689.

114. John L. Martin, "The Impact of AIDS on Gay Male Sexual Behavior Patterns in New York City," *American Journal of Public Health* 77 (1987): 578–581.

115. John B. McKinlay and Sonja M. McKinlay, "The Questionable Contribution of Medical Measures to the Decline of Mortality in the United States in the Twentieth Century," *Milbank Memorial Fund Quarterly* 55 (1977): 425. I want to thank Daniel M. Fox for bringing this article and its hypothesis to my attention.

116. Thomas McKeown, R. G. Record, and R. D. Turner, "An Interpretation of the Decline of Mortality in England and Wales during the Twentieth Century," *Population Studies* 29 (1975): 391–422.

Legitimation through Disaster: AIDS and the Gay Movement

Dennis Altman

This chapter is about a paradox and its political impact. Although the AIDS epidemic has occurred in a period when social conservatives have been politically dominant in most Western societies—increasing the stigma against homosexuals and homosexuality—it has also translated into much greater recognition of the homosexual community and a homosexual movement, in most Western democracies. (Most of the examples discussed in this chapter will be drawn from the United States and Australia, although similar tendencies can be seen in other Western countries.)

Central to understanding the paradox described above is the fact that when AIDS was first recognized as a new disease, it was conceptualized as a disease of urban male homosexuals. We now know enough of the natural history of the syndrome, however, to realize that it almost certainly existed in central Africa, and maybe in Haiti as well, before it was first reported by the Centers for Disease Control (CDC) in 1981. But the fact that AIDS was linked in its original conceptualization to gay men—and that in most Western countries male homosexual sex remains to date the largest single source of transmission—is crucial to understanding the paradox.

It is not, of course, homosexuals who are at risk for AIDS but rather those who practice certain forms of "unsafe" sex. This distinction between behavior and identity, which often seems academic, is in fact vital to a rational understanding of AIDS.[1] Because the media and the public generally do not make these distinctions, "gay" and "AIDS" have become conflated, so that the public perception of homosexuality becomes largely indistinguishable from its perception of AIDS. This, in turn, has two consequences: (1) It causes unnecessary discrimination against all those who are identified as gay (including, in some cases, lesbians), and (2) it also means that people who are not perceived (and do not perceive themselves) as engaging in high-risk behaviors can deny that they are at risk of HIV infection.

In the early stages of the contemporary homosexual movement—which developed out of the whole social, political, and cultural ferment of the late 1960s—many of its demands could be summarized with the slogan "Get the State Off Our Back!"[2] As the gay movement matured in the 1970s, however, it made more concrete demands of governments, pressing for antidiscrimination ordinances and for financial support for gay organizations and activities. But, in large part, the gay movement retained an adversarial relationship with government, a relationship made possible because of the movement's emphasis on self-assertion ("coming out") and challenging social stigma.

All this changed with the appearance of AIDS. Demands for government-funded research were first made by New York's Gay Men's Health Crisis, the first community-based AIDS organization. And the demands have not stopped there: Governments are asked to support research, patient care, services, and education programs. Inevitably such demands involve gay participation in the processes of government—policy-making, membership on liaison committees, day-to-day contact with bureaucrats, and so forth.

But the process has been two-way. Governments have understood that to research the disease, to provide the necessary services, and to bring about the behavioral changes (primary prevention) believed to be the most effective strategies against the spread of the disease, contact with the most affected groups is required. AIDS has thus forced governments to recognize organizations they had previously ignored, and this has resulted in strengthened gay organizations, often with the help of state resources. Ironically, the conservative Reagan administration has had more contacts with organized gay groups than any of its predecessors, largely because of AIDS. In a number of other countries gays have been accorded some official recognition in formulating official AIDS strategies, and their organizations subsidized; in the Australian state of Victoria, for example, the government fostered the development of a Gay Men's Community Health Centre. Even Great Britain, where the Thatcher government has hardly been sympathetic to gay demands, belatedly helped to fund the Terence Higgins Trust, which was established in 1982 to provide care for and information on AIDS.

Faced with a new epidemic disease, public health authorities have had to find ways to control its spread, minimize its consequences, and care for those who are sick. In the absence of either a cure or a vaccine for AIDS, there is clearly considerable room for divergence on how best to respond, epitomized by the difference between the measures taken by the city of San Francisco and the Australian state of Queensland.[3]

I want to stress at the outset one crucial difference between these two cases—namely, that San Francisco was prepared from early on in the course of the epidemic to devote considerable resources to AIDS, *and to develop a partnership between government and community-based organizations in the use of these resources.* As two researchers note, the city developed "a relatively coordinated set of services for AIDS patients and citizens in major risk groups, from outpatient care to housing and counseling to prevention through community education."[4]

Through large-scale city support for the largely gay-based AIDS Foundation and the Shanti Project, a number of programs were developed to provide care and support for AIDS patients; large-scale educational and counseling programs were also established for groups perceived as at-risk.[5] As a consequence, hospitalization costs for AIDS patients in San Francisco were lower than in other cities, where homecare facilities were less freely available; moreover, the level of public knowledge about the medical facts of the disease was considerably higher.[6]

Where San Francisco has been a pacesetter for the rest of the United States, the state of Queensland has lagged behind the Australian federal government, even refusing to cooperate with the National Advisory Committee on AIDS (NACAIDS) because of the presence on the committee of openly gay members. The Australian system of universal health insurance and the Queensland tradition of free hospitals have meant that basic medical services are available to all. In dealing with communities affected by AIDS, however, the state has shown itself to be punitive and uncooperative. A conservative state, Queensland has draconian drug laws and (like two other Australian states) has retained the criminal status of homosexuality; these attitudes are reflected in the government's response to the epidemic.

In 1984 the Queensland government legislated to make the transmission of AIDS a criminal offense unless the person was in a marital relationship and voluntarily ran the risk of being infected. National attempts to implement anti-AIDS educational programs have been resisted by Queensland, whose premier has publicly opposed any attempt to make condoms more widely available. The crucial point here is that the Queensland government to this day refuses officially to cooperate with either gay community groups or with the (not exclusively gay) Queensland AIDS Council (QAC). The federal government has therefore made special arrangements to bypass the state and provide financial assistance to the QAC.

Both the San Francisco and Queensland governments exercise limited jurisdiction; in both cases, ultimate responsibility for crucial aspects of health policy rests with the federal government. In the United States, where there is no equivalent to the universal national health insurance system found in almost every other Western country, the Reagan administration's determination to cut back on health-care spending has placed particular strains on local governments and community organizations; many individuals with AIDS in the United States (and almost certainly many more with AIDS-related complex [ARC]) do not have access to even minimum medical care.[7] Partly because of its unwillingness to accept federal responsibility for health, and partly because of the pressures of right-wing moralists, the United States has failed to develop any coordinated national response to the epidemic—despite calls for action from a number of organizations, and the reality that the epidemic has hit the United States far harder than any other Western country.[8]

The most serious problem in the United States has been the reluctance to mount a national program of AIDS-prevention education similar to that in a number of European countries. Even though a report by the U.S. Surgeon General C. Everett Koop—a conservative—stressed the need for large-scale education, virtually nothing has been done in large areas of the United States; in most states, what education programs exist are run mostly by gay community organizations, using their own resources. Squeamishness regarding open discussions about sex and drug use, and politicians' fear of the right have been major factors in limiting these campaigns.

Australia shares some of the United States' moralism (though there are also significant differences; fundamentalist Protestantism is less important, but Australia's Catholic church is even more conservative than the United States'). Nonetheless, the greater direct role of the federal government, in addition to the part played by a national advisory structure with community representation, have meant that Australia, like most of northern Europe, has embarked on a national education campaign, employing the image of "the Grim Reaper" in television advertisements to create widespread awareness of the threat of AIDS transmission. The campaign led to criticism from all quarters: Some gay groups felt it was not nearly specific enough, while the right condemned what they called "a condom culture."[9]

THE PROBLEMS OF PREVENTION: PUBLIC HEALTH VERSUS DISCRIMINATION

As a generalization, the response of gay groups and those working in local AIDS education and advocacy programs has been to stress large-scale education about primary prevention, while conservative medical, political, and religious figures have emphasized widespread testing for the HIV antibody and restrictive legislation. The issue of testing for HIV antibodies among high-risk populations (i.e., is it a useful tool in AIDS prevention?) has been a major debate in most Western countries. AIDS organizations have generally argued that large-scale testing is undesirable and that mandatory testing of high-risk groups will, in the words of Surgeon General C. Everett Koop, compel "those infected with the AIDS virus [to] go underground out of the mainstream of health care and education."[10] As the National Gay and Lesbian Task Force (NGLTF) argued:

> The experience of the gay community—the only group where significant prevention and risk-reduction programs have taken place—demonstrates that education and counseling, *not* testing, are critical to changing behavior. Not everyone needs or desires to know his/her antibody status. No one should be forced into that position, particularly given the potentially severe social, legal and economic ramifications of testing.[11]

The NGLTF's antitesting position is further strengthened by the fact that test results often obtain false positives for the presence of HIV antibodies.[12]

It is easy to portray this dispute over testing as one that pits public health advocates against proponents of gay rights.[13] In reality, the dispute centers on different conceptions of public health: Those who oppose mandatory testing are concerned that the fear of discrimination resulting from seropositive results will force those most at risk to avoid needed testing, counseling, and contact with support services. This argument has been used against Reagan administration proposals on testing, and against state legislation that requires the reporting of names of those who test positive.[14] It is vital to understand the extent to which discrimination (real and perceived) against "AIDS carriers" is a factor, and how it is strengthened every time a politician or religious figure talks of quarantine or isolation.

Even enlightened governments have aroused fears of discrimination against homosexuals in the name of AIDS prevention. In Sweden major disagreements have emerged over the provisions for confidentiality in HIV-antibody testing, with the national gay organization expressing apprehensions about the consequences. At this writing a similar dispute has erupted in Australia between Victoria's AIDS Council and the (Labour) state government, which, in marked contrast to the Reagan administration, has enabled and even encouraged gay participation in resolving the dispute.

Of course, certain sorts of discrimination are justified in the interests of public health, and reasonable people can disagree about the balance—as was true in the protracted debate in San Francisco concerning the gay bathhouses.[15] But few diseases in recent history have led to as many stringent proposals to restrict the rights of those affected, and even fewer have led to claims for discrimination against *all* members of "high-risk" groups, whether or not they were actually ill or contagious. Fear of AIDS has elicited a welter of irrational reactions based on the stereotyping of homosexuals.[16] The U.S. Justice Department has ruled that persons with AIDS may be dismissed from their jobs because of fear of transmission, even where such fears are not medically supported;[17] some state courts and legislatures, however, have taken an opposite position. Fear of AIDS was invoked by the state of Georgia in its successful defense of its antisodomy law before the Supreme Court in 1986. A number of governments (including the United States) have sought to make evidence of HIV-antibody-free (noncarrier) status a requirement for immigration or even entry; in West Germany this provision has led to a bitter dispute between the Interior and Health ministries.

AIDS AND GAY RIGHTS: PROGRESS OR REVERSAL?

Fear of and hostility toward those with AIDS most clearly overlap with more generalized homophobia in the attempts by some politicians and a number of fundamentalists to use the epidemic to argue against homosexual rights. In the eyes of the religious right, AIDS is literally viewed as a God-given opportunity to reverse social attitudes toward homosexuality, which have grown more tolerant over the past decade; in English-speaking countries particularly, fundamentalists have invoked fire-and-brimstone rhetoric to argue that AIDS is evidence of God's wrath. It seems likely that some of President Reagan's reluctance to commit his administration to the battle against the epidemic has had much to do with his unwillingness to antagonize the fundamentalists in the Republican constituency; latest victim of right-wing attacks is Surgeon General C. Everett Koop, who has been bitterly assailed for his espousal of widespread AIDS-prevention education.[18]

The greatest danger of discrimination can occur where the religious and political right combine to organize antihomosexual campaigns invoking the fear of AIDS. For example, in California's November 1986 elections a group associated with Lyndon LaRouche proposed a measure to quarantine those who test antibody positive; it was defeated after gay and medical groups mounted a major campaign against it—supported by almost all mainstream politicians.[19] Even though there is no good medical argument for a large-scale quarantine—let alone the extraordinary practical difficulties it would involve—this will undoubtedly not be the last time quarantine measures are proposed. (Introducing a bill for notification of all HIV-positives, one New Zealand member of parliament (M.P.) said: "As far as I'm concerned, they should be monitored and bloody well isolated."[20]

These extreme examples, however, need to be balanced against the ways in which the increased visibility of gays owing to AIDS has also increased recognition that they constitute a legitimate community; one study in California suggests increased support for gay civil rights over the past decade, despite fear of AIDS.[21] Nevertheless, the political balance still seems unclear. New York City finally adopted an antidiscrimination ordinance in 1986 protecting homosexuals, despite concern about AIDS, and decriminalization was achieved by a free parliamentary vote in New Zealand in 1986; on the other hand, Western Australia rejected decriminalization largely because of AIDS-related hysteria.[22] Several U.S. cities, including Los Angeles and San Francisco, have adopted specific ordinances against AIDS-related discrimination. That these are necessary is suggested by the rise in AIDS-related cases before various state and city human rights commissions over the past year.[23]

Gay groups have quickly learned which aspects of the political system are most amenable to pressure; in the United States, at a national level, this has involved working through the courts (a vast number of AIDS-related cases are already working their way through the judicial system) and, especially, sympathetic members of Congress. The first hearings on AIDS were those organized by Rep. Henry A. Waxman (D.-Calif.) in 1983 and Rep. Ted Weiss (D.-N.Y.) in 1984; not surprisingly both men have large and well-organized gay constituencies. They were subsequently supported by other congressional members, almost all of whom also have strong gay organizations in their districts. Openly gay politicians, in addition, have run successful, or nearly so, campaigns for national office: San Francisco City Council member Harry Britt was almost elected to Congress in 1987. Congressman Gerry E. Studds "came out" as a result of the scandal following his initial election, and has since been reelected; he has more recently been joined by Congressman Barney Frank, also from Massachusetts; there are, or have been, openly gay state legislators in Minnesota and Massachusetts.

In the executive branch of government—except for some local jurisdictions, especially in California—gay participation in policy-making has been informal and, to that extent, dependent on personal networks. In other political systems, where legislatures are far more dependent on executives, the possibilities for political intervention (available in the United States through congressional initiatives) are far less viable. Thus, in Australia, direct lobbying of the federal Health Department has been much more important than contact with parliamentarians; as early as 1984 the government allowed gay participation in policy-making when it established a ministerial advisory committee on AIDS and included representatives of gay-community groups; it followed this action with government support (and funding) for a national association of AIDS organizations designed to allow direct contact between the federal government and the AIDS-prevention movement. There is, in Australia, a parliamentary committee on AIDS, but its role vis-à-vis making policy is minor compared to the roles played by the National Advisory Committee or the more medically oriented Federal AIDS Task Force.[24]

Two points need be made: First, the recognition of homosexual rights is fragile, and can easily change. (It is unlikely, for instance, that it would survive a change of federal government in the Australian case.) Second, recognition and incorporation into the system itself have presented new problems for the gay movement.

THE CONSEQUENCES OF COOPERATION BETWEEN GAY ORGANIZATIONS AND THE STATE

Among the groups most affected by AIDS, only the homosexuals have been able to mobilize and articulate political demands. The public's perception of the disease therefore continues to be more closely linked with homosexuals than its epidemiology suggests. In the United States this is further complicated by racial divisions and intravenous drug use, as a far higher proportion of AIDS cases that are not sexually transmitted are found among blacks and Hispanics than among whites.[25] Even now one feature of AIDS organizations is the underrepresentation of people of color, including homosexuals. Even in countries where this is not a problem, the dominance of AIDS as an issue makes the gap between gay women and men increasingly more difficult to bridge; although many lesbians are heavily involved in AIDS work, most gay women cannot identify with AIDS as a central issue in the way true for many gay men.

No AIDS organization is exclusively gay, and few are as restrictive in their nomenclature as the Gay Men's Health Crisis (GMHC, which ironically has a considerable heterosexual clientele and corps of volunteers). Even so, AIDS has mobilized more gay men into political and community organizations, although not into specific demonstrations and marches, than any other event in the short history of the gay movement. In every major city of the United States, Canada, Australasia, and most of northern Europe, the appearance of AIDS has led thousands of gay men (and others) to volunteer in programs of care, support, counseling, and education. But this in turn creates several problems: It reinforces the public's misperception of the causal link between AIDS and homosexuality; it forces other issues off the gay movement's agenda and monopolizes its attention; and it creates new tensions as dependence on government and the emergence of a new class of AIDS experts leads to growing strains within the movement.

One could in fact posit that AIDS has created a shift in the leadership of the gay movement, accentuating the trend toward leaders who can claim professional expertise instead of activist credentials—a move already under way during the late 1970s. This has been most obvious in the rise to prominence of openly gay medical doctors, who have been able to use their professional skills and sexual identity to claim a certain legitimacy in the eyes of government; groups like the American

Physicians for Human Rights have become prominent within the gay movement largely because of the epidemic. But the new leadership also includes those skilled in legislative and bureaucratic lobbying, and one consequence of this shift has been to reduce the representativeness of leadership in terms of class, race, and age.

Observing the gay movement as a participant, I have found that AIDS has changed the movement in ways none of us could have anticipated in the much headier days of the 1970s. Obviously the stakes are higher: However important law reform was, it does not compare with the urgent need to respond to an epidemic that in some cities (New York, San Francisco, Houston, Copenhagen, Sydney) was striking nearly every gay man. In response, new people have come into the movement; many gay men who had hitherto regarded gay politics as irrelevant, have become the front-line activists because of AIDS.

But many experienced activists have found that AIDS has turned them into professionals; the people who run the large organizations, such as GMHC, the Terence Higgins Trust, the San Francisco AIDS Foundation, the AIDS Council of New South Wales, and so forth, spend much of their time now dealing with government bureaucrats, health-system managers, and various authorities whom they had once denounced as "the enemy." Unconsciously, certain forms of co-optation inevitably take place; governments fund jobs, trips, and conferences, and those who take part begin to see things differently. Thus, a new tension develops within the rank-and-file, many of whom came into AIDS work as volunteers concerned to look directly after the sick and dying, who feel estranged from the new bureaucrats their own movement seems to have spawned.

Despite very different political, medical, and cultural contexts, both New York and Melbourne have undergone similar developments. In 1987 a bitter exchange erupted between GMHC and its critics, who accused the former of timidity, political cowardice, and an inability to cope.[26] Although the tone in Melbourne is different, almost all of the issues present in the New York clash emerged at a May 1987 public meeting organized by the Victorian AIDS Council to canvass the community regarding some proposed legislation. Similarly, one observer of the Terence Higgins Trust claimed that the criticisms of GMHC were equally applicable in Britain.[27] This is hardly surprising: The social and political ramifications of AIDS are enormously complex, requiring unprepared community groups to create institutions that can keep pace with the rapidly escalating caseload, political complexity, and administrative problems in an atmosphere of considerable emotional and political tension.

There is evidence that gays in the United States are becoming increasingly militant about AIDS, and that the tendency of the past few years for co-optation into the system is being superseded by a recognition of the limits of such an approach. The attacks on GMHC presaged a new anger at conferences held in 1987—for instance, Duke Comegys's widely reported call for nonviolent civil disobedience to put pressure on governments[28] (Comegys is cochairman of the Human Rights Campaign Fund, a gay political action committee).

NATIONAL DIFFERENCES

One of the fascinating social aspects of the AIDS epidemic is the different responses of various societies and governments. As a gross generalization, the most effective responses have been observed in those areas where the gay movement already existed as a legitimate and recognized pressure group; this would be true of San Francisco, the Netherlands, and Scandinavia, and to a lesser extent, Switzerland and several Australian states, where governments have been willing to work alongside gay community groups to deal with the epidemic. (The earliest official response came from the already existing San Francisco City Office of Lesbian and Gay Health.) With the partial exception of hemophiliacs, other affected groups were too unorganized and socially stigmatized to be able to exert any meaningful pressure for government action, although more recently drug-treatment professionals have played a role in AIDS politics. (At a conference in Stockholm in October 1986, I observed obvious tensions between gay activists and social workers with a drug-user clientele.)

Canada (although not each province), Great Britain, New Zealand, West Germany, and some other areas of the United States (the rest of California, New York, Massachusetts, Washington, D.C., etc.) were slower to respond but have basically moved toward the San Francisco model of large-scale education and service programs in cooperation with community groups. Even so, as Daniel M. Fox has pointed out, "Without a national program, community-based organizations are unlikely to emerge or to be influential in cities with small, politically weak gay populations."[29] Other parts of the United States and most of Mediterranean Europe still typify what my editors at the *Village Voice* called "malign neglect." The oddest case is France, where despite a considerable caseload and a leading role in medical research, virtually no government action has been forthcoming from either Socialist or conservative ministers, and where even the gay movement, in decline throughout the 1980s, has failed to mobilize around AIDS. (In an overview of the French gay world written in 1985, Alain Sanzio spoke of "the persistent refusal of the gay community to recognize the reality of AIDS.")[30] Reports of a similar form of denial are made about Italy, where, so far, the majority of cases are found among intravenous drug users.[31]

Of course, other factors besides the existing strength of the gay movement have affected the extent to which AIDS organizations have been included in policy-making; Australia's apparent lead has a lot to do with the concern of the Labour Health Minister, Dr. Neal Blewett, who was greatly influenced by his fact-finding visit to San Francisco in early 1985 (his New Zealand counterpart has been less willing to endorse official gay participation in decision making). Although hardly a surprising assertion, nominally left-wing governments have generally been responsive to gay demands on AIDS-related issues (although there are some exceptions such as Greece, whose Socialist government has a very bad record on gay issues, and Switzerland, whose conservative government took the lead in national AIDS-education campaigns). Differences in political culture, too, are significant; Denmark's response appears more in alignment with its gay groups than does Sweden's, and the explanation seems to have more to do with cultural differences than with differences in the strength of the gay movement in the two countries. Where governments are themselves influenced by traditional morality this will, of course, be reflected in their policies; Italy's Christian Democrat health minister, Carlo Cattin, assailed any suggestion that he should support "publicity for anal intercourse and condoms."[32]

Nor should we forget Alexis de Tocqueville's comments on volunteerism: "Wherever, at the head of some new undertaking, you see the government in France or a man of rank in England, in the United States you will be sure to find an association."[33] Tocqueville would hardly be surprised that the largest community response to AIDS has come in Anglo-Saxon societies. The differences in the extent to which gay communities themselves have mobilized around AIDS reflect deeper variations in national political cultures and their attitudes to volunteerism and interest-group organization. (The American irony is that groups such as the GMHC or AIDS Project–Los Angeles are almost perfect examples of Reaganite volunteerism, but right-wing moralists have prevented the White House from acknowledging their roles.)[34]

NEW PERCEPTIONS OF HOMOSEXUALITY

It is difficult to speak of the impact of AIDS without speaking of the changing perceptions of homosexuals, so intertwined are the two in the public imagination. AIDS seems to have heightened both the stigma and the respectability of homosexuals; in unraveling this apparent contradiction, we can come to terms with certain crucial social changes.

The common assumption is that AIDS has been responsible for reversing, or at least halting, a gradual social acceptance of homosexuality as an "alternate life-style," an acceptance that had grown out of changes in sexual mores and the commercialization of sexuality during the 1970s. It is not hard to point to the hostile rhetoric, increased anti-gay violence, and the quite considerable discrimination directly linked to AIDS.[35] Evidence of increased violence directed against homosexuals, much of it linked to AIDS, was recognized by a special congressional hearing in late 1986.[36]

The reality may well be that the response to AIDS thus far has largely been a reflection of the extent to which preceding gay-rights struggles had achieved a place in the political process for gay organizations; AIDS has thus highlighted a process already under way. The point has often been made that the epidemiology of AIDS would have been very different in most Western countries had it not been for the expansion of gay sexual networks in the 1970s. Equally, the response of governments would have been very different—and almost certainly slower and more repressive—if this expansion had not also been accompanied by the growth of gay political organizations that provided a basis for the development of community-based groups in response to the epidemic. Thus, the paradox I set out at the beginning of this chapter is no such thing; shorn of its emotional and voyeuristic content, the politics of AIDS follows closely the assumptions of interest-group politics in most Western societies. At the level of conventional liberal political analysis, the case of AIDS bears out the adage that the squeaky wheel gets the oil.

AIDS has brought issues of central concern to the gay movement onto the mainstream political agenda: at an enormous price the gay movement has become a recognized actor in the politics of health policy-making. Thus, while I agree with Allan M. Brandt that "the AIDS epidemic threatens to undo a generation of progress toward gay rights,"[37] such a development is not inevitable. Political will and mobilization can have a large effect on the social impact of the disease.

NOTES

1. Dennis Altman, *The Homosexualization of America* (Boston: Beacon, 1983), ch. 2.

2. Dennis Altman, *Homosexual: Oppression and Liberation* (New York: Avon, 1972); for the relationship between gay liberation and earlier gay organizations, see John d' Emilio, *Sexual Politics, Sexual Communities* (Chicago: University of Chicago Press, 1983).

3. Dennis Altman, "The Impact of AIDS," *British Medical Bulletin* 44 (1987).

4. Peter Arno and R. Hughes, "Local Responses to the AIDS Epidemic: New York and San Francisco" (Paper presented at the Annual Meeting of the APHA, Washington, D.C., November 1985).

5. For an overview of the city's response, see K. Leishman, "A Crisis in Public Health," *Atlantic,* 1985, 18–41.

6. See A. Scitovsky, M. Cline, and P. Lee, "Medical Care Costs of AIDS Patients in San Francisco," in *AIDS: Public Policy Dimensions,* ed. J. Griggs (New York: United Hospital Fund, 1987), and L. Tempshok, D. Sweet, and J. Zich, "A Three-City Comparison of the Public's Knowledge and Awareness About AIDS," *Psychology and Health* (forthcoming).

7. See S. Waldman, "The Other AIDS Crisis," *Washington Monthly,* 1986, 25–31.

8. See Institute of Medicine and National Academy of Science, *Confronting AIDS* (Washington, D.C.: National Academy Press, 1986); P. Lee and P. Arno, "AIDS and Health Policy," *AIDS: Public Policy Dimensions,* ed. J. Griggs.

9. "Bishops Condemn 'Condom Culture' in AIDS Campaign," *Melbourne Herald,* 20 May 1987.

10. *Surgeon General's Report on AIDS* (Washington, D.C.: U.S. Public Health Service, 1986), 30.

11. National Gay and Lesbian Task Force, news release, Washington, D.C., 5 February 1987.

12. See S. McCombie, "The Cultural Impact of the AIDS Test," *Social Science and Medicine* 23 (1986): 455–459.

13. See e.g., G. Bell, "AIDS in Australia," *Sydney Bulletin,* 17 March 1987; Gawenda, "AIDS: Reaping Responsibility," *The Age* (Melbourne), 2 May 1987.

14. See Mark Vandervelden, "Colorado Legislature Approves Mandatory AIDS Reporting Law," *The Advocate,* 26 May 1987.

15. See Dennis Altman, *AIDS in the Mind of America* (Garden City, N.Y.: Anchor/Doubleday, 1986), 146–155.

16. See P. Tatchell, *AIDS: A Guide to Survival* (London: Gay Men's Press, 1986), 97–101; M. Somerville, "Structuring the Legal and Ethical Issues Raised by AIDS," in *AIDS: Social Policy, Ethics and the Law* (Monash: Monash University Centre for Human Bioethics, 1986).

17. "Frighten and be Fired," *The Economist,* 28 June 1986.

18. See "Facing the AIDS Crisis," *Newsweek,* 9 June 1987.

19. "LaRouche Initiative Stopped Dead," *New York Native,* 17 November 1986, 6.

20. "Jones Plans Introduction of AIDS Law," *Wellington Dominion,* 30 May 1987.

21. A. Sniderman, B. Wolfinger, D. Mutz, and J. Wiley, "Values under Pressure" (Paper delivered at the Annual Meeting of the American Political Science Association, August 1986).

22. "AIDS Bogy Foils Labor Bill," *Weekend Australian,* 20 June 1987.

23. See "The AIDS Epidemic and Business," *Business Week,* 23 March 1987, 62.

24. See Margaret Duckett, *Australia's Response to AIDS* (Canberra: Department of Health, 1986).

25. See R. Goldstein, "The Hidden Epidemic: AIDS and Race," *Village Voice,* 10 March 1987.

26. "See the Open Letter" by Larry Kramer, *New York Native,* 26 January 1987, and responses in the 9 and 16 February issues.

27. Simon Watney, "The Politics of AIDS," *City Limits* (March 1987).

28. "Gay Health Conference; *The Advocate,* 28 April 1987.

29. Daniel M. Fox, "AIDS and the American Health Polity," *Milbank Quarterly* 64 (1986): 7–33.

30. A. Sanzio, "Splendeurs et misères des gais 80 . . ." *Masques* 25–26 (1985): 59.

31. W. Franklin, "Italian Fast-Tracking," *The Advocate,* 17 March 1987, 32.

32. Lionel Poverb, "La mitre on la copote?" *Gai Pied Hebdo* 258 (Paris), 21 February 1987.

33. Alexis de Tocqueville, *Democracy in America,* abr. ver., ed. Andrew Hacker (New York: Washington Square Press, 1964), 181.

34. See Altman, *AIDS in the Mind of America,* 178.

35. See R. Meislin, "AIDS Said to Increase Bias against Homosexuals," *New York Times,* 20 January 1986.

36. "Gays Testify on Homophobic Violence," *The Advocate,* 11 November 1986.

37. Allan M. Brandt, *No Magic Bullet,* rev. ed. (New York: Oxford University Press, 1987), 194.

AIDS and the American Health Polity: The History and Prospects of a Crisis of Authority

Daniel M. Fox

In 1981, when AIDS was first recognized, the American health polity was changing more rapidly than it had in a generation. The individuals and institutions that make up the health polity had a growing sense of discontinuity with the past. They were poorly prepared to take aggressive, confident action against an infectious disease that was linked in the majority of cases to individual behavior, was expensive to study and treat, and required a coordinated array of public and personal health services.

The unconventional phrase *health polity* emcompasses more individuals, institutions, and ideas than the words ordinarily used to describe health policies and politics. A polity is broader than a sector or an industry. It includes more people than providers and consumers of health services, more institutions than a health-care delivery system. It is more than an aggregation of policies. The *Oxford English Dictionary* defines polity as "a particular form of political organization, a form of government . . . an organized society or community." I use the phrase *health polity* to describe the ways a community, in the broad sense of the *OED* definition, conceives of and organizes its response to health and illness.

My thesis is that when the AIDS epidemic began, a profound crisis of authority was transforming the American health polity. The roots of this crisis reached back in time, some for decades, others for just a few years. They included changes in the causes of sickness and death and, therefore, concerted efforts to adapt facilities and payment mechanisms in order to address them; ambivalence about the recent progress of medical research, reflected in slower growth in research budgets and efforts to make scientists more accountable to their financial sponsors and the media; a growing belief that individuals should take more responsibility for their own health and that public health agencies should encourage them to do so; a sense that the cost of health care was rising uncontrollably and should be contained; and an increase in the power of the private sector and of the states within the health polity. Everyone who worked in the health sector knew that a crisis was occurring; so did attentive consumers of print and television news. Uncertainty about priorities, resources, and, most important, leadership pervaded the health polity. The AIDS epidemic is an additional element in an ongoing crisis.

I write first as a historian and then as an advocate. This essay has three parts, the first two of which are analytical, contemporary history. First I describe the origins of the crisis of authority. I then describe how the crisis has influenced the polity's response to AIDS. In the third part, I identify shortcomings in the American health polity's response to illness; flaws that have been revealed more clearly by this epidemic. The original version of this chapter was written in the spring and summer of 1986 and published in December of that year in *The Milbank Quarterly* supplement, "AIDS: The Social Consequences of an Epidemic." By the time I revised it in January 1988 for publication in this book, the response of the American health polity to AIDS had changed considerably. The centrist coalition that had dominated American social policy from the 1930s to the 1970s was resurgent. The crisis of authority, however, is far from ended.

THE HEALTH POLITY IN 1981

THE DECLINING IMPORTANCE OF INFECTIOUS DISEASE

The most profound change affecting the health polity in the late 1970s and early 1980s was a major shift in patterns of illness, a shift with consequences for every individual and institution within the polity. Chronic disease had become the leading cause of disability and death. For half a century many people in the health polity had advocated changes in the array of institutions for treatment, in professional education, and, most important, in the financing of health care to take account of the growing prevalence of chronic illness. But the institutions of the health polity accommodated slowly to the new epidemiological situation. Most physicians, hospital managers, and, most important, Blue Cross and health insurance executives behaved as if infectious disease, injury, and the acute phases of chronic illness were the major causes of sickness and death. Most of the resources allocated to the health polity were therefore spent to manage acute episodes of illness and their aftermath. Nevertheless, by the late 1970s the burden of chronic, degenerative disease in an aging population was stimulating a profound reallocation of resources, new assumptions about the responsibilities of individuals and institutions, and considerable concern about rising costs.[1]

In the 1970s, moreover, physicians, health officials, and journalists frequently described infectious diseases as problems that had been, or soon would be, solved by scientific progress and an improved standard of living. They usually defined the most pressing health problems as cancer, heart disease, mental illness, and infant mortality among the poor. In contrast, almost everyone knew the history of success in the struggle against infectious diseases during the past century. Smallpox would soon be the first infectious disease to be eradicated; measles would be the next target.[2] Controlling an infectious disease now seemed to be a routine process of discovering its cause and cure. It was no longer necessary, in the United States at least, to crusade for proper sanitation, housing, and diet in order to reduce the incidence of infectious disease. There was considerable evidence that, from the early nineteenth century until at least the 1930s, changes in diet and living conditions had, in fact, been more important than medical intervention in bringing most infectious diseases under control.[3] As a result of rapid scientific advance since the 1940s, moreover, many diseases that had once been leading causes of death had become brief, if unpleasant, episodes of illness. According to leading medical scientists, this success proved that research in basic science should have higher priority than efforts at care and cure.[4] By the early 1980s infectious disease accounted for "less than 5 percent of the costs estimated for all diseases in the United States."[5]

Sexually transmitted diseases (STDs) were now accorded lower priority than ever before as threats to health. Syphilis and gonorrhea were amenable to drug therapy. Public health professionals now considered treatment a method of controlling venereal disease. The availability of treatment, whether in public health clinics or the offices of private physicians, created opportunities for education as well as cure.[6] Although public health agencies still conducted vigilant surveillance, physicians reported a smaller number of their cases than they did in the past, in large measure because they perceived venereal disease as less of a threat to the community.[7]

Just a few years later, some people would recall with nostalgia the general attitude toward infectious disease in the late 1970s. In 1986, for instance, a third-year resident, who had entered medical school at the end of the 1970s, lamented that "many of today's residents spent their formative years in medical training during an era when the ability of the scientific community to solve health care problems seemed limitless."[8] The chief of the infectious disease bureau of a state health department recalled that, before the AIDS epidemic began, he had been considering a job with the World Health Organization because his work in the United States had become routine. In 1987 the chief of the infectious disease division at a major medical school, talking about AIDS to first-year students, lamented that he had chosen his specialty because he liked the idea of helping patients to recover quickly from their illnesses.

INCREASING PRIORITY OF CHRONIC DEGENERATIVE DISEASE

For more than half a century a growing number of experts had urged that more attention and resources be allocated to chronic degenerative disease. In the 1920s and 1930s a few academic physicians had insisted that chronic disease—then often called "incurable illness"—would become more prevalent as the average length of life increased in the United States. They urged their colleagues to accord higher prestige and priority to long-term and home care, but without much success.[9]

Chronic disease attracted increasing attention in the 1950s. The privately organized Commission on Chronic Illness issued what were later regarded as landmark studies (1956–1959), and some medical specialists began to shift their emphasis from infectious to chronic disease. Among the first to do so were specialists in tuberculosis, who broadened their emphasis to diseases of the respiratory system after streptomycin was introduced as a cure for tuberculosis in the late 1940s.[10] The new specialty of rehabilitation medicine gained widespread publicity as a result of its success during and after World War II and the vigorous support throughout the 1950s that it received from the Eisenhower administration and Congress.[11] By the late 1950s the Hill-Burton Act had been amended to encourage the construction of facilities for long-term care and rehabilitation.

Nevertheless, priority within the health polity continued to be accorded to acute rather than long-term care—either for infectious disease or for acute episodes of chronic illness. There were several reasons for this. Physicians' prestige among both their colleagues and the general public continued to rest on their ability to intervene in crises rather than on their effectiveness as long-term managers of difficult cases. Moreover, most of the money to purchase health services was paid by Blue Cross and commercial insurers on behalf of employed workers and their dependents, whose greatest immediate need was for acute care. Organized labor had little incentive to negotiate for fringe benefits for people too old or too sick to work. Since the inception of group prepayment for medical care in the 1930s, Blue Cross and commercial companies had resisted covering care for chronic illness, most likely because they feared that it would lead to adverse selection of risks and undesirably high premiums. Leading spokesmen for voluntary insurance argued that employee groups, even large groups of employees in the geographic areas covered by "community rated" plans, were too small to carry the large financial risks of chronic disease. Nevertheless, a constituency for long-term care of chronic illness was first created in the 1950s by the campaign for Social Security disability insurance and then in the early 1960s by efforts to create what in 1965 became Medicare.[12]

In the 1960s debates about national policy focused attention on unmet needs for health services in general and especially on care for the chronically ill. Some advocates of health insurance for the elderly under Social Security, enacted as Medicare in 1965, emphasized the need for long-term as well as acute care. Nevertheless, Medicare insured more comprehensively against the costs of acute episodes of illness than for outpatient, nursing home, or home health care.[13] Medicaid, however, which had been conceived mainly as a program of acute care for recipients of categorical public assistance, quickly became a major payor for nursing home and home health care for the elderly. By 1967 there was little controversy about the inception of the Regional Medical Program, which dispensed federal grants to diffuse the results of academic research about the major chronic diseases—heart disease, cancer, and stroke.[14]

Federal leadership in shifting priority to chronic degenerative disease continued during the Nixon administration. In 1970 President Richard M. Nixon declared war on cancer.[15] Two years later an amendment to the Social Security Act nationalized the cost of treating end-stage renal disease by covering kidney transplants and dialysis under Medicare.

INDIVIDUAL RESPONSIBILITY FOR HEALTH

By the 1970s there was considerable evidence that progress in controlling and preventing disease, especially chronic disease, could be achieved by changing personal behavior—"life-styles" was the euphemism—more effectively and economically than as a result of medical research and practice. Accordingly, health professionals and the media admonished individuals to modify their behavior in order to prevent or delay the onset of heart disease, stroke, and some cancers. To the surprise of many cynics, these pleas were effective.[16] Millions of people stopped smoking, drank less, exercised more, and ate less salt and fewer fatty foods. Preventing chronic disease had become a popular cause and, for some entrepreneurs, a lucrative one. For the first time since the nineteenth century, manufacturers of food products advertised that they improved health, often with the sanction of medical scientists. Manufacturers of healthier bread, cereals, and even stimulants, in turn, promoted exercise. Some of the new emphasis on individual behavior was fueled by concern to reduce or shift the cost of health services. But much of it was associated with a spreading interest in fitness, and with the belief that individuals should exert more control over their own bodies.

This promotion of individual responsibility occurred at the same time as increasing emphasis on the rights of patients, particularly their right to be treated with dignity and only after giving informed consent. Some health educators urged individuals to take more responsibility for their own health status in part so that they could demand more timely and efficient attention from the individuals and institutions of the health polity.[17] Critics of this point of view described it as another instance of "blaming the victim," of making individuals responsible for the physiological results of inadequate income and education.[18] The new emphasis on individual responsibility for health strengthened existing oversimplifications of cause and effect in the spread of disease. Individuals could be held responsible for behavior they engaged in before it was known to be dangerous. Moreover, individuals could be artificially abstracted from the social groups that formed their values and influenced their behavior.

Reflecting the new emphasis on individual behavior, state and local public health agencies joined campaigns to persuade individuals to reduce smoking and substance abuse. Even vaccination became a matter of individual choice. Public health officials, who in the past had insisted that children be required by law to be vaccinated, now educated parents to make prudent choices.

Control of environmental pollution and occupational hazards were important exceptions to the increasing individualization of public health services. Public officials at the local, state, and federal levels exercised collective responsibility and evoked hostility from industry. Assisted and sometimes provoked by voluntary groups, public health officials called attention to the hazards of lead-based paint, fertilizers, chemical dumps, and atomic wastes. For reasons that may relate to a dichotomy between environmental and personal health services that arose around the turn of the century, the emphasis on collective rights and responsibilities in protecting people from diseases with environmental origins was not translated into other areas of public health practice. Diseases were increasingly categorized as subject either to individual or to collective action.

THE UNFULFILLED PROMISE OF SCIENCE

Another reason for urging individuals to take more responsibility for their own health was widespread frustration, articulated particularly by some members of Congress, at the inability of medical science to keep some of its implied promises of the 1940s and 1950s. The great advances against infectious disease of the 1940s, especially the development of effective antibiotic drugs, had been widely publicized as the beginning of a permanent revolution in medicine. During the 1950s the budget of the National Institutes of Health and the expenditures of voluntary associations that sponsored research grew faster than ever before. Members of Congress, philanthropists, the press, and the general public expected that the causes of and cures for chronic diseases would soon be found because of research on basic biological processes.[19] But medical scientists proved to be better at basic research and at devising new technologies for diagnosis and for keeping very sick patients alive than at finding cures. This technology was disseminated rapidly because third-party payors eagerly reimbursed hospitals for purchasing it—which they did at the request of growing numbers of physicians in each medical specialty. The Regional Medical Program, as it was originally conceived, proved to be redundant. But the vast expenditure for technology had little impact on either mortality from particular diseases or on the growing morbidity from chronic illness. In the absence of new miracle drugs, the responsibility of individuals to reduce their risks was accorded even greater importance.

In addition, by the 1970s scientists sometimes seemed to be losing their privileged status within the health polity. Their success in the struggle against disease was no longer taken for granted, and they were frequently admonished to propose ways to solve practical problems and to be more accessible and forthcoming to representatives of the press and television. Moreover, scientists were no longer assumed to be virtuous as well as effective. Some years earlier, what was called the "bioethics movement," largely a coalition of philosophers, theologians, and some physicians, had begun a strenuous critique of medical scientists, especially clinical investigators. To many participants in this movement, protecting patients and research subjects from harm was the highest ethical goal. For some ethicists, autonomy took precedence over beneficence as goals.[20] Their concern with autonomy was embodied in federal regulations for the protection of human subjects in research. Similarly, the venerable antivivisectionist controversy was reactivated by a new animal rights movement. In part as a response to external criticism of science, but also because of general economic problems, research priorities and budgets were scrutinized more carefully than ever before by federal officials and the Congress.

For a generation the resources allocated to the health polity grew because everyone assumed that the nation's health would improve if more money was spent for research, hospitals, physicians' services, and educating health professionals. Public subsidies helped to create an increasing supply of hospitals, professionals, and research facilities. Blue Cross/Blue Shield and commercial insurers, using the premiums paid by employers and employees, stimulated demand for care. After 1965, when Medicare and Medicaid were established, the federal government became the largest third-party payor. In the early and mid-1970s there was broad agreement that access to basic medical care for the poor and the elderly was a diminishing problem,[21] that the next problems to solve were improving the quality of care and expanding the coverage of insurance and public-entitlement programs. But the consensus that had unified the health polity since World War II was now eroding.[22]

FROM COMPREHENSIVE SERVICES TO COST CONTROL

The broad coalition that had dominated the health polity since the 1930s broke apart in the 1970s. The labor movement, weakened by declining membership, ceased to lobby forcefully on behalf of broad social policy. Executives of large corporations, who for thirty years had provided their employees with generous health insurance benefits, found it increasingly difficult in the economic conditions of the 1970s to pay the cost of health care by raising the price of goods and services. The comprehensive first-dollar insurance coverage available to workers in the largest industries began to be described as a luxury that must be sacrificed in order to avoid increasing unemployment. Community rating, which had been endorsed by labor and business leaders in the 1940s as a way to increase equitable access to comprehensive health care, had been sacrificed to "experience rating," which shifted costs to the groups that could least afford to pay them. Furthermore, generous health insurance benefits seemed to encourage unnecessary surgery and excessive hospital stays. Evidence that numerous hospitals and physicians inflated their charges because third parties would pay them provided business, labor, and government leaders with additional justification for cost-containment measures. As tax revenues declined in the recessions of the 1970s, the federal government and the states changed the emphasis of health policy from providing access to more comprehensive services to cost control.

Advocates of cost control also argued that generous subsidies and reimbursement policies had created an oversupply of physicians and hospitals. Many of them wanted to reallocate the resources of the health sector to take account of the increasing incidence and prevalence of chronic illness. They contrasted excess capacity to provide acute care with the lack of facilities for long-term care.

THE CRISIS OF AUTHORITY

The new emphasis on cost control and reallocating resources was evidence of a profound change in the distribution of authority within the health polity. Since World War II authority in health affairs, as in social policy generally, has been increasingly centralized in the federal government, although considerable power remained with state government and with employers. Centralized authority was frequently displayed in programs that required local initiative to meet federal standards; for example, the hospital construction program created by the Hill-Burton Act of 1945 and the community mental health and neighborhood health centers of the 1960s. In 1978 a political scientist, surveying health policy since the mid-1960s, wrote that "in no other area of social policy has the federal government been so flexible, responsive, and innovative."[23]

But the federal role in social policy generally, but especially in health, narrowed after 1978. National health insurance, which many people had believed to be imminent a few years earlier, was politically moribund by the late 1970s.[24] In Congress and federal agencies, active discussion took place about containing health care costs through tax policy and new reimbursement strategies, which would encourage competition and offer incentives for physicians to use fewer resources.[25] Prepaid group practices, which for half a century had been the favorite strategy of liberals for increasing access to medical care, were renamed Health Maintenance Organizations (HMOs) by the federal government and used as a mechanism to control costs.[26] Diagnosis Related Groups (DRG), a mechanism to control hospital costs by setting prices based on the intensity of resource utilization, were devised by researchers at Yale University in the mid-1970s and were initially implemented in New Jersey.[27]

At the same time many state health departments or rate-setting commissions became, for the first time, active managers of the health industry. The goal of state and regional health planning changed from promoting rational growth to encouraging shrinkage or consolidation. Regulation—a word once associated mainly with the states' responsibility to implement health codes and to license professionals—was now used more often to refer to setting reimbursement rates and issuing certificates of need for construction and new equipment. Other states, however, chose to withdraw from active regulation of health affairs. Their leaders adopted the rhetoric of deregulation and competition that was heard with increasing frequency in discussions of national economic and social policy.

Business leaders began to claim new authority in the health polity. They perceived the cost of health benefits as an impediment to competition with foreign firms and a stimulus to dangerously high rates of inflation. In the United States, unlike other industrial nations, health insurance was linked to employment and was, therefore, a cost of production. A growing number of employers were choosing self-insurance in order to reduce costs. Many of them took advantage of a 1978 amendment to the Internal Revenue Code that permitted individual employees to select from a menu of benefits that often included less generous health insurance.[28] Responding to pressure from employers, Blue Cross and commercial insurance companies began to write policies with larger deductibles and copayments, to scrutinize claims more rigorously, to require second opinions and screening before hospital admissions, and to reduce beneficiaries' freedom to choose among physicians.

The health polity was experiencing a crisis of authority. Assumptions about the balance of power in the health polity that had been accepted since the New Deal (though often grudgingly) were now challenged. In health affairs, as in social policy generally, increasing centralization was no longer regarded as inevitable. Many members of Congress and federal officials were eager to devolve authority over health affairs to the states and the private sector; business leaders were taking more initiative. Devolution would soon be accelerated by the Reagan administration. The health polity in 1981, when AIDS was first recognized, was more fragmented than it had been at any time since the 1930s.

THE HEALTH POLITY RESPONDS TO AIDS

THE MODERN RESPONSE TO EPIDEMIC DISEASE

The health polity had, however, devised a set of responses to epidemics during the twentieth century, and these responses had been increasingly effective in controlling infectious disease.[29] At the beginning of the AIDS epidemic there seemed no reason to doubt that the problems posed by this new infection could be solved promptly and efficiently by applying the well-tested methods of surveillance, research, prevention, and treatment in a coordinated effort involving the federal government and the states. These methods had recently been used, with comforting success, to control Legionnaires' disease and toxic-shock syndrome. Hardly anybody had noticed that during the preparations in 1976 for an epidemic of influenza that did not occur, some senior administration officials raised strong ideological objections to direct federal intervention.[30] Nevertheless, in 1981, despite the crisis of authority in the health polity, AIDS did not seem to be an unusual challenge.

Widely shared assumptions about recent history generated confidence in the standard public health responses to epidemics. For a generation scientists had rapidly identified new infectious agents and devised tests for their presence, vaccines against them, and drugs to treat their victims. Most physicians and hospitals dutifully reported most cases of life-threatening disease, and public health officials held these reports in strict confidence. Although mass screening programs were sometimes controversial and were only partially effective in identifying new cases, there were widely accepted techniques for managing them. Since the early 1970s, moreover, it seemed possible to prevent disease through education and advertising. Finally, despite the problems of high costs and fragmented authority, more Americans than ever before had access to medical care as a result of insurance or public subsidy.

Seven years after AIDS was first diagnosed, many public health officials remain confident that the syndrome will eventually be controlled by the conventional techniques for responding to epidemic disease. In support of this position they note that there have been no documented breaches of confidentiality in reporting or screening and that scientists have identified the infectious agent, devised a test for antibodies to it, report progress in the search for a vaccine, and, in AZT (Azidothymidine, tradenamed "Retrovir"), devised the first effective pharmacological intervention. Furthermore, these officials observe that many gay men have modified their sexual practices in response to education; that no one is known to have been denied treatment for AIDS because of inability to pay for it; and that in several major cities innovative programs of care are being offered to AIDS patients.

Other observers dispute this optimism, claiming that the conventional epidemic-controlling methods are inadequate to address AIDS.[31] They point to events or policies that appear to proceed from hostility or insensitivity to gay men and intravenous drug users. Many gay men, for instance, fear their privacy is threatened by reporting and screening policies that offer confidentiality, which could be breached, instead of guaranteeing anonymity. The Reagan administration was, until 1986, reluctant to request funds from Congress for research on and services for dealing with the epidemic; President Reagan did not even mention AIDS publicly until January 1986. Despite education in "safer" sex, much of it financed by public funds, the percentage of gay men who have positive antibodies to the human immunodeficiency virus (HIV) continues to increase. Also, public agencies in many cities and states have been reluctant to reach out to drug users in illegal "shooting galleries" or to provide them with sterile needles. Many third parties are reluctant to pay the additional costs of treating patients with AIDS. Although programs to create separate hospital units and community facilities for AIDS patients have been presented by their sponsors as positive steps, some critics view them as the beginning of tacit quarantine measures against modern-day lepers.

Without denying the persistence of discrimination against gays, and the blacks and Hispanics who are disproportionately represented among intravenous drug users, I believe the conventional responses to epidemics were now inadequate mainly because of the crisis of authority in the health polity. A polity that is focused increasingly on chronic degenerative disease, that embraces cost control as the chief goal of health policy, and in which central authority has been diminishing cannot forcefully address this epidemic. In the following paragraphs I describe how this crisis of authority has influenced the actions of the health polity in surveillance, research, paying treatment costs, and organizing services for persons with AIDS.

Surveillance Disagreements over surveillance policy have highlighted problems of cost and fragmented authority. Until 1987 the definition of a reportable case of AIDS used by the Centers for Disease Control (CDC) excluded many cases of illness related to HIV infection. Because most states have adopted the CDC's definition, the incidence and prevalence of AIDS and AIDS-related complex (ARC) can only be conjectured. The absence of accurate information has impeded accurate study of the onset and duration, as well as the cost, of the AIDS continuum. Surveillance policy, on the surface a straightforward problem in public health practice, in fact understates the severity and the cost of the epidemic.

Moreover, legal standards for the confidentiality of case reports vary among the states. By the end of 1987, nine states routinely collected the names of HIV-positive people. Two of these states, Colorado and Idaho, were using the names to trace sexual contacts.[32] Moreover, because most states classify AIDS as a communicable disease, case reports are not protected as strongly by statutes as they are for sexually transmitted diseases. They can, for example, be subpoenaed, although there is no evidence that they have been.

The lack of uniformity among the states in standards of confidentiality is an old problem made worse by the absence of national leadership in health affairs. On the one hand, surveillance policy has always been the responsibility of state governments, except for Indians, immigrants, and the military. On the other, standards of confidentiality affect civil liberties, an area of policy over which all three branches of the federal government had, until recently, been exerting increasing authority for a generation.[33]

The lack of consensus about standards to protect confidentiality increases the fear of many gay men that they will be stigmatized and persecuted. This fear, already intense, grew after the publication of a survey commissioned by the *Los Angeles Times*, according to which "most Americans favor some sort of legal discrimination against homosexuals as a result of AIDS."[34] Fear became rage when columnist William F.

Buckley, Jr., wrote in the *New York Times* that "everyone detected with AIDS should be tattooed on the upper forearm, to protect common needle users, and on the buttocks, to prevent the victimization of other homosexuals."[35] The fear is so intense it embraces the entire range of public policy: the irrational—Lyndon Larouche's proposal to screen every American for HIV antibodies; the dubiously effective—bills in several states to quarantine AIDS patients; the debatable—proposals to identify children or school employees with AIDS to school officials; and the traditional—the implementation of such STD-control techniques as the tracing of contacts.

Very little has been written or said to date about the effect AIDS has on the stigmatization of intravenous drug users. Unlike homosexuals, they do not organize to assert their rights, and they do not receive much public sympathy when they claim to do no harm by their private behavior. Drug users are generally stereotyped as pariahs who alternate between preying on innocent victims and receiving treatment and support at public expense. Many of them, furthermore, are also stigmatized because they are black or Hispanic. Addicts who die of AIDS may use fewer public funds than those who survive to receive treatment for their drug problems. Although several landmark civil liberties cases in the past have involved addicts, their rights—unlike those of gay men—have not yet been a subject of litigation during the AIDS epidemic.

Research The history of research on AIDS was strongly influenced by the disinclination of the Reagan administration to assert central authority in the health polity.[36] In 1985 the Office of Technology Assessment, a congressional agency, reported that "increases in funding specifically for AIDS have come at the initiative of Congress, not the Administration." Moreover, "PHS [Public Health Service] agencies have had difficulties in planning their AIDS related activities because of uncertainties over budget and personnel allocations."[37] In January 1986 President Reagan called AIDS "one of the highest public health priorities" but at the same time proposed to reduce spending for AIDS research by considerably more than the amount mandated by the Gramm-Rudman-Hollings Act.[38] In 1986 and 1987 Congress continued to appropriate more funds for research than the administration requested— in the last days of the 1987 session, for instance, increasing the AIDS budget of the National Institutes of Health (NIH) to $448 million from $253 million the previous year.[39] Throughout the Reagan administration, budget officials had deliberately understated the NIH budget request, knowing Congress would add to it. But the congressional increases for AIDS were greater than for other NIH programs.

As a result, at least in part, of the administration's reluctance to fund AIDS research during the first several years of the epidemic, voluntary contributions and state appropriations for laboratory and clinical investigation have been more important than in other recent epidemics. Foundations to sponsor medical research that had been established in New York City and, after Rock Hudson's death from AIDS, in Los Angeles merged to form the American Foundation for AIDS Research. In several cities, community-based organizations raised funds for research within and outside gay communities using techniques similar to those invented many years earlier by the National Tuberculosis Association and the National Foundation for Infantile Paralysis. The states of California and New York appropriated funds for research. These appropriations may be the first significant state expenditures for research related to a particular disease—except, perhaps, mental illness—since the early years of this century.

Similarly, state and local health departments, frequently in collaboration with community-based organizations, took the initiative in programs to prevent AIDS through public education. If the epidemic had occurred in the 1960s or even the early 1970s, the federal government might have established a program of grants for community action against AIDS. Consistent with the social policy of those years, such a program would have included guidelines for citizen participation. In the 1980s, in the absence of federal initiative, the leaders of community-based organizations in each major city combined goals and strategies from the gay rights, handicapped rights, and antipoverty movements of the recent past. Because they do not receive federal funds, some community groups have been free to move beyond educational programs and mobilize political action on behalf of patients with AIDS.[40] However, without a national program, community-based organizations are unlikely to emerge or to be influential in cities with small, politically weak gay populations.

Cost of Treatment Because the epidemic began when government and private payors were restraining growth in the health sector, responsibility for the costs of treating patients with AIDS became a controversial issue. Many groups within the health polity had incentives to publicize and even to exaggerate high estimates of the costs of treating patients with AIDS. Prominent hospital managers were uncomfortable with the new price-based prospective reimbursement and under pressure to offer discounts to Health Maintenance and Preferred Provider organizations. They encouraged speculation by journalists that the cost of treating patients with AIDS was 40 to 100 percent higher per day than the average for patients in their institutions. Many insurance executives embraced the highest estimates, perhaps because they wanted the states or the federal government to assume the burden of payment. A few insurance companies tried to obtain permission from state regulatory agencies to deny initial coverage to persons at risk of AIDS.[41] Officials of the federal Health Care Financing Administration (HCFA) avoided discussing the cost of treating AIDS. Both the administration and Congress have ignored suggestions that the two-year waiting period for Medicare eligibility be waived for persons with AIDS who qualify for Social Security Disability Insurance. When persons with AIDS qualify financially for the less generous disability provisions of the Supplemental Security Income program, they are eligible to receive Medicaid: The states have become the payors of last resort.

The actual costs of treating patients with AIDS are difficult to estimate because responses to the initial research on the subject are heavily political. The authors of the first systematic study, conducted by the Centers for Disease Control in 1985, estimated that the cost of hospital care between diagnosis and death averaged $147,000.[42] They derived this figure by using charges as a proxy for cost and multiplying them by an average length of stay, which was unusually long because it was disproportionately weighted with data from New York City municipal hospitals, which treated large numbers of intravenous drug users with multiple secondary infections and few home or community alternatives to hospitalization. The CDC study then compared hospital expenditures for AIDS with those for lung cancer and chronic obstructive pulmonary disease and found they were "similar," despite the obvious differences in the course, duration, and incidence of these diseases. Whatever the authors intended, the exaggerated estimates alarmed insurers (now prohibited by insurance regulators in several states from denying coverage to victims of AIDS), public officials, hospital executives, and the media. Other studies conducted in San Francisco alarmed some hospital executives because their estimates of the cost of hospitalization, between diagnosis and death—$27,857—were so low that it undercut their demand for higher reimbursement for AIDS patients.[43]

By early 1988 AIDS was usually presented as being about as expensive as other fatal illnesses. The major policy problem was now generally perceived as meeting the increasing burden of payment in the public sector—on Medicaid, state indigent-care programs, and public hospitals. Moreover, as the proportion of intravenous drug users with AIDS and HIV infection grew, concern about public burden was augmented by the traditional complaint of liberals and minority group leaders that programs for the poor are poor programs.[44]

Patient Services In no previous epidemic have variations in lengths of hospital stay and in how services for patients are organized in different cities been so widely discussed. Most of the variation in the utilization of services seems to be a result of the availability of nonhospital services—particularly ambulatory medical care, skilled-nursing facilities, housing, hospices, and home health care. A few city and state health departments have tried to coordinate services. The San Francisco health department, allied with voluntary associations in the gay community, organized a network of inpatient, outpatient, and support services.[45] In order to achieve similar goals in a different political environment—one that is larger, more competitive among institutions, and has no tradition of coordination by consensus—the New York State Health Department created a program of "managed care." In this program, state officials are selecting hospitals that agree to meet specified criteria for managing a continuum of services within and outside the hospital.[46] Each hospital receives a higher reimbursement rate based on its proposal. By early 1988 the state had designated ten hospitals as care-managing centers. Further, every hospital in the state has received a higher rate of reimbursement for each AIDS patient treated since 1984.[47]

The New York State Health Department requires that its AIDS Centers, like the first such center San Francisco General Hospital, dedicate beds for AIDS patients. The rationale for the requirement, according to a principal author of the New York program, is that patients "will be treated better" if they are clustered. He defined "treated better" to mean that, as in San Francisco, AIDS patients would be served by nursing and social service staff who had volunteered for their roles, and that there would be greater attention for continuity of care. In addition, the dedicated beds in San Francisco, combined with case-management services, seemed to be related to shorter lengths of stay and lower utilization of intensive care.

Many hospital administrators and physicians in New York were enraged by the requirement to dedicate beds. They insisted that segregated patients and their hospitals would be stigmatized, and that dedicated beds created new burdens for nurses who were already overworked and in short supply. Perhaps most important in their view, the Health Department was intruding on the domain of physicians and hospital staff. In the final regulations, a compromise was arranged that, Health Department officials hoped, would lead most of the designated centers to dedicate beds. In fact, many teaching hospitals in New York already clustered their AIDS patients for convenience in managing them. This dispute, like so many others during the epidemic, was less about AIDS than about the changing distribution of authority in the health polity.

In August 1986 the Robert Wood Johnson Foundation made the first awards in a $17.2 million program to encourage case management for AIDS patients. Funds were granted to applicants from ten of the twenty-one Standard Metropolitan Statistical Areas with the most cases of AIDS. Announcing the program, in January 1986, a foundation official described the federal government as if it were another philanthropic organization: "If an anticipated federal-grants initiative for similar purposes materializes, the Foundation and the Department of Health and Human Services are planning to coordinate the two programs as closely as possible."[48] In 1985 Congress had appropriated $16 million for AIDS Health Services Projects in the four cities with the greatest number of cases. But the Reagan administration initially sequestered these funds. For the first time since the 1950s a foundation program served as a surrogate for, rather than as an example to, the federal government. By late 1987 the Federal Health Resources and Services Administration had funded service projects in most of the cities in the Robert Wood Johnson Foundation's program.

The absence of national policy to organize and finance treatment for patients with AIDS may be appreciated by state and local officials who prefer to avoid responsibility for treating these patients. After a generation in which access to health services was gradually improved as a result of federal programs, geographic inequities may be increasing more rapidly for persons with AIDS than for victims of other diseases. In other words, AIDS patients in states or cities with relatively unresponsive health departments and no Robert Wood Johnson Foundation money may receive considerably less or lower-quality care than patients in other jurisdictions. The programs funded by the Robert Wood Johnson Foundation may be emulated elsewhere because, according to evidence from San Francisco, coordination reduces the length of hospital stays and the utilization of intensive care. But earlier discharge from hospitals can also be combined with inadequate outpatient, nursing home, and home care. In many places, that is, superficial or cynical emulation of the policies of San Francisco or New York could produce results similar to what has happened when mental patients were deinstitutionalized.

Historical precedents abound for superficial or cynical distortion of strategies to improve health and social welfare in the United States. Since the 1930s officials of many state and local agencies have accepted the policies urged by experts with national visibility only under court order or when adopting them was a precondition for receiving federal funds. The possibility that these officials will resist pleas and even incentives to coordinate services for AIDS patients is enhanced by the unwillingness of the Reagan administration to insist on particular actions by state governments and by the recent retreat of the federal courts from mandating states to improve the care of particular classes of patients.

The public officials and staff members of voluntary associations who coordinate treatment for patients with AIDS have benefited from the gradual reorganization of services to emphasize chronic illness. Like tuberculosis, the most lethal disease of the nineteenth century, AIDS is an infectious disease that requires services outside the hospital. Reimbursement incentives offered by Medicare and private insurance since 1981 have stimulated a substantial increase in the number of home health care agencies and skilled-nursing facilities. Techniques for case management have been elaborated and tested in the past few years under waivers from HCFA and by Blue Cross plans and commercial insurance companies. Moreover, recent interest in substituting palliative for heroic measures in treating patients whose illnesses are terminal has increased reimbursement for, and thus the availability of, hospice services.

Furthermore, AIDS, like tuberculosis a century ago, must increasingly be treated as a chronic illness rather than as a series of discrete acute episodes. Some persons with AIDS are living longer as a result of the introduction of AZT. Other chemotherapeutic measures will no doubt create increasing demand for long-term-care services. AIDS is increasingly a chronic illness among children, requiring a coordinated pattern of services for as yet-indeterminate lengths of time.

AIDS is, to date, the only disease for which institutions are receiving grants and special reimbursement to coordinate inpatient and out-of-hospital services. The only comparable disease-specific case management is for end-stage renal disease—mainly for the procurement and distribution of organs. It is too soon to know if the interest groups organized around other diseases and conditions—people with brain injuries or multiple handicaps, for example—will demand similar services.

What is certain, however, is that the response of the American health polity to the AIDS epidemic has been shaped by fundamental changes that were occurring simultaneously. The most important of these changes, which I describe earlier, were according priority to chronic degenerative disease, emphasizing the responsibility of individuals for their own health, and controlling expenditures for health services. With the narrowed federal role in health care, a crisis of authority was transforming the health polity. The future of the AIDS epidemic will be shaped not only by the number and distribution of cases and by the results of research, but also—and perhaps most important—by how that crisis is resolved. If the polity continues to respond to AIDS as it did until 1986, the epidemic will likely mark yet another incidence of the gradual decline in collective responsibility for the human condition in the United States. On the other hand, the resurgence of the political center in the health polity which began in 1986 could transform the country's response to the epidemic.

By early 1987 there were several signs that incremental improvement in access to and coverage for health services was a serious political issue for the first time since the mid-1970s. In 1986 Congress required employers to permit employees to continue their health benefits for eighteen months after termination. More than a dozen states had enacted schemes to pay the health care costs of people who were uninsured or underinsured. In 1987 a bipartisan coalition in Congress expanded the administration's modest proposal to cover the catastrophic costs of illness under Medicare.

This general revitalization of the centrist, or incrementalist, coalition, which had dominated health policy for a generation, quickly influenced policy for paying the costs of AIDS. Congress responded to testimony about the high cost of AZT, the first moderately effective therapy for some AIDS patients, with an appropriation of $30 million to the states to subsidize the costs of the drug. The administration responded promptly and favorably to requests by several states for waivers to pay for noninstitutional services for persons with AIDS that are not usually covered under Medicaid. The Intragovernmental Task Force on AIDS Health Care Delivery, which convened in January 1987, recommended federal loan guarantees for long-term-care facilities (including hospices) for people with AIDS. The Health Care Financing Administration issued a report by the RAND corporation that predicted that AIDS would place an increasing burden on the Medicaid system. The report was reinforced by an independent study concluding that "public teaching hospitals in states with restrictive Medicaid programs will be most adversely affected" by the burden of AIDS costs. In the fall of 1987 the National Center for Health Services Research and Technology Assessment contracted for the preparation of methods and instruments to measure and project more accurately the national cost of the disease, the cost-effectiveness of alternative ways of organizing services and treating the disease, and the relationship between the costs of AIDS and those of other diseases. In this environment of renewed interest in national policy, researchers who work on AIDS policy have been reporting calls from staff members of leading candidates for the 1988 presidential nominations.[49]

AIDS AND THE FUTURE OF THE HEALTH POLITY

A POLEMICAL INTERPRETATION OF RECENT HISTORY

I describe next how the American health polity might reconsider its response to AIDS or to any other life-threatening disease. Between the late 1970s and the late 1980s the health polity broke sharply with long-term trends in American social policy. For most of the century there was a gradual shift from assigning responsibility to care for the sick to individuals and families toward collective responsibility and entitlement; individualism was considered a weak basis for social policy in an industrial society. For most of the century authority in the health polity was gradually centralized in national institutions—notably the federal government, large insurance companies, international labor unions, and professional associations; fragmentation was considered inconsistent with a just and efficient society. The centralization of authority in national institutions, however, was never complete in any area of social policy: State and local institutions, both public and private, continued to exert enormous power. A health insurance system based almost entirely on employment and retirement from it created considerable insecurity and inequity. But the trend was clear: Until the late 1970s those who opposed centralization, particularly the ideological right, considered themselves a minority group.

The AIDS epidemic coincided with a concerted effort within the polity to reverse the trends toward centralization in social policy. Authority within the polity was therefore devolving to the states and to private corporations. The AIDS epidemic provides evidence that this reversal of social policy threatened public security against illness. I summarize that evidence and its implications in my concluding paragraphs.

THE PERSISTENCE OF THE UNEXPECTED

AIDS should provide convincing evidence that, despite the achievements of biomedical scientists, epidemics of diseases of mysterious origin and long latency will continue to occur, even in industrial countries. Some of these diseases will be infectious; most will probably be linked in some way to behavior or location or work. Science will continue to comprehend nature incompletely. The individuals and institutions who comprise the health polity should therefore accept the need to study and treat a greater variety of diseases than anyone can now imagine. Pressure to contain costs should be offset by a sense that there are limits to how much health care resources can be reduced in a society concerned about its survival.

The epidemic should also lead to better understanding of some practical implications of the platitude that all diseases are social as well as biological events. In the years before the AIDS epidemic the health polity accorded priority to biological factors in disease because its members were optimistic about the progress of medical science. The social basis of disease was not so much denied, as some critics charged, as it was ignored because of the health polity's enthusiasm about the results of laboratory research. However precisely social factors in disease can be identified, they do not contribute as effectively to diagnosis or therapy as does the study of diseased tissue. The AIDS epidemic, however, makes it difficult to deny that many pathogens only cause disease when people facilitate their transmission. As a result of AIDS there may be increased willingness to speak openly about sexual behavior and to provide more systematic education about it. There is already evidence that, in some schools, teachers are being more explicit about the risks of sexual behavior in response to students' fears about AIDS.[50] The media have been more explicit and accurate in reporting about AIDS than about any disease in the past that was linked to sexual behavior.

THE LIMITS OF INDIVIDUAL RESPONSIBILITY

The epidemic also offers evidence that contradicts the assumption that it is desirable or even possible to substitute individual for collective responsibility for social welfare. For more than a decade it has been fashionable among some politicians and policy intellectuals to assert that, given proper incentives, individuals can provide adequately for their own health and welfare. A plausible extension of this argument is that removing people who have positive HIV antibodies from insurance pools would, in the short run, save money for other people in those pools. Proponents of individualizing risk do not seem to care that removal of such individuals would also prevent those with positive antibodies who do *not* develop AIDS from subsidizing health care for other people.

Individualizing risk reinforces a shortsighted view of what constitutes rational social policy. Consider a society in which everyone who is considered a poor risk is denied insurance or forced to enroll in a group composed entirely of people with expensive afflictions. In such a society, the premiums for the oldest and sickest people would be prohibitively high, forcing them to seek public assistance or charity. Because most people are likely to become very old, very sick, or both, the consequences of creating smaller, more homogenous risk pools would be widespread pauperization. The political response to such a perverse policy might be broader support for a federally financed program of insurance against the costs of catastrophic illness.

AIDS also challenges the wisdom of offering incentives to apparently healthy young people to choose the least comprehensive health insurance. The beginning of the epidemic coincided with the decision of many employers to offer their employees so-called flexible-benefit plans. Under these plans, employees who considered themselves to be in excellent health could substitute other benefits, or in some instances cash, for the most expensive health insurance. There are no data about how many AIDS patients, most of them in their thirties and forties and with no previous history of serious illness, chose such substitutions.

The epidemic emphasizes the limitations of social policy that links entitlement to health insurance to employment rather than to membership in society and that provides benefits as a result of bargaining rather than entitlement. Since World World II most Americans of working age have obtained health insurance from their employers or their unions. Federal income tax laws encouraged the link between insurance and employment and prohibited firms from discriminating among workers at different levels of pay in awarding benefits. The tax laws cannot, however, remedy disparities in the coverage offered by different firms. Moreover, state governments have been reluctant to mandate coverage in large measure because, under federal law, mandates encourage firms to shift to unregulated self-insurance—and have done so mainly in response to pressure from members of new provider groups (e.g., psychologists) who wanted to be reimbursed. As a result, the extent and duration of coverage vary enormously among workers with different employers. AIDS, which at the present time mainly affects people of working age, including intravenous drug users (many of whom do not work at all), reveals the limits of an insurance system that has not been compelled to offer a set of adequate minimum benefits.

The epidemic has also exposed the fragility of personal-support networks that are frequently promoted as substitutes for services that are provided, at higher social cost, by insurance, philanthropy, or through public policy. People who are at risk of contracting AIDS may be only slightly more isolated than everybody else. Americans increasingly live in small households, or alone; in the future families and friends may be less frequently available during crises than ever before. Most of us may need sympathetic case management by professionals during our catastrophic illnesses.

THE REASSERTION OF CENTRAL AUTHORITY

Finally, the AIDS epidemic may demonstrate that the American health polity best serves the public interest when institutions within it struggle to assert central authority, when they do not accept fragmentation as the goal as well as the norm of health affairs. The unwillingness of the federal government to exert strong leadership in response to AIDS has been criticized by members of Congress, journalists, and patients since the beginning of the epidemic. In the absence of federal assertiveness, however, the health departments of several cities and states have coordinated the response of the health polity to AIDS. These health departments have tried, in different ways, to counter fragmentation by linking their traditional responsibility for surveillance with their more recent mandate to manage the health system. To the extent that similar linkage of the responsibilities of public health officers occurs elsewhere, it may partially substitute for the abdication of federal leadership and, perhaps, serve as a model for future national administrations.

These lessons about policy and authority could be drawn from the history to early 1988 of the response of the American health polity to AIDS. If they are not, we may recall the 1980s as a time when many Americans became increasingly complacent about the consequences of dread disease and unwilling to insist that the individuals and institutions of the health polity struggle against them.

NOTES

This chapter is an updated version of an article first published in the *Milbank Quarterly* 64, supplement (1986): 7–33. It is based on published and unpublished sources, interviews, conversation, and observation. I have indicated my obligation to written sources in citations in the text. I have not, however, ascribed particular comments—even quotes—to particular people. Some of my interviews were formal, either on or off the record. On many occasions, however, I benefited from conversations that were not, at the time, regarded by the people I was talking to or by myself as data for an essay in contemporary history and advocacy of social policy. Sometimes the conversations were privileged as a result of my participation in research bearing on the making of policy. I list here, alphabetically, the names of some of the people who have in conversations helped to shape my views about the health polity's response to the AIDS epidemic: Dennis Altman, Drew Altman, Stephen Anderman, Peter Arno, David Axelrod, Ronald Bayer, Joseph Blount, Allan M. Brandt, Cyril Brosnan, Susan Brown, Brent Cassens, Ward Cates, James Chin, Mary Cline, Peter Drottman, Ernest Drucker, Reuben Dworsky, Ann Hardy, Russell Havlack, Brian Hendricks, Robert Hummel, Mathilde Krim, Sheldon Landesman, Philip R. Lee, Richard Needle, Alvin Novick, Gerald M. Oppenheimer, Mel Rosen, Charles E. Rosenberg, Barbara G. Rosenkrantz, William Sabella, Stephen Schultz, Roy Steigbigel, Ann A. Scitovsky, and David P. Willis.

1. Daniel M. Fox, "Health Policy and Changing Epidemiology in the United States: Chronic Disease in the Twentieth Century," in *Is This the Way We Want to Die?* ed. Russell Maulitz (New Brunswick, N.J.: Rutgers University Press, forthcoming).
2. Louise B. Russell, *Is Prevention Better Than Cure?* (Washington, D.C.: Brookings Institution, 1986).
3. Thomas McKeown, *The Modern Rise of Population* (New York: Academic Press, 1976).
4. Lewis Thomas, *The Lives of a Cell: Notes of a Biology Watcher* (New York: Viking, 1974).
5. Dorothy P. Rice, T. A. Hodgson, and A. W. Kopstein, "The Economic Cost of Illness: A Replication and Update," *Health Care Financing Review* 7 (1985): 61–80.
6. J. M. List et al., eds., *Maxcy-Rosenau Public Health and Preventive Medicine,* 12th ed. (Norwalk, Conn.: Appleton-Century-Crofts, 1986).
7. R. L. Cleeve et al., "Physicians' Attitudes toward Venereal Disease Reporting," *Journal of the American Medical Association* 202 (1967): 941–946.
8. R. M. Wachter, "The Impact of the Acquired Immuno-Deficiency Syndrome in Medical Residency Training," *New England Journal of Medicine* 314 (1986): 177–180.

9. Fox, "Health Policy and Changing Epidemiology," in *Is This the Way We Want to Die?* ed. Maulitz.

10. W. Bruce Fye, "The Literature of Internal Medicine," in *Grand Rounds*, ed. Diana Long and Russell Maulitz (Philadelphia: University of Pennsylvania Press, 1988).

11. Edward Berkowitz, "The Federal Government and the Emergence of Rehabilitation Medicine," *Historian* 43 (1981): 24–33.

12. Edward Berkowitz, *Disabled Policy* (New York: Cambridge University Press, 1987); Sherry I. David, *With Dignity: The Search for Medicare and Medicaid* (Westport, Conn.: Greenwood Press, 1985).

13. Theodore R. Marmor, *The Politics of Medicare* (Chicago: Aldine, 1973).

14. Daniel M. Fox, *Health Policies, Health Politics: The British and American Experience* (Princeton: Princeton University Press, 1986).

15. Richard A. Rettig, *Cancer Crusade: The Story of the National Cancer Act of 1971* (Princeton: Princeton University Press, 1977).

16. John H. Knowles, ed., *Doing Better and Feeling Worse: Health in the United States* (New York: W. W. Norton, 1977).

17. Lowell S. Levin, A. H. Katz, and E. Holst, *Self-Care: Lay Initiatives in Health* (New York: Prodist, 1976).

18. Robert Crawford, "You Are Dangerous to Your Health: The Ideology and Politics of Victim Blaming," *International Journal of Health Services* 7 (1977): 663–680.

19. Stephen P. Strickland, *Politics, Science and Dread Disease: A Short History of United States Medical Research Policy* (Cambridge: Harvard University Press, 1972).

20. Edmund D. Pellegrino, "The Reconciliation of Technology and Humanism: A Flexnarian Task 75 Years Later," in *For the Good of the Patient: The Restoration of Beneficence in Medical Ethics,* ed. Edmund D. Pellegrino and David C. Thomasma (New York: Oxford University Press, 1988).

21. Ronald Anderson and L. A. Aday, *Health Care in the United States: Equitable for Whom?* (Beverly Hills, Calif.: Sage, 1977).

22. Daniel M. Fox, "The New Discontinuity in Health Policy," in *America in Theory: Humanists Look at Public Life,* ed. D. Donoghue, L. Berlowitz, C. Menand (New York: Oxford University Press, 1988).

23. Lawrence D. Brown, "The Formulation of Federal Health Care Policy," *Bulletin of the New York Academy of Medicine* 54 (1978): 45–58.

24. Daniel M. Fox, "Chances for Comprehensive NHI Are Slim in the U.S.," *Hospitals* 52 (1978): 77–80.

25. Jack A. Meyer, ed., *Market Reforms in Health Care: Current Issues, New Directions, Strategic Decisions* (Washington, D.C.: American Enterprise Institute, 1983).

26. Lawrence D. Brown, *Politics and Health Care: HMOs as Federal Policy* (Washington, D.C.: Brookings Institution, 1983).

27. John D. Thompson, "Epidemiology and Health Services Administration: Future Relationships in Practice and Education," *Milbank Memorial Fund Quarterly* 56 (1978): 253–273.

28. Daniel M. Fox and Daniel C. Schaffer, "Tax Policy as Social Policy: Cafeteria Plans, 1978–85," *Journal of Health Politics, Policy and Law* 12 (1987): 609–664.

29. Harry F. Dowling, *Fighting Infection: Conquests of the Twentieth Century* (Cambridge: Harvard University Press, 1977).

30. Arthur M. Silverstein, *Pure Politics and Impure Science: The Swine Flu Affair* (Baltimore: Johns Hopkins University Press, 1981).

31. Dennis Altman, *AIDS in the Mind of America* (Garden City, N.Y.: Anchor/Doubleday, 1986); Randy Shilts, *And the Band Played On: Politics, People and the AIDS Epidemic* (New York: St. Martin's Press, 1987).

32. Intergovernmental Health Policy Project, *AIDS: A Public Health Challenge: State Issues, Policies and Programs* (Washington, D.C.: U.S. Department of Health and Human Services, 1987).

33. Lawrence Gostin, W. J. Curran, and M. Clark, "The Case against Compulsory Case Finding in Controlling AIDS . . . ," *American Journal of Law and Medicine* 12 (1987): 7–53.

34. E. R. Shipp, "Physical Suffering Is Not the Only Pain that AIDS Can Inflict," *New York Times,* 17 February 1986.

35. William F. Buckley, Jr., "Crucial Step in Combating the AIDS Epidemic: Identify All the Carriers," *New York Times,* 18 March 1986.

36. Peter S. Arno and Philip R. Lee, "The Federal Response to the AIDS Epidemic," in *AIDS: Public Policy Dimensions,* ed. J. Griggs (New York: United Hospital Fund, 1987).

37. U.S. Congress, Office of Technology Assessment, *Review of the Public Health Service Response to AIDS* (Washington: OTA, 1985).

38. C. Norman, "Congress Likely to Halt Shrinkage in AIDS Funds," *Science* 231 (1986): 1364–1365; "AIDS Research Funding," *Blue Sheet: Health Policy and Biomedical Research News of the Week,* 26 February 1986.

39. W.B., "AIDS Funds Increased; Helos Meanne Blunted," *Science* 239 (1988): 140.

40. Richard F. Needle et al., "The Evolving Role of Health Education in the AIDS Epidemic: The Experience of Nine High-Incidence Cities" (Report prepared for the Centers for Disease Control, 1986).

41. Randy Shilts, "Insurance Denied? Industry May Screen for AIDS Virus," *Village Voice,* 3 September 1985.

42. AIDS cost studies are referenced and summarized in Daniel M. Fox and Emily Thomas, "AIDS Cost Analysis and Social Policy," *Law, Medicine, and Health Care* 15 (1987–1988): 186–211.

43. Ibid.

44. Ibid.

45. Peter S. Arno and R. G. Hughes, "Local Policy Response to the AIDS Epidemic," (Unpublished paper, 1985); Peter S. Arno, "The Non-profit Sector's Response to the AIDS Epidemic: Community-based Services in San Francisco," *American Journal of Public Health* 76 (1986): 1325–1330.

46. State of New York, Department of Health, *Request for Applications for Designation of AIDS Centers* (Albany, 24 March 1986).

47. Susan Dentzer, "Why AIDS Won't Bankrupt U.S.," *U.S. News and World Report,* 18 January 1988, 20–22.

48. Robert Wood Johnson Foundation, press release, "AIDS Health Services Program," January 1986.

49. Fox and Thomas, "AIDS Cost Analysis."

50. Sara Rimer, "High School Course Is Shattering Myths about AIDS," *New York Times,* 5 March 1986.

Notes on Contributors

Dennis Altman is senior lecturer in politics at La Trobe University in Melbourne, Australia. He is the author of *AIDS in the Mind of America: The Social, Political, and Psychological Impact of a New Epidemic.*

Allan M. Brandt is associate professor of the history of medicine and science at Harvard Medical School, and in the department of history of science, Harvard University. He is the author of *No Magic Bullet: A Social History of Venereal Disease in the United States since 1880.*

Elizabeth Fee is associate professor of health policy at the Johns Hopkins School of Hygiene and Public Health. She is the author of *Disease and Discovery: A History of the Johns Hopkins School of Hygiene and Public Health* and editor of *Women and Health: The Politics of Sex in Medicine.*

Daniel M. Fox is professor of humanities in medicine at the State University of New York at Stony Brook. His most recent books are *Health Policies, Health Politics: The Experience of Britain and America, 1911–1965* and (with Christopher Lawrence) *Photographing Medicine: Images and Power in Britain and America since 1840.*

Diane R. Karp, an art historian, has served as curator at the Philadelphia Museum of Art and on the faculty of Temple University. She is the author of *Ars Medica: Art, Medicine, and the Human Condition.*

David F. Musto is professor of psychiatry and history at Yale University. He is the author of *The American Disease: A History of Narcotics and Addiction in America* and many papers on drug use and addiction.

Gerald M. Oppenheimer is associate professor of health sciences and nutrition at Brooklyn College, and staff associate in the G. H. Sergievsky Center, Faculty of Medicine, Columbia University. He has published papers on AIDS and health insurance, epidemiology, and the history of medicine.

Dorothy Porter is researching the history of public health in nineteenth- and twentieth-century Britain. With Roy Porter, she has recently written a history of illness in eighteenth-century England, entitled *Sickness, Suffering, and the Self.*

Roy Porter is senior lecturer in the social history of medicine at the Wellcome Institute for the History of Medicine in London. His books include the recently published *Mind-Forg'd Manacles: A History of Madness in England from the Restoration to the Regency.*

Guenter B. Risse is professor and chairman of the Department of History and Philosophy of the Health Sciences at the University of California at San Francisco. His books on the history of medicine include the recently published *Hospital Life in Enlightenment Scotland: Care and Teaching at the Royal Infirmary of Edinburgh.*

Charles E. Rosenberg is professor of history at the University of Pennsylvania. His books include *The Cholera Years: The United States in 1832, 1849, and 1866* and, most recently published, *The Care of Strangers: The Rise of America's Hospital System.*

Paula A. Treichler is associate professor of medical humanities in the University of Illinois College of Medicine at Urbana. She is coauthor of *A Feminist Dictionary* and coeditor of *For Alma Mater: Theory and Practice in Feminist Scholarship.*

Index

Compositor:	G&S Typesetters, Inc.
Text:	10/13 Sabon
Display:	Sabon
Printer:	Maple-Vail Book Mfg. Group
Binder:	Maple-Vail Book Mfg. Group